speak to me in nuclear medicine

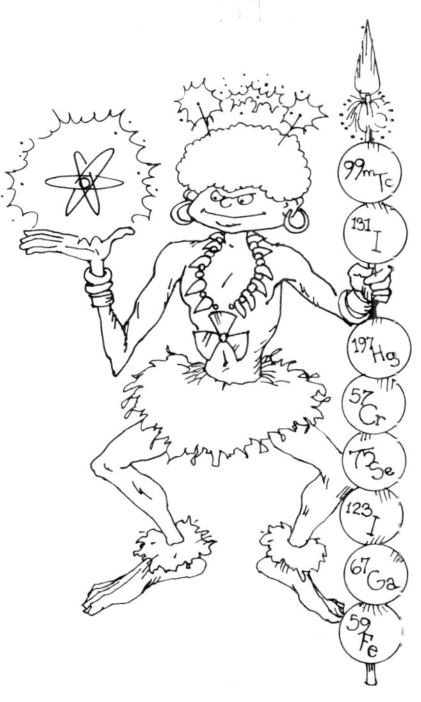

speak to me in nuclear medicine

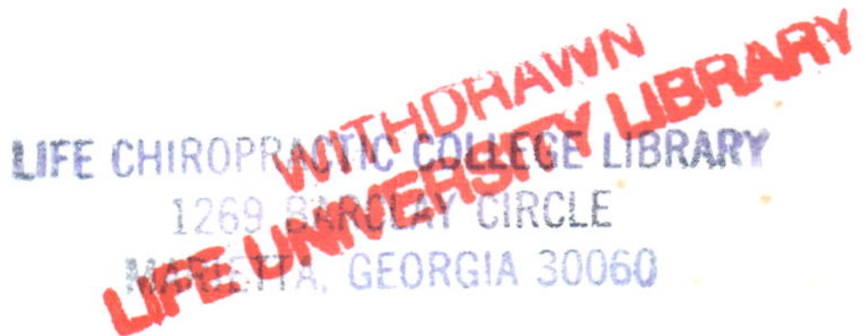

PHILIP SHTASEL, D.O.

Director, Division of Nuclear Medicine; Associate, Department of
Radiology, Metropolitan Hospital, Philadelphia, Pennsylvania

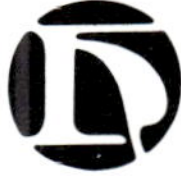

Medical Department
Harper & Row, Publishers
Hagerstown, Maryland
New York, San Francisco, London

Cover and text designed by Maria S. Karkucinski

*Composed in Helvetica, linotype, by American Book–Stratford Press
Lithography and printing by Murray Printing Company, Inc.*

76 77 78 79 80 81   10 9 8 7 6 5 4 3 2 1

Library of Congress Cataloging in Publication Data
Shtasel, Philip, 1925–
    Speak to me in nuclear medicine.
    Bibliography: p.
    Includes index.
    1. Radioisotope scanning.   I. Title
[DNLM: 1. Nuclear Medicine. WN440 S561s]
RC78.7.R4S57   616.07'575   76–3671
ISBN 0–06–142383–1

to: t + 3 + b

Lypt: Nick Nardello

contents

8 ETC. Etc. etc.
chapter

index

foreword

If ever there were a textbook that tells it like it is, this is that book. No dry, pedantic style, no endless lists of clinically useless facts of physics, no rose-colored glasses "evaluation" of an "exciting new discipline"—instead, a sober, yet pleasant, down-to-earth description of a field that has been around for forty years, told by a master of that discipline in an easy-going style that's sure to please.

Doctor Shtasel's method—based on many years of experience as a practicing radiologist—is unique. Rather than describe test results in various disease states, he approaches nuclear medicine procedures from the standpoint of the clinician— what kind of information does such-and-such a procedure give? how useful is it in providing that information? how is the test done? how does it compare with other tests? and what improvements are on the horizon?

More to the point, Doctor Shtasel lets the reader know just where any procedure fits into the infinite scheme of things, information which is difficult to come by in standard textbooks on nuclear medicine. This comes from the nature of Doctor Shtasel's approach to clinical problems as a general radiologist. He utilizes each special discipline to its best advantage—angiography, nuclear medicine, ultrasonography, tomography, etc.—and is not emotionally committed to any one. As a result, the reader can expect to get, and does get, a fair shake. Doctor Shtasel also brings to bear a broad knowledge of the relevant literature, and a critical eye for the nuances of practice.

His style—from the title on the cover to the last page—will come as somewhat of a shock to the reader, as it did to me. Whoever heard of a textbook reading the way people actually talk? In this, I believe, lies the key to its appeal, since it makes the learning process as easy as a curbstone consultation, which is what this book really is. All you have to do is sit back and listen.

I know of no other book which will give the student, the house officer, and the practicing physician as much information about nuclear medicine in such a palatable and profitable way as this book.

N. DAVID CHARKES, M.D.
Professor in Radiology (Nuclear Medicine)
and Associate Professor of Medicine,
Temple University Medical School,
Philadelphia, Pennsylvania

August 1, 1975
Wynnewood, Pa.

preface

Not too long after establishing shop in a remote corner of the X-ray Department—the usual humble beginnings of those who ply the art—we received from a well-respected staff member the following request, yea, demand: "Speak to me in Nuclear Medicine! I must learn your language!" That directive has been repeated many times. It reflects the desire and need of the general medical community to know what we are doing. We consider this community to be the Noncritical Medical Masses, which I define to be those persons related in any way to the healing arts but possessing no expertise in Nuclear Medicine. However, when supplied with the information they desire, this noncritical group will go "critical,"* thus providing a new relationship between the general medical community and the nuclear medicine man which has explosive potentials for improved patient diagnosis and management.

If a poll were directed to medical students, house staff, family physicians, most specialists, and even nurses, technologists, and paramedical groups asking "WHAT THE WORLD NEEDS NOW?," another text on nuclear medicine would undoubtedly finish an undistinguished last. Yet, our daily experiences suggest the contrary *if* this text were directed exclusively to this group. It was just these daily experiences of fielding his/her† questions that confirmed the need of a reference source for the nonnuclear specialist.

Questions came from all floors and all offices. Our area of competence seems to cross almost all others; the typical day includes discussions, explanations, and suggestions to members of all our staffs. After many such days merged into years, it became apparent that the nonspecialist's overall purview of the parameters of nuclear medicine—its basic science, diagnostic indications, limitations, hazards, expectations, and priorities—was far more limited than was his general knowledge in most other areas. Intrinsic and extrinsic factors contribute to this situation.

Intrinsic: Since nuclear medicine is the youngest of all of the major disciplines, many practitioners may never have received any didactic exposure to the subject. For others, the rate of growth and ever increasing scope of activity rendered their background obsolescent. No good reference source is available at the level required. The encyclopedic text or specialty journal is not only beyond the need but intimidating in its depth and range. The nonsubscription periodical, on the other hand, often resorts to generalization and simplification, leaving the uninformed misinformed.

The extrinsic factor has to do with restrictions which are not imposed on any other specialty, regulations which may on occasion introduce confusion. The practice of nuclear medicine is under the direct control and supervision of city, state, and federal authorities. The community hospital assumes a low pecking-order position on the nuclear Totem. Nuclides described so glowingly and with

---

* In nuclear parlance a critical mass is defined as the condition necessary to create an atomic explosion. With that definition we have concluded all the nuclear physics this text contains.

† Having established that we respect that the masses are bisexual, we will henceforth eliminate the "he/she" designation simply because it is too cumbersome. In its place we will alternate the gender of pronoun equally and without bias.

so much potential by the university-complex department may not be available at the community level for years.

Similar stratification exists with respect to instrumentation. Technology, always a model ahead of this year's budget, leaves a smaller department at a disadvantage.

The noncritical masses often request that which cannot be done in their hospital. In concern, frustration, and even contumely, they demand, "Well, what can you do here?"

I hope to answer those and other questions in this book. A reference for the nonspecialist is long overdue. We consider this group to be any and all who have need for or interest in our specialty but who have neither background nor competence in the subject or, even more importantly, do not aspire to maximum informational acquisition. Their desire stops short of board eligibility. They simply require a tour book to guide them through "It's a great place to visit, but I wouldn't want to live here" kind of thing. It need not encompass everything everyone ever wanted to know, but enough about a lot.

Having thus made the first decision that a source was indicated, I was faced with the task of deciding what the nonspecialist needed and desired. The analogy to the gourmet became tempting: It was not so much what was on the menu, since they all look so much alike, as it was how the items were to be prepared and served. The specialty of the house had to be organ scanning, our meat and potatoes. Instrumentation, technique, radiopharmaceuticals, dosimetry, and other such ingredients are for the chef and need not be the concern of the diner. The menu will be *a la carte* so that a gamut of *in vitro* side dishes will be available to the discriminating or catholic taste. The weight watchers dessert of nuclear therapy may also be enjoyed.

In each appropriate chapter, three basic tables appear, to be used according to the needs and desires of the reader. The information in Table I is categorized as "WHY, WHAT, HOW, and YEA or NAY." It is basic and summarizes the potentials of the diagnostic scope, the tools to accomplish the measurement, the procedural generalities, and the order of merit of a particular technique.

Tables 2 and 3 are expansions of Table I. They are "More Abouts—What and How."

That, dear diary, is how it all began. The Lord, my staff, said "Speak to Me." So I spoke.

acknowledgments

I had always thought that those breathless, eye-fluttering, voice-choking "Thank you, without you it couldn't have been done" utterances by Oscar recipients were some dutiful exercise in feigned humility. Then I got involved in this. The thark-yous that follow are neither dutiful nor demanded but are offered with utmost sincerity and gratitude—because each in his/her way really was integral in this becoming reality.

My most belated recognition is to Doctor Harold Isard who opened the door so many years ago and to Doctor Bernard Shapiro who took me through it and has been a constant guide since.

My sincere appreciation to the members of the Philadelphia Nuclear Community for general help and stimulation.

My repetitive gratitude to my associates Doctors Robert R. Rosenbaum and Lewis Halin for pulling the extra oar as I "did my thing." Add Howard Foster, a tireless resident who performed above and beyond the call in sorting and sifting.

A real big one to the First Team: Jesse Dixon, who saw it start, Eugene Boyer, my scanning right arm, and Marci Lesser who catalyzed an "also ran" into a pennant contender.

A tip of the cap to Doctor José Morales for a good idea?

A blanket gracias to the Staff of Metropolitan Hospital who supported me all the way and to the nice people at Harper & Row for patience and understanding.

To Ms. Dee Watson, who must be the world's most patient, pleasant, willing and noncomplaining virtuoso of the keyboard (typewriter): that old but still unbeatable cliché—"words fail me." Just know how important you were.

Lastly, Doctor N. David Charkes, a superb physician but an even greater person and friend. No short descriptive (or to use his word—"cutesie") sentence could say it. So, again, the inadequate—Thanks!

introduction

"Tradition." That's what the Fiddler called it. It explains why the Star Spangled Banner precedes a football game, why a toast precedes a drink, and why chapters on nuclear and molecular physics, mathematics and electronics, and instrumentation and radiobiology precede the clinical chapters in most nuclear medicine texts. But, after much soul-searching and some throwing of caution to the winds we have decided that the game can stand on its own without the anthem, the drink without the toast, and the text without those certifiers of erudition—the basic sciences. Well, almost.

Some irreducible minimums must be included. To drive home a new car one need not know the mechanics of the engine, but it is critical to know how to turn on the ignition, activate the windshield wiper, and identify the correct petrol. So too, here, the Why of each chapter will be unique to the organ system discussed. But since the basic How and What refer to the instrumentation and pharmaceuticals that apply to all, rather than repeat them throughout, the following will suffice as a noncritical mass tour down the main highways and byways of the basics required to dig this nuclear scene.

Three tables appear in each of chapters 1 through 7. In the first and third, reference to instrumentation (How) is made. It will suffice here to simply identify the two basic types of scanning equipment now in use and broadly contrast their differences. The two generic terms for this photographic hardware are scanner and camera.

"Scanner" is an acceptable abbreviation for rectilinear scanning device. It embodies a crystal on a moving arm. The crystal detects the emission of radioactive decay and by moving in a continuing, progressive, linear pattern across the entire area of examination plots out the location of the radiation as sequential isolated points in the field of view. These thousands of data points become the composite picture image.

The camera, in contradistinction, images an entire field of view with a large stationary crystal and just as faithfully records the location of the radiation.

The advantages and disadvantages of each are beyond our discussion here. When either is available the hardware is chosen appropriate to the task. In many problems the choice is immaterial. However, if rapidly changing events require documentation by picture images, the camera is essential. This type of study is frequently referred to as a "flow." It is a dynamic event and is captured only when a series of short-exposure images can be obtained sequentially in a space of seconds. Obviously, the time-consuming point-by-point plotting of the rectilinear mode is inappropriate for flow studies. Other situations are better served by the scanner.

The scanner is advantageous when the part to be examined is larger than 12 inches, situated deep in the body, or when the pharmaceutical agent employed exceeds 400 keV. The camera "sees" areas only as large as the diameter of its crystal face, exhibits superior resolution closer to its surface, and has diminished efficiency with radionuclides of high photon energy. (However, recent modifications, such as a moving table and focusing devices, are improving the versatility of the camera and diminishing the need for two distinct instruments.)

It is often helpful that the patient be advised of these instruments before study.

Although he will be informed of them at the time of examination, it will be by a "stranger," frequently the technologist ("not even a Doctor"), rather than by his own trusted physician. A descriptive word or two goes far to allay the understandable anxiety experienced by many. The patient should know that these instruments are large and bulky. It is normal and proper that the scanner move backward and forward across her body, often making a clattering or clicking sound. The face of the camera fits snugly against his body; the scanner head does not even touch. It is most reassuring to be so forewarned.

The radiopharmaceuticals (What) appropriate to the problem are also listed. Whereas such elements as iodine, mercury, chromium, and gold have a familiar ring, a name that may be totally unknown to most assumes front and center position—technetium!

Although technetium has become, at least for this historic moment, the almost universal radiopharmaceutical, it is little known outside of the domain of nuclear medicine. This is understandable since it must be produced artificially (technetium —from the Greek—means artificial) from radioactive molybdenum, which in turn must be produced from stable molybdenum. The technetium obtained (^{99m}Tc) is metastable, thus the addition of m to the superscript mass number, and in six hours half of it decays to ^{99}Tc. Appropriately compounded ^{99m}Tc can be chemically manipulated into multiple valence states that manifest different reactions and biologic properties. The pertechnetate form (TcO_4^-) is obtained in the usual elution process of the ^{99}molybdenum to obtain ^{99m}Tc. An analogy has been drawn between the molybdenum-technetium process and the acquisition of milk from a cow. Thus, the manipulation of the molybdenum generator is referred to as "milking" the generator ("cow") to produce Tc ("milk"). In the pertechnetate form Tc behaves very much like iodine and accumulates in similar anatomic locations, e.g., thyroid, salivary glands, choroid plexuses, and GI tract. Its nuclear superiority to iodine resides in its shorter half-life, which permits the use of large doses and thus results in improved images obtained in less time, and in its decay emissions being in an energy range ideally suited to present instrumentation.

That concludes the How and What and should suffice when used in conjunction with the tables as a basic introduction to the instrumentation and pharmaceuticals of nuclear medicine, but perhaps we should end with several pointers on how to look at a scan. The picture is a composite of information employing the white-to-black scale produced by capturing the decay emissions and translating their energy into light pulses that expose film, be it x ray, Polaroid, or 35–70 mm. When the record is a negative, such as with x-ray or 35–70-mm film the presence of activity is recorded as black and its absence as white. The Polaroid image is a "positive" and the tones are reversed—activity is white, nonactivity black. Each organ is imaged uniquely, utilizing—when possible—the physiologic parameter exclusive to the system, e.g., the phagocytic potential of the reticuloendothelial system to capture colloidal particles in the imaging of the liver, the ability of the thyroid to extract and store iodide. Physical principles are often employed, e.g., the embolization of the capillary bed of the lung to identify the integrity of its perfusion. Included in each chapter will be a discussion of how the particular scan is obtained and how to look at it.

This then is our Bill of Fare.

Bon Appétit.

speak to me in nuclear medicine

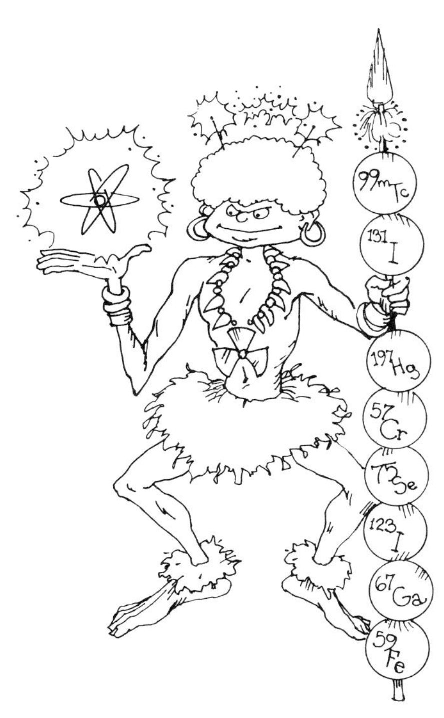

If ever a technologic breakthrough wagged the diagnostic tail, it must be in the nuclear imaging of the heart and vessels. It goes without repetitive dogma that every day in every way the advent of newer radiopharmaceuticals and forging of harder hardware constantly improved the overall investigative potential, but there are advances, and there are Advances. One of the latter, the gamma camera, made this chapter worth writing.

All subsequent discussion will deal only with imaging as opposed to the more inclusive possibilities of physiologic monitoring with radionuclides, *e.g.,* determination of left ventricular ejection fractions and cardiac output, detection of left intracardiac shunts with inhaled gases, and circulation time. These and other similar determinations are still beyond the abilities of the routine nuclear department and thus violate our ground rule of only describing that which is applicable to the critical nuclear masses. Thus, setting aside this category of physiologic monitoring, reference to older texts will quickly affirm that with respect to imaging, the cardiovascular system has been treated no

differently from the other systems. Static images were the thing. And this methodology was appropriate for depicting those large blood pools whose size and contour remain static. It was thus possible to detect the configuration of the intracardiac volume, and when this was contrasted against the roentgen contour a judgment with respect to pericardial effusion placenta could be localized and its position in could be made. Similarly, the isolated vascular the uterus established. These techniques comprised the isotopic 1–2 punch for the system. The chapters on cardiovascular imaging were very short.

The static approach was fine for imaging the cardio but a bomb for imaging the vascular. In order for a vessel segment to be imaged it must be depicted at the specific moment in history

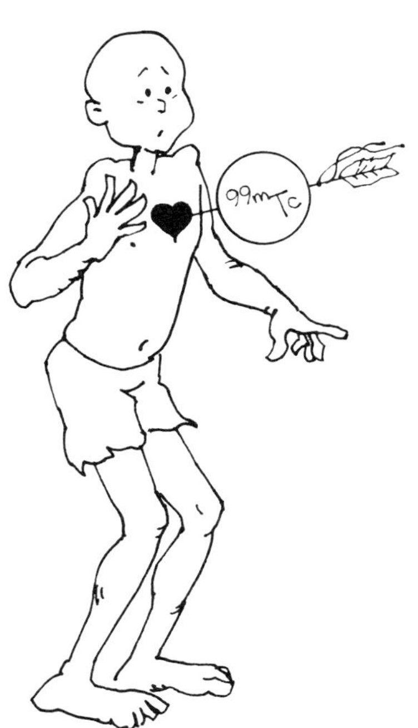

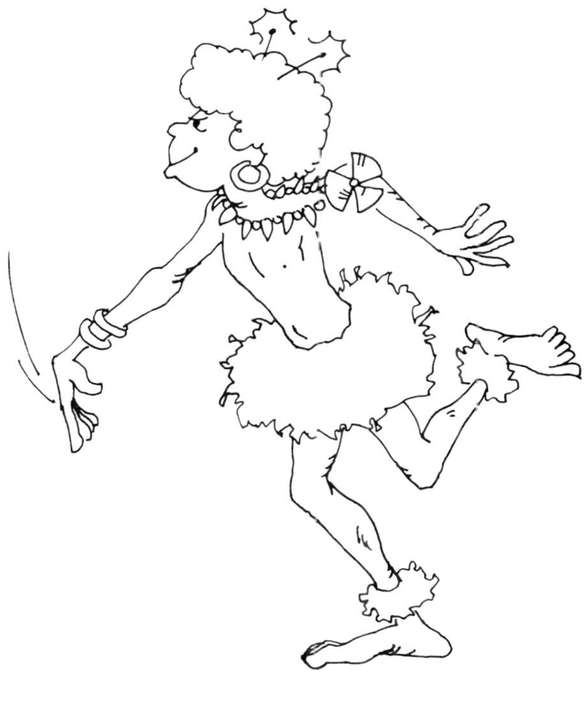

chapter 1

vessels and heart

when the radiopharmaceutical that is carried by the blood moves through it for the first time. As the nuclide leaves the major vessels and perfuses all the tissues, the "background" assumes activity and the particular vessel of interest may no longer be definable from the surrounding structures. The specific period of best definition is in the order of seconds. To be meaningful images must be obtained during that increment of time, usually 10–20 sec, when the bolus of nuclide first reaches the area of concern and before extensive surrounding perfusion occurs. This is imaging the "flow" or dynamic scanning.

The gamma camera provided the potential for this type of picture by making rapid sequential exposures possible. The "flow" could thus be recorded. The "snap-shot" became the "flickers," and nuclear angiocardiography was born. In the early postnatal period, less than 10 years ago, practitioners of the art in a somewhat self-conscious defense described their baby, nuclear angiocardiography, in mildly deprecating terms such as "poor man's angiography." The series of picture images shown on every appropriate and even on some inappropriate occasions by the doting parents of their new infant was greeted by the untrained eye with a traditional response—"only a father could love it." And indeed these representations did not have the sharp, crisp, exquisite detail of x-ray angiography. But what they lacked in splendor they more than compensated for in multiple pluses:

1. The technique is not invasive of arterial structures. All studies are performed by a peripheral venous puncture.
2. The time of examination is in the order of seconds to minutes.
3. Iodinated contrast media are avoided.
4. Radiation exposure is dramatically reduced.
5. The costs in time, material, personnel, and money are a fraction of those for contrast procedures.

As the infant grew into childhood, its parents with the help of adoring relatives (the pharmacologist and instrument maker) learned how better to show off their offspring. The addition of computer technology permitted storage and manipulation of the raw camera data. Particular radionuclides offered enhanced imaging of particular vascular areas. The poor man's label was no longer appropriate, and like all other things in our inflated society had to be upgraded to at least "middle class angiography."

WHAT

blood pool: heart–placenta

The choice of agent for the heart pool study is not particularly critical. Technetium 99m sodium pertechnetate is quite suitable. However, for the placental pool ^{99m}Tc human serum albumin is preferable since it will not accumulate in the bladder or cross the placenta. Indium 113m is also a good agent in placental localization.

vascular flow

Again, at least for now, ^{99m}Tc as pertechnetate is Mr. Everything (for a more detailed discussion of this radionuclide, go directly back to What in the Introduction). If the dynamic imaging is part of another procedure, *e.g.*, the flow portion of a renal or brain study, and a chelating-type agent is chosen, that agent is equally appropriate for the rapid-sequence phase.

myocardial

The final word is not yet in on the agent of choice. Nor is the final word yet in on the technique of choice, *i.e.*, intravenous or intraarterial routes of injection.

Until all down state counties are heard from, the various pharmaceuticals that have been studied are listed under their route of injection.

Intravenous

Potassium 43
Cesium 129
Cesium 131
Oleic acid I 131
Gallium 67
Rubidium 81
Ammonia 13
Tetracycline labeled with technetium 99m
Thallium 201
Phosphates labeled with technetium 99m

Most experience has been gained with ^{43}K and ^{129}Cs. However, thallium (^{201}Tl) is just becoming commercially available, and initial reports are most favorable. Also, great words are being heard about the phosphates labeled with technetium, particularly the pyrophosphates. Although these agents were originally and exclusively considered for bone imaging, they appear capable of localizing in myocardium.

Intraarterial (Coronary Artery)

Xenon 133
$H_2^{15}O$
Albumin microspheres labeled with
technetium 99m
Strontium 85
Iodine 131

Here, too, no single choice is head and shoulders or myocardium and pericardium above the others. Xenon and labeled oxygen are wash-out procedures; the use of microspheres permits imaging.

peripheral

When the venous system is to be imaged, similar to contrast angiography, introduction of the nuclide is by the venous route in the foot, and ^{99m}Tc, either as pertechnetate in saline or as albumin microspheres, is preferred. Microspheres may also be tagged with ^{113m}In.

When the venous system is to be imaged for the possibility of thrombus formation, fibrinogen labeled usually with a radionuclide of iodine is injected several hours or days prior to imaging. Streptokinase and urokinase labeled with ^{99m}Tc have also been used successfully for the detection of deep vein thrombosis.

When the arterial side is to be investigated, intraarterial injection of ^{99m}Tc or ^{113m}In microspheres is employed. A translumbar aortic puncture site is common.

HOW

blood pool—heart and placenta

No patient preparation is required. The radioisotope is injected intravenously and scanning is initiated almost immediately. Usually, a supine position is preferred. The time of examination varies with the scanning instrument and pharmaceutical. Total time is about 4–5 min for pericardial effusion studies done by dynamic flow and static imaging with the camera. If only a static blood pool is imaged by rectilinear modes, increase the time to 15–20 min.

The procedure for placental localization by imaging is quite similar to the pericardial sequence. Performed by camera with dynamic and static components, placental localization requires 5–10 min. Rectilinear images are 2–3 times slower.

If, however, the "point-count" system of localization is employed the little mother-to-be should be warned that a "hop scotch" board will be drawn on her abdomen. This technique requires that the entire abdomen be divided into a 9- or 12-box grid and each box counted by a probe that just touches the skin. The count rate is then plotted, and the highest count area wins the placenta.

Obviously, it is vital to ascertain the position of the cervical os relative to the placenta. Each laboratory establishes it own method for determining the location of the os. If external approximation is practiced (as is most usual), nothing need be said to the patient. If, however, direct and exact localization is performed by the placement of a point source of radioactivity directly over the os, the patient should be warned that this is coming. The order of merit of these techniques is good to excellent. For effusion problems in which the volume exceeds 150–200 cc, the detection accuracy is 90+%. If, however, the volume is less, don't bet the mortgage money, since accuracy falls off sharply. If the choice rests between nuclear and special radiologic techniques, *e.g.,* carbon dioxide or angiography, scan every time, but—if available—sophisticated sonography is the way to go.

The same order of yea or nay is suggested for the placenta: nuclear over all else except sound.

flow studies

Each study requires custom tailoring as to position and time sequence to image the desired vessel or area, but all are similar in mode of administration and time of examination. An IV route is always taken. However, an effort is made to keep the injected volume as a contained bolus, and multiple techniques exist to accomplish this end. Perhaps the most popular (it was at least the first) is still distinguished by the name of its originator, the Oldendorf method. Injection into the basilic antecubital vein is performed just below a blood pressure cuff, which is inflated to exceed the patient's systolic pressure. The cuff is then snapped off, and the injected material— at least in theory—travels rapidly towards the heart. Although the technique does not cause any discomfort, it should be described since most patients find the procedure unusual. The time of examination rarely exceeds 2–3 min. No preparation is necessary. The order of merit takes

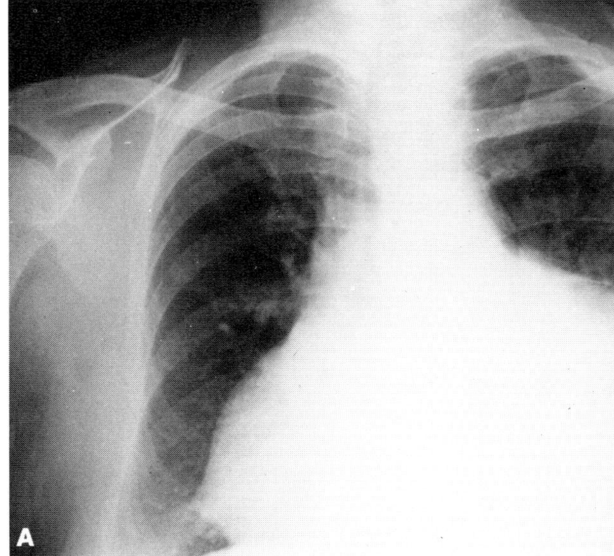

Fig. 1-1. Pericardial effusion

A. X ray. The cardiac silhouette is grossly distorted and presents a typical "water bottle" contour.

B. Scan. The cardiac blood pool imaged with ^{99m}Tc (white) is significantly smaller in volume than the x-ray comparison. A wide clear space (halo) surrounds the heart and separates it from the pulmonary perfusion and intraabdominal organ activity.

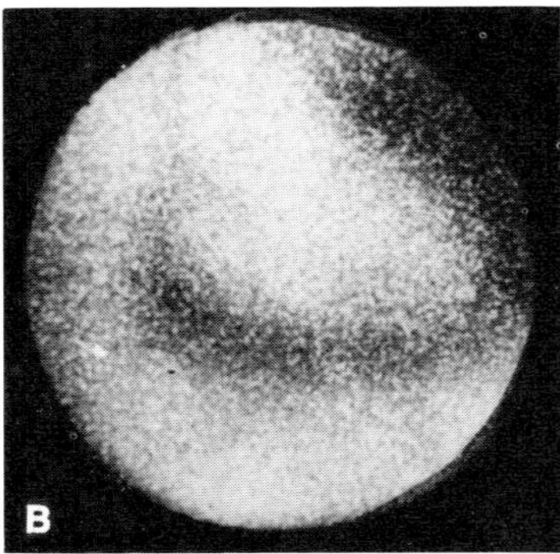

the full four-star rating. No other available technique can so quickly, easily, and economically accomplish the same end.

myocardial

If perfusion studies are to be performed at the same time as the coronary angiography, all of those things that the patient should know about that procedure apply to the imaging phase. The radioactive nuclide is injected by catheter, and pictures are obtained. The angiographer is the first pilot on this mission.

If the IV method is employed, nothing special is to be anticipated. Screening is performed, depending on the radionuclide, at any time from 5 min to days after injection.

The jury is still out as to the final order of merit, but hearts are beginning to beat more rapidly because of the enthusiastic reports being heard about thallium and pyrophosphate imaging.

peripheral vascular

Here, too, the technique is a function of the imaged structure. If peripheral arterial perfusion is performed, the radiopharmaceutical is injected intraarterially, usually by a translumbar aortic puncture. This, too, is usually done at the time of contrast roentgen study, and scanning is at the back end of that evaluation.

Two methods of imaging the venous system are now in vogue: isotopic venography and thrombosis detection. Venography is identical to roentgen venography except that a radiopharmaceutical rather than a radiopaque agent is injected into a vein on the dorsum of the foot. When prospective studies for thrombus formation are performed, the radionuclide is injected at the time of surgery and the lower extremities monitored on a scheduled post-operative routine.

Neither method is particularly attractive at this time. Unless the patient is allergic to contrast media, x-ray venography can be done with the same effort and setup and will produce far superior vascular definition. Perhaps isotopic venography has merit as a routine study employing ^{99m}Tc albumin microspheres or ^{99m}Tc MAA (macroaggregated human serum albumin) as an accompaniment of lung scanning. The isotope could be injected into the foot and a venogram obtained prior to the lung images. If the findings are abnormal and require further definition, the contrast venogram can then be done.

With respect to the detection of thrombus formation the labeled fibrinogen studies seem useful in identifying forming thrombi; with thrombosis, the sensitivity appears less. Thus, it may eventually be utilized to monitor the

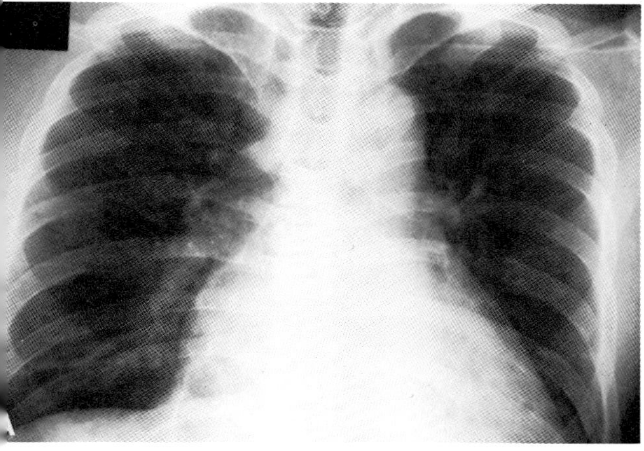

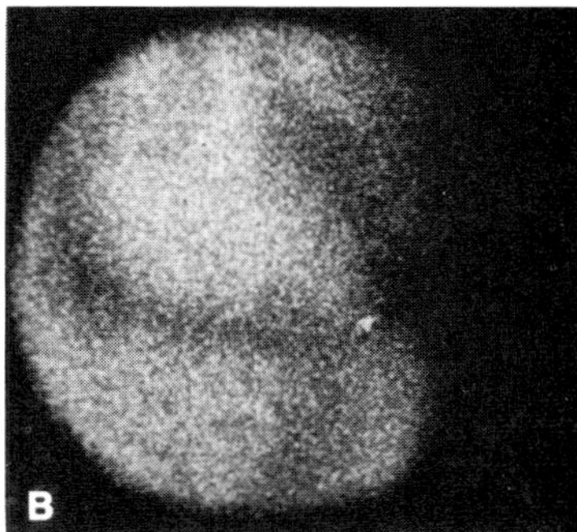

Fig. 1-2. Cardiac hypertrophy—no effusion
A. X ray. The cardiac silhouette is enlarged. The right and left borders tend to bulge, suggesting an early "water bottle" contour.
B. Scan. The cardiac blood pool imaged with ^{99m}Tc closely approximates the x-ray image.

postoperative patient for the development of thrombi rather than evaluate the subject with established phlebitis.

WHY

pericardial effusion

Recognition and detection of fluid in the pericardium is often a vexing matter. Frequently, the initial suggestion of this possibility originates with a chest x ray and the identification of a cardiac contour change: the classic "water bottle" heart configuration. When the volume of the effusion exceeds 200 cc the search is usually successful. However, lesser volumes are less well detected. This relationship is fortunately self-serving since the smaller volumes rarely cause detectable roentgen changes so that the search for an undetectable volume is gratefully never initiated. We will probably never know the number of effusions that go unsuspected and which, even if suspected, might well go undetected.

The diagnosis is dependent on establishing a discrepancy between the cardiac image on x ray and the actual cardiac blood pool contour on scan. The radionuclide image will show only the chamber volume. When the effusion is massive the incongruity of the contour of the blood pool and the x ray silhouette will readily establish the diagnosis (Fig. 1-1). With smaller effusions the detection becomes less obvious and other signs are employed. When there is no effusion the activity of the intracardiac pool is in close proximity to the activity of the intrapulmonary and intrahepatic blood pools. These areas are normally separated only by the thickness of the myocardium and diaphragm. As the separation increases with the interposition of fluid in the pericardium, the image of the pools defines this separation by a "halo," or clear zone, and the heart activity no longer merges with that of the liver and lungs.

Difficulties arise, as above noted, in the detection of small effusions. The scan image is not readily superimposed on the chest x ray to compare contours. Techniques to provide one-to-one x-ray and scan geometries for comparison must be performed by rectilinear instruments. Such comparisons are difficult and tedious to obtain and when finally done are open to question. The intercomparison of a chest x ray and a pericardial scan by camera technique in which the image size is approximately 1 in. in diameter needs no editorial comment.

Minimal separations of the heart pool when they exist must be differentially considered. Myocardial hypertrophy may cause a halo (Fig. 1-2). Amyloidosis can be confusing, as can myocardial tumors or pericardial cysts. So, if ultrasonics are available, we recommend that diagnostic direction. However, if ultrasonics are unavailable, by all means scan, but be appraised of its limitations.

placental localization

Fortunately, third trimester bleeding is not frequently a problem. Estimates are that 2–4% of all pregnancies experience some late bleeding, and of this group approximately one-fourth are due to abnormal implantation sites.

If radiation hazard to the fetus were not a deterrent, placental localization would be relatively easy. The high-volume blood pool lends itself to ready detection (Fig. 1–3). However, most radiopharmaceuticals cross the placental barrier and result in a "hot baby." This was particularly troublesome when ^{131}I was the investigating nuclide. Lugol's iodine solution was required to block the fetal thyroid. Even the short-lived agents such as technetium and indium must be used judiciously. It is this concern that creates the diagnostic difficulty since low doses decrease the accuracy of localization, particularly if implantation is on the posterior uterine wall. Difficulty is also encountered in the differential consideration between a low-lying and a marginal implantation (Fig. 1-4). However, the study is valuable and highly accurate. Older point-count grid techniques have been generally replaced by scan procedures. Dynamic flow imaging over the pelvis usually identifies the placental pool within seconds, but here, too, with mock sadness we must doff our diagnostic caps in the direction of ultrasonics. If this modality is available, it is to be preferred. Its accuracy in localization is at least equal to that of imaging, and the fact that the desired information can be obtained without adding a radiation burden to mamma and baby makes it no contest.

flow

Organ Perfusion. In recent years, flow evaluations have been incorporated into the static portions of certain organ studies so that it is now almost routine to perform a perfusion scan of the brain at the time of radioisotopic injection and obtain the "conventional" images later. Similarly, perfusion of other organ systems has proven and is proving valuable in the detection of renal hypertension and in the evaluation of the vascularity of an intrarenal mass, the relative vascularity of a defect in the liver, any abdominal mass, thyroid nodules, and so forth. Each of these applications will be fully discussed in the chapter dealing with the particular organ.

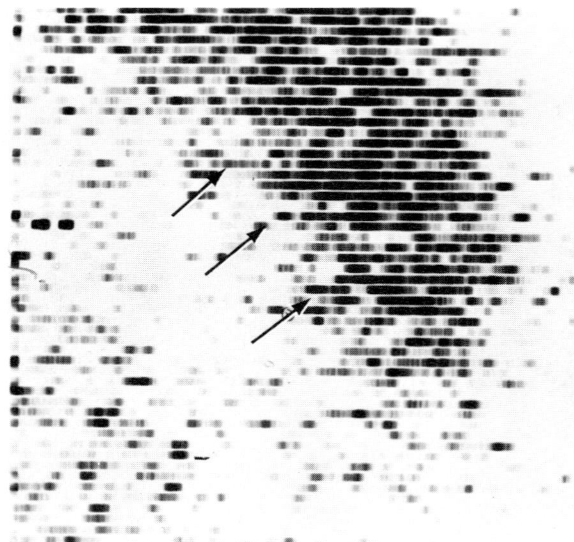

Fig. 1-3. Normal placental implantation. Scan. An ovoid or semilunar collection of activity appears high in the left uterine fundus following the IV injection of ^{131}I human serum albumin. The *x* is at the umbilicus. The cervix marker is not seen.

Fig. 1-4. Placenta previa
A. Scan, 18 sec. Following injection of 2 mCi ^{99m}Tc placental activity is localized along the left uterine wall. The activity extends to the marker (arrow) placed 2 cm above the symphysis pubis—the anticipated site of the cervix.
B. Line sketch of A. The placental blood pool is black. The rim of activity on the right is perfusion of the uterine wall.

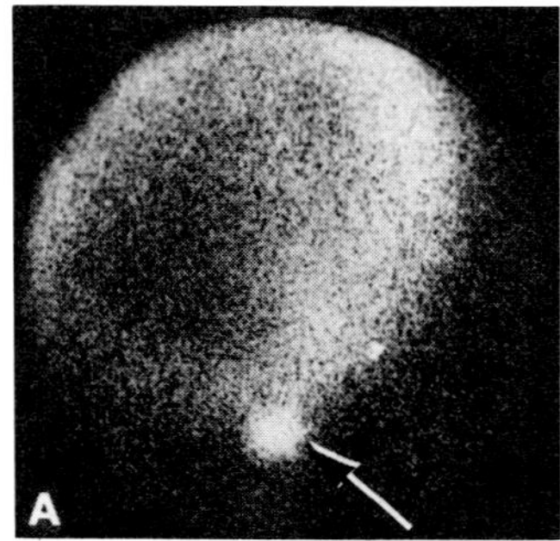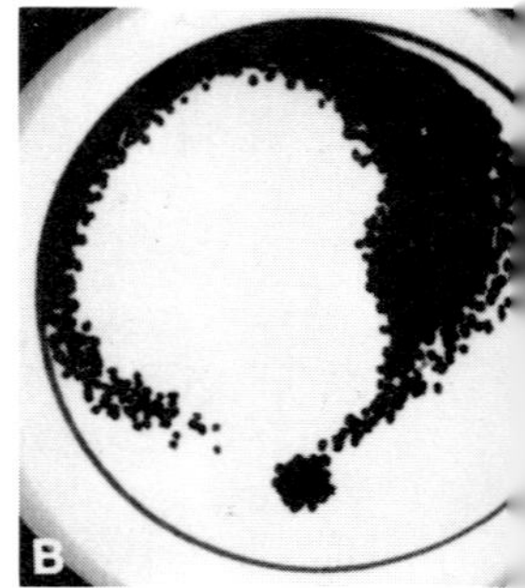

Vascular Perfusion (Radioisotope Angiography).
It is perhaps a misrepresentation to suggest
that isotopic angiography (venous and arterial)
is capable of visualizing any and all vascular
structures with sufficient clarity and detail to
permit some judgment and opinion with reference
to them. As in all scanning, visualization is
dependent on a higher concentration of activity
in the structure of interest than in its surrounding
area or background. In static imaging, attempts
are made physiologically or physically, or both,
to extract, incorporate, block, phagocytose, to
do anything that will keep the "target" (*i.e.,*
thyroid, brain, or kidney) "hotter" (*i.e.,* more
radioactive) than the "nontarget" region (*i.e.,*
the surrounding structure, or background). This
condition has been described as the target:
nontarget ratio, and the ability and quality of
imaging is dependent on this relationship.

Dynamic imaging utilizes time as its gimmick.
At some particular increment there is a greater
concentration of radioactivity within a vessel
segment than around it. However, as the bolus is
propelled, it becomes diluted, more importantly,
it becomes distributed throughout the vasculature, thus affectively raising the activity of all of
the background structures. Thus, only the major
vessels can be successfully identified and
evaluated individually. Abnormalities in smaller
structures may be appreciated by identifying the
altered vascularity of the area they supply but
not by direct visualization of the vessel itself.
An occlusion of the superior vena cava is
distinguishable by direct evidence; an infarction
of the middle cerebral artery is diagnosable by
inference.

Having thus identified the general deficiencies, weaknesses, exceptions, deletions, and the
like and with the ground rules established, we
can discuss radioisotope angiography more
specifically.

VENOUS. Superior Vena Cava. Historically
(1966) isotope angiography was born with
superior vena caval imaging. The superior vena
cava is the ideal vessel for these purposes. Any
upper extremity injection will drain into the cava
without significant attenuation of the bolus. Its
position is also ideal for camera visualization
and there is sufficient time between the first
appearance of activity and the loss of definition
secondary to pulmonary perfusion to track out
the cava and right heart in excellent detail (Figs.
1-5 and 1-6).

Surprisingly little attention was given to this
technique for several years. Sporadic reports
describing complete obstruction and collateral
flow have appeared, but the procedure has yet
to be adapted as a routine evaluation for
mediastinal disease. We will delineate our
reasons for urging that radionuclide cavography
become such a routine.

The superior vena caval syndrome is as a
rule a relatively clear-cut clinical entity that
offers little diagnostic difficulty. The patient
usually has a past history of malignancy, usually
pulmonary. Signs and symptoms are characterized by edema of the face, neck, and upper
extremity, dilated veins over the upper half of
the body, and—frequently—acute dyspnea and
cyanosis. Immediate and heroic measures,
usually with radiation therapy, are required.

This was the type of patient originally being
studied by isotopic cavagraphy. The images
were dramatic reflections of the obstructive
anatomy. The collateral pathways were
catalogued via the internal mammary, azygos,
hemiazygos, vertebral, intercostal, and long
thoracic routes (Figs. 1-7 and 1-8). But the
obvious question was inevitably asked, "Who
needs those little Polaroids when the patient's
picture is so clear?" Except to perhaps monitor
the effects of therapy on the obstructive pattern,
the criticism is valid. However, logic suggests
that there must be intermediate stages between
the normal and full-blown syndrome which, if
recognized, could meaningfully affect therapy.
And indeed, there are.

Firstly, it is helpful to extend the search
beyond the cava *per se* and consider the entire
inflow tract, *i.e.,* the subclavian and innominate
veins in addition to the cava. The technique
should be identified as a "mediastinal flow."

Secondly, the injection should be made
simultaneously in each arm so that both the right
and left venous pathways are imaged. It is not
uncommon for obstruction to begin in the left
innominate vein, and obviously this would be
missed if injection were only right-sided. It is
needless to add *vice versa* if only a left-sided
instillation is employed.

Thirdly, a mediastinal flow study should be a
part of the routine evaluation of any and all
pulmonary neoplasms, proven or suspected. It is
only by this routine that early and preclinical
evidence of mediastinal invasion or nodal
involvement, or both, will be appreciated and
appropriate measures instituted. The data thus
derived can be obtained in no other way in many

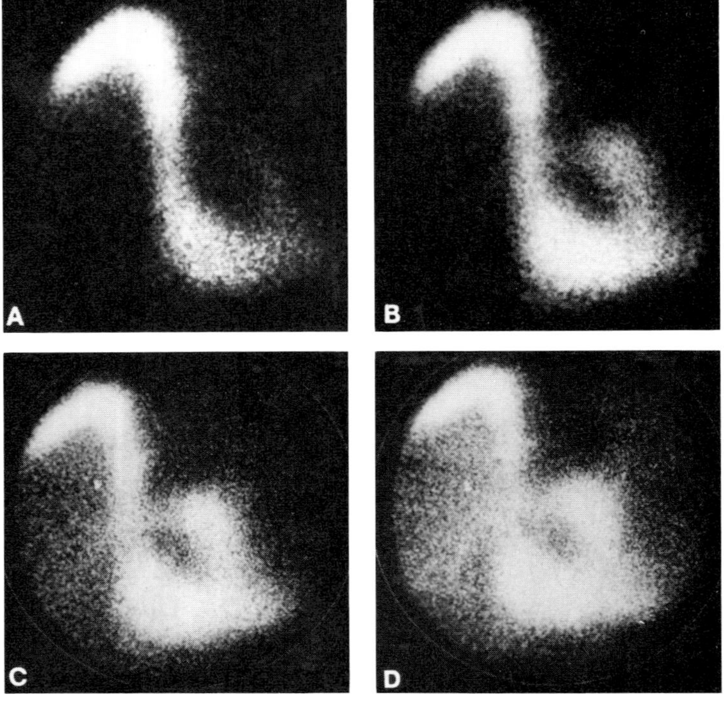

Fig. 1-5. Normal mediastinal flow (right injection). A 10-mCi bolus injection of ^{99m}Tc was made in the right anticubital fossa. Sequential images were obtained with the patient supine.
- **A.** 6–9 sec. The right subclavian vein, the right innominate vein, the superior vena cava, and the right atrium are identified. The innominate–caval axis is vertical.
- **B.** 9–12 sec. The bolus has moved into the right ventricle and the pulmonary conus.
- **C.** 12–15 sec. The right pulmonary artery can be seen as a horizontal band crossing the cava. Early pulmonary perfusion is present.
- **D.** 15–18 sec. Further pulmonary perfusion. Early left cardiac opacification is beginning, and the ventricle can be seen.

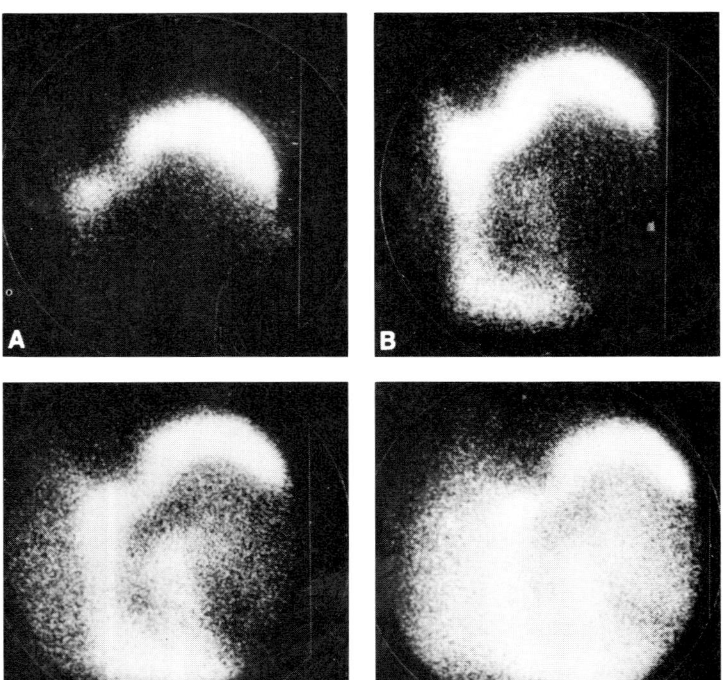

Fig. 1-6. Normal mediastinal flow (left injection). Similar to Figure 1-5, but injection is made into the left anticubital vein.
- **A.** 8–11 sec. The left subclavian vein and left innominate vein are identified. A "notch" is often present in the innominate vein.
- **B.** 11–14 sec. Forward progress to the superior vena cava and right atrium. The left innominate notch disappears.
- **C.** 14–17 sec. Activity in the right ventricle, pulmonary conus, and lungs.
- **D.** 17–20 sec. Extensive pulmonary perfusion obscures the definition of the mediastinal structures.

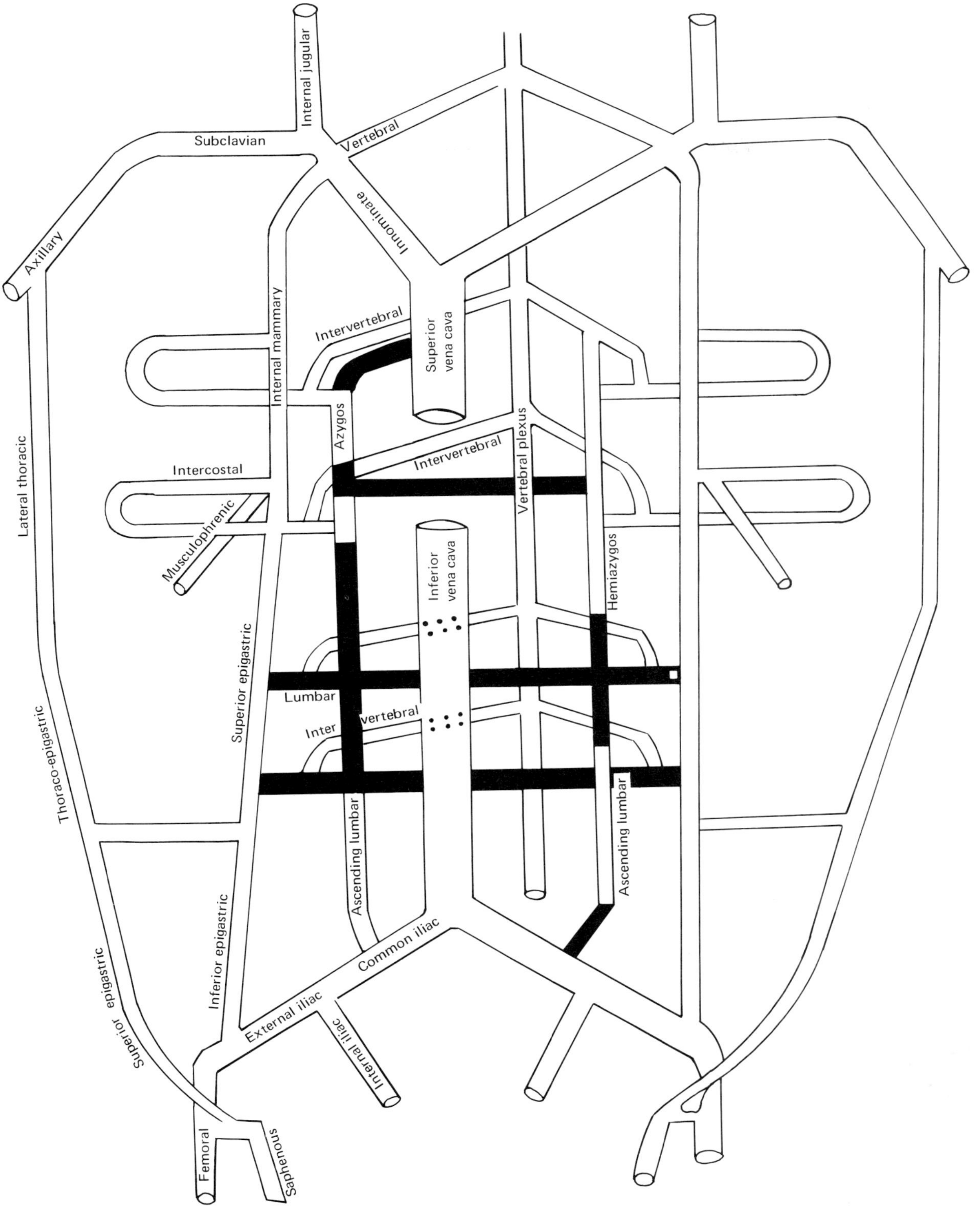

Fig. 1-7. Collateral systems. A composite, schematic representation of the four principal collateral systems in superior vena caval obstruction. (McIntire FT, Sykes EM. Ann Intern Med 925–960, 1949)

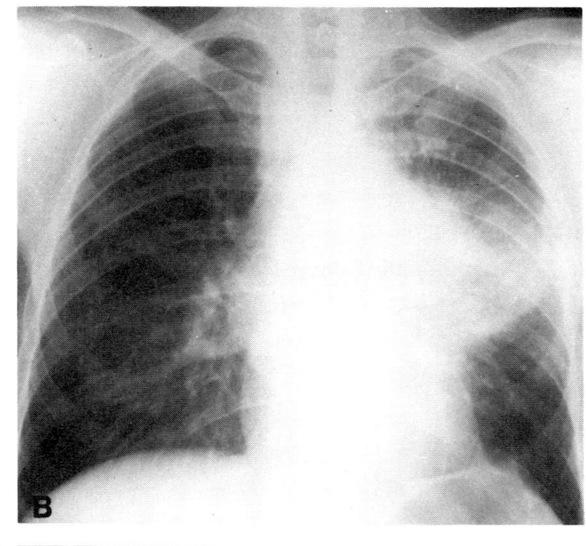

Fig. 1-8. Superior vena caval obstruction
Diagnosis: Epidermoid carcinoma of lung
  A. Scan, 6–9 sec. An incomplete obstruction of the
      left innominate vein and a prominent intercostal
      collateral pathway (arrows)
  B. X ray. Large mass lesion left lung
Diagnosis: Oat cell carcinoma
  C. Scan, 8–11 sec. The superior vena cava is
      obstructed (arrow). Prominent right intercostal
      collaterals exist.
  D. X ray. Right paramediastinal mass
Diagnosis: Epidermoid carcinoma
  E. Scan, 7–10 sec. There is obstruction of both the
      right and left innominate veins. Collateralization on
      the right is by way of the lateral thoracic (arrow)
      and intercostal routes. On the left, the internal
      mammary vein is seen (arrow).
  F. X ray. Right paramediastinal mass and atelectasis
Diagnosis: Squamous cell carcinoma

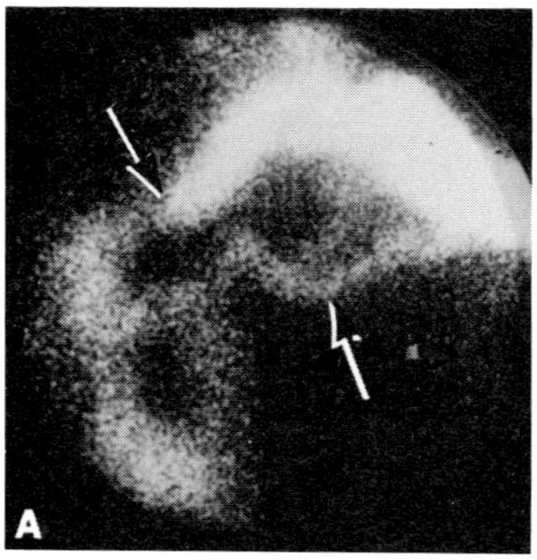

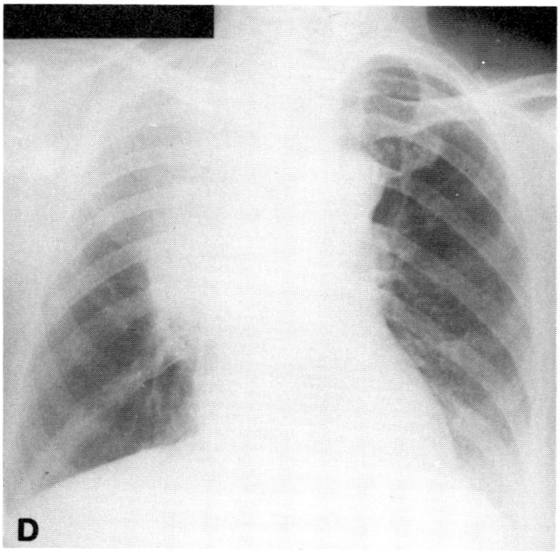

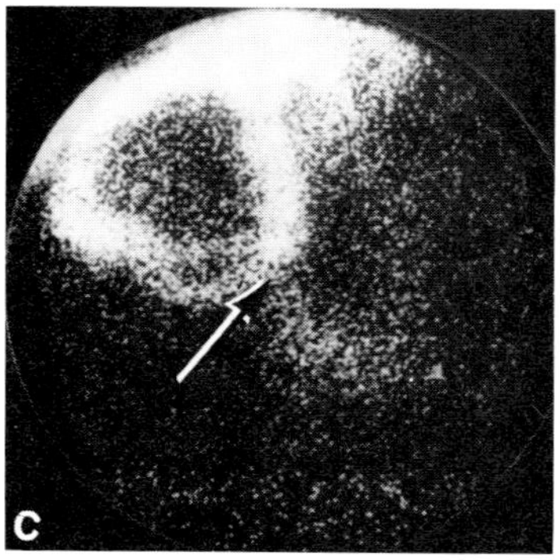

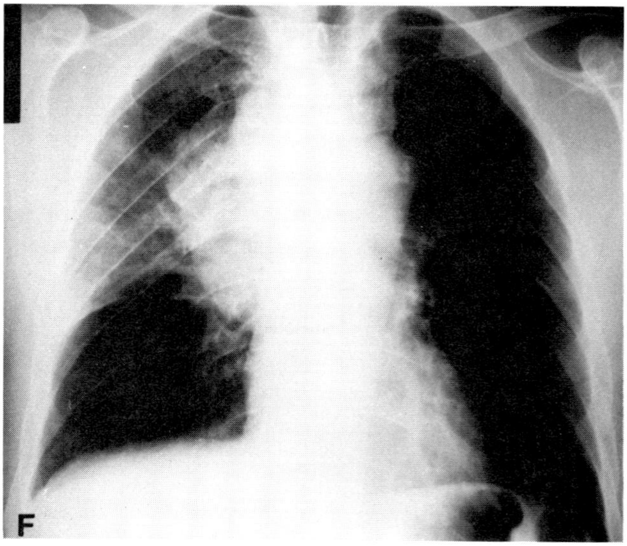

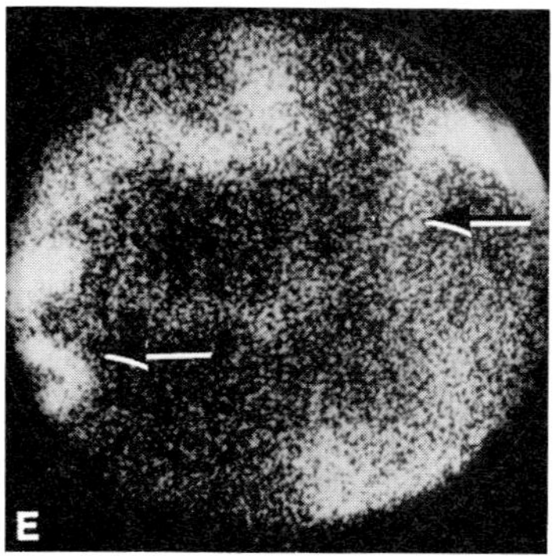

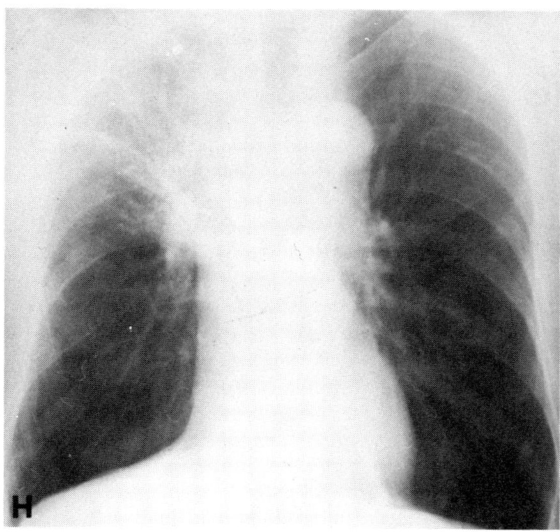

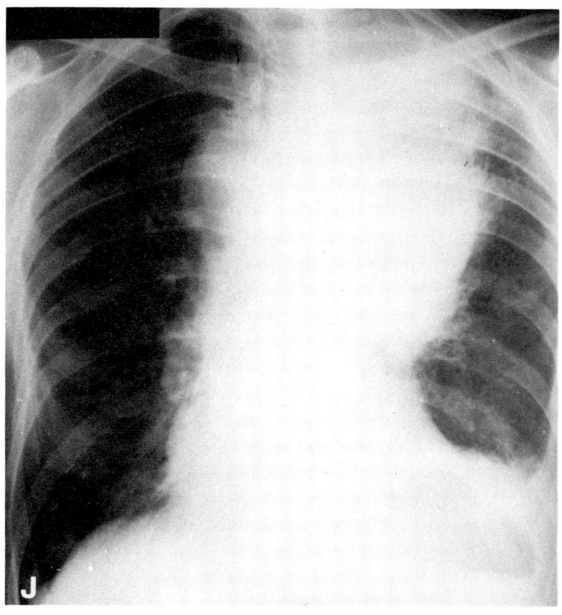

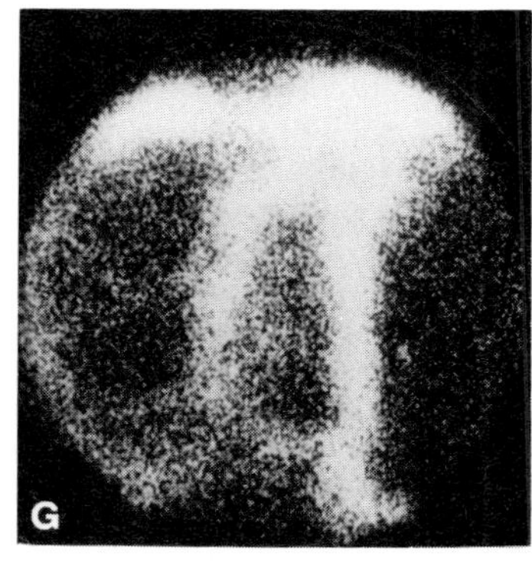

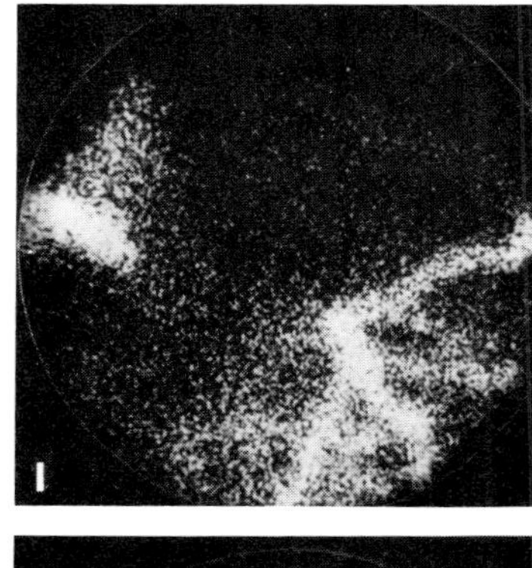

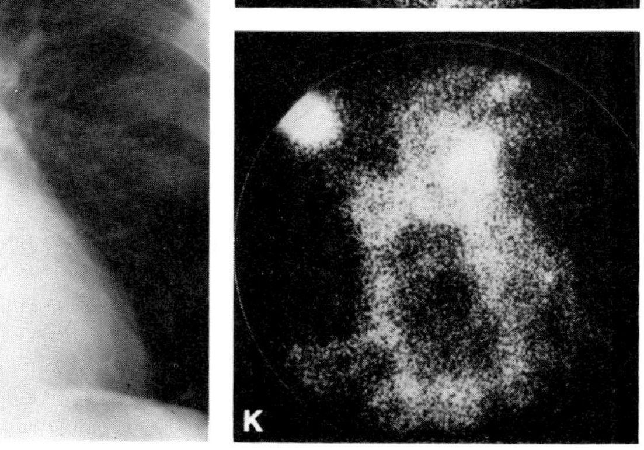

Fig. 1-8 continued.

G. Scan, 15–18 sec. Collateralization is predominantly by the azygos–hemiazygos system. There are also lateral thoracic–inferior vena caval routes.

H. X ray. Mass and atelectasis of right upper lobe

Diagnosis: Oat cell carcinoma

I. Scan, 11–14 sec. Total obstruction with all collateral routes employed

J. X ray. Left paramediastinal and upper lobe mass

Diagnosis: Oat cell carcinoma

K. Scan, 9–12 sec. Total obstruction with all collateral routes

L. X ray. Right upper lobe mass

cases, or only by the traumatic intervention of mediastinoscopy in others.

A very short and hopefully painless anatomic discussion will establish the basis for our enthusiasm. As part of the thoracic wall the anterior and posterior mediastinal boundaries are firm and unyielding. The lateral boundaries are elastic and provide routes of expansion or movement. The mediastinal components are for the most part protected against extrinsic pressure. The trachea, although displaceable, is rarely compressible because of its cartilagenous rings. The esophagus is in a somewhat-protected position posteriorly and its mobility and elasticity diminish the risk of impairment by extrinsic sources. The arterial structures are relatively immune because of their muscular walls and high gradient of pressure. Thus, only the large mediastinal veins with their thin walls and low-pressure system reflect extrinsic pressure. Their anterior position enhances their vulnerability by permitting compression against the sternum.

Thus, the setting of our drama. Enter now the villain—adenopathy. The right anterior mediastinal and right lateral–paratracheal chains are in direct proximity to the right innominate vein, the arch of the azygos, and the superior vena cava. These two groups receive all of the drainage from the right lung, the lower portion of the left lung, the lower trachea, the proximal bronchi, the thoracic esophagus, the diaphragmatic and mediastinal pleura, the heart and pericardium, and the thymus (Fig. 1-9). It can therefore be anticipated that nodal enlargement can and will produce pressure changes on the adjacent venous structures.

The earliest changes we have recognized manifest themselves as mild indentations on the cava which result in a loss of its vertical contour. Rather than the absolutely straight upstanding citizen it is, a slight wobble develops. Obviously, the degree of wobble varies with the extent of pressure and from the almost indistinguishable wobble progression produces a clearly atypical contour that presents in one of two general signs, either as sinusoid or as a frank displacement. The former we call the "undulating cava" (Fig. 1-10), the latter the "listing cava" (Fig. 1-11). It has been our experience that when this undulation or listing is present in cases of pulmonary neoplasm it is secondary to mediastinal adenopathy and the problem is inoperable. Obviously, undulation will be present from any cause of adenopathy so

that positive changes can be anticipated in any states that classically enlarge mediastinal nodes, *e.g.*, Hodgkin's, sarcoid, or leukemia. When the displacement occurs without the undulation and the primary chest pathology is not pulmonary neoplasm, the change may not signify adenopathy, but may simply reflect extrinsic pressure without invasion. Undulation and listing are not the only manifestations of extrinsic pressure. A "skip area" of activity may reflect the same mechanism. This sign probably reflects a greater degree of pressure or perhaps simply reflects the particular anatomic site of stress. The "skip" is identified as a focal defect of activity in the continuity pattern of the vessel and is more commonly seen in the innominate vein than in the cava (Figs. 1-12 and 1-13). Often the skip is associated with a wobble. Any combination may occur, *e.g.*, only undulation, only pinch in one vessel, pinch in more than one vessel, pinch plus undulation.

All of these patients are studied because their chest x rays are positive. The x rays, however, do not identify whether or not there is actual mediastinal invasion or extension, as defined by changes on the mediastinal vessels since there is no predictable correlation between the roentgen defect and the isotopic flow. Minimal x-ray changes may be associated with extensive vascular change. Contrary-wise, massive lesions may show a normal cava (Fig. 1-14). Additionally, the site of x-ray involvement is not always the side of vessel encroachment.

Our experience has shown that when the x-ray lesion is a pulmonary neoplasm and there is any scan documentation of venous encroachment—from undulation to skip to complete obstruction—the same prognostic inference exists for all: inoperable. Thus, the study becomes an invaluable addition to the work-up of the pulmonary neoplasm patient. There is one important note of caution: one anatomic site in which this skip or pinch may be normal and should not be confused with adenopathy or tumor mass exists at the entrance of the superior vena cava into the right atrium. At this point, the pericardial reflection produces an inconstant shallow indentation on the cava which looks identical to the defect of pressure (Fig. 1-15). Differentiation is made essentially on the location of the skip. If it is high, particularly at the junction of the innominate–right or innominate–left, or both, beware that complete obstruction may be imminent. If the pinch is just

Fig. 1-14. X ray positive—scan negative
Diagnosis: Epidermoid carcinoma
A. Scan. Normal flow
B. X ray. Mass lesion with atelectasis (right upper lobe)
Diagnosis: Epidermoid carcinoma
C. Scan. Normal flow
D. X ray. Mass in right suprahilar region
Diagnosis: Squamous cell carcinoma
E. Scan. Normal flow
F. X ray. Right suprahilar mass (left upper lobe mass)

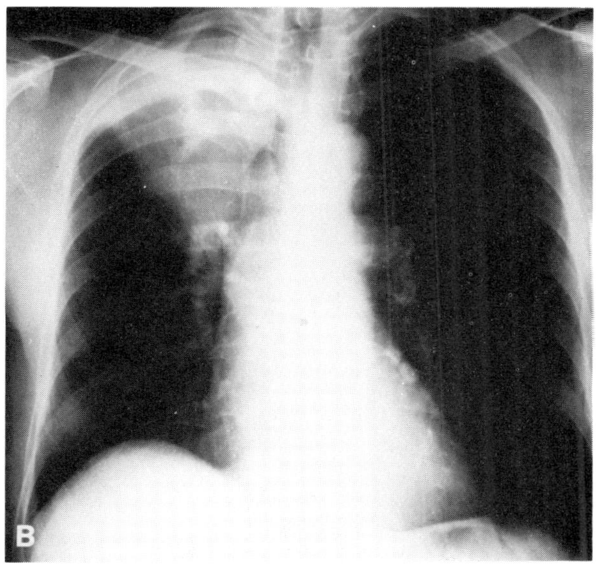

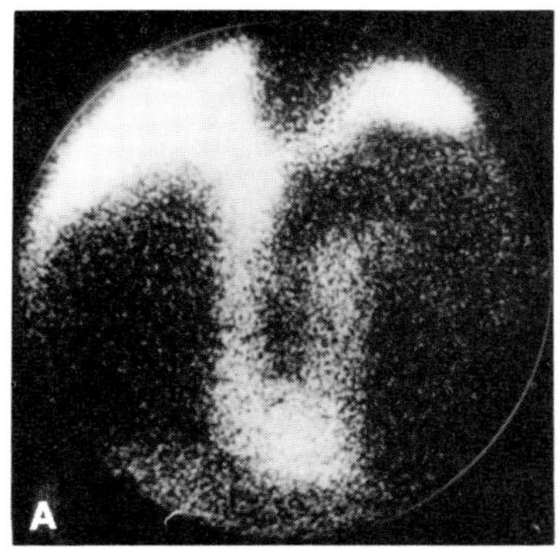

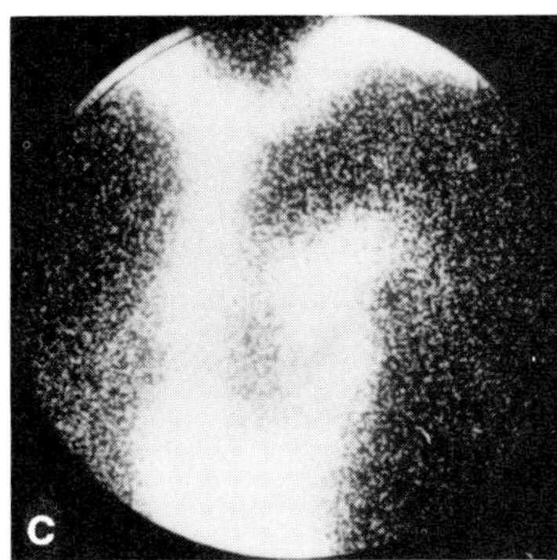

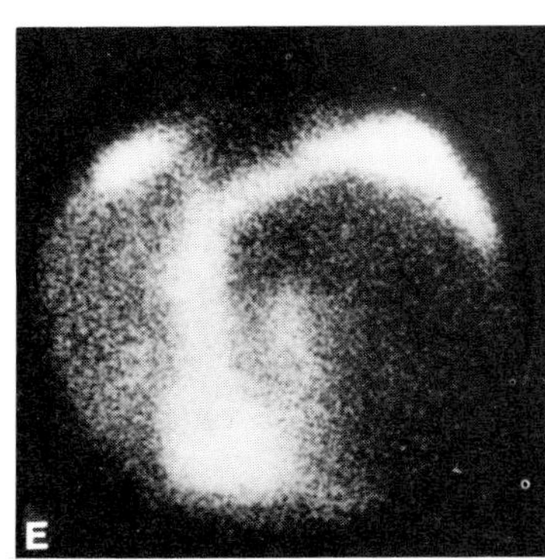

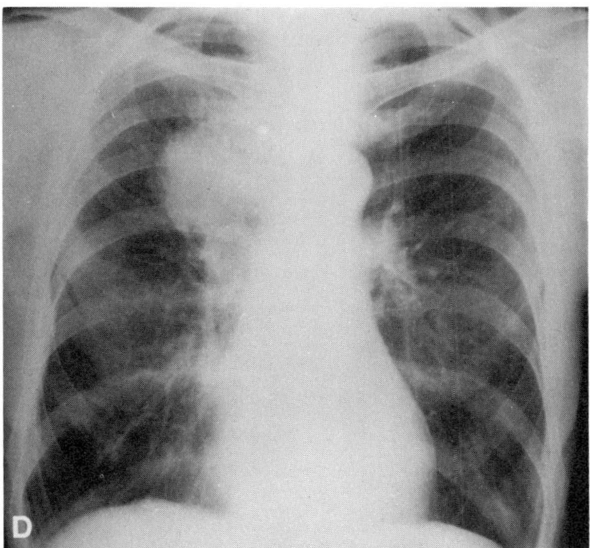

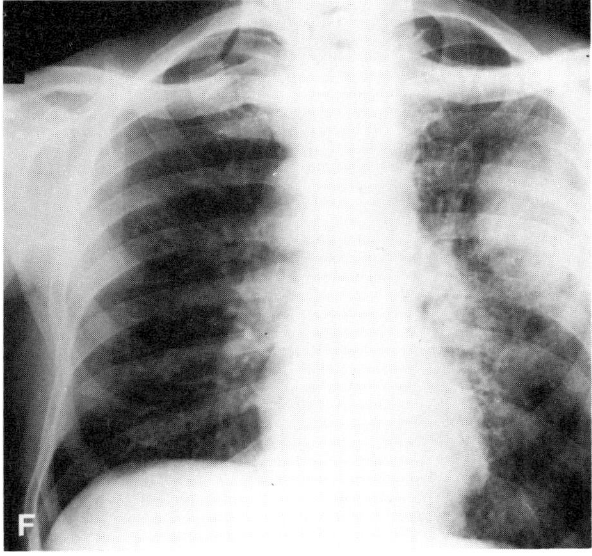

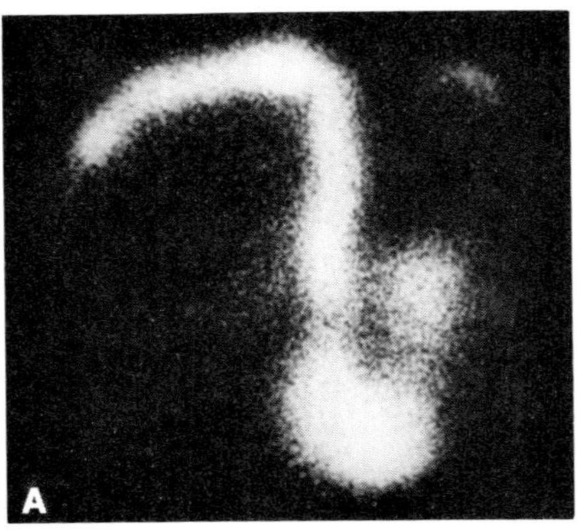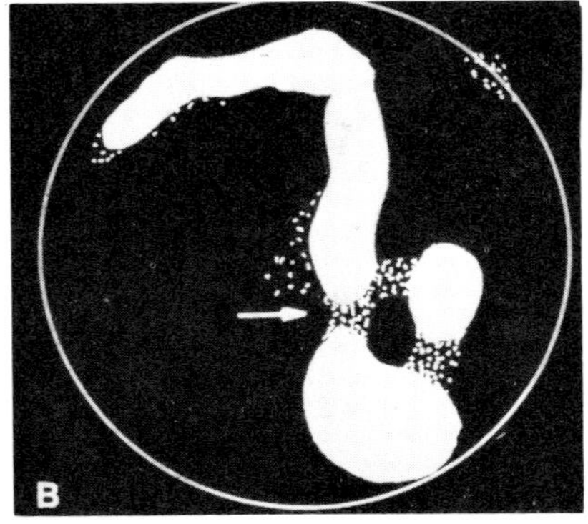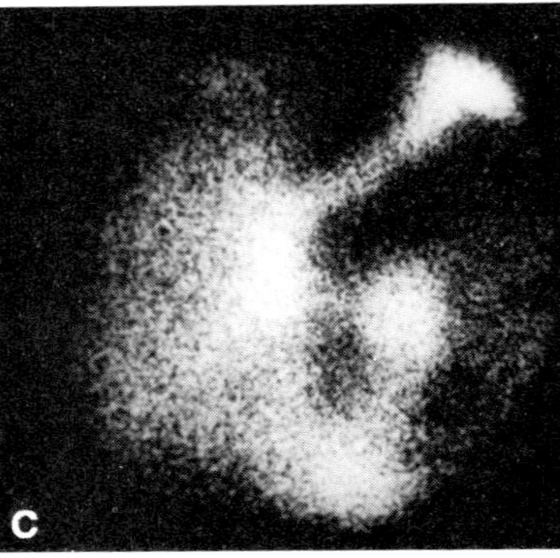
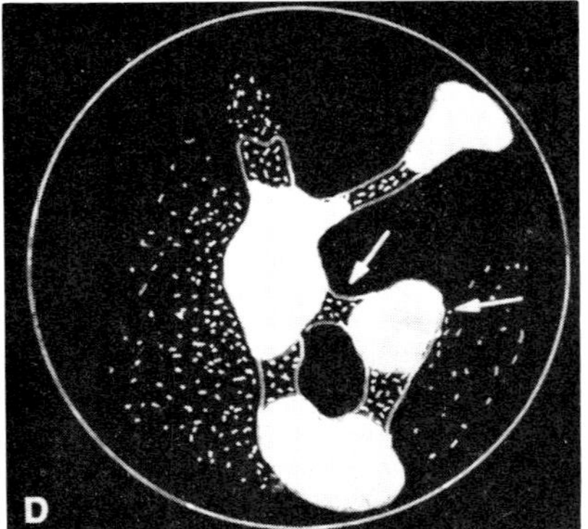

Fig. 1-15. Normal superior vena cava—pericardial defect
- **A.** Scan, 0–3 sec. There is a defect "pinch" at the lower portion of the superior vena cava.
- **B.** Line sketch of **A.** Arrow is at the site of defect.
- **C.** Scan, 3–6 sec. The "defect" is obscured by activity in the lungs. The pulmonary conus and right pulmonary arteries are clearly defined.
- **D.** Line sketch of **C.** Arrows identify the pulmonary conus and right pulmonary artery.

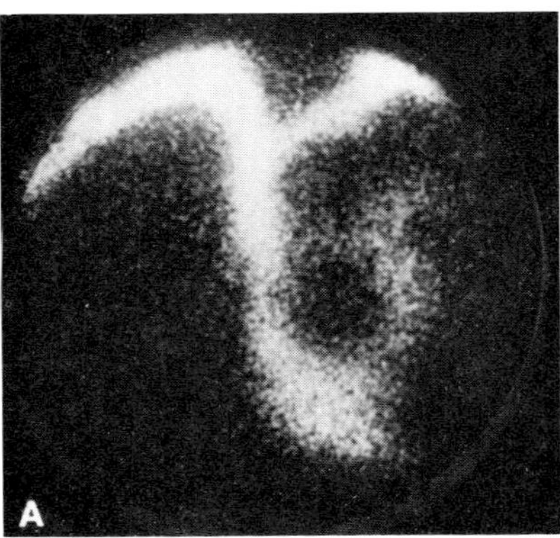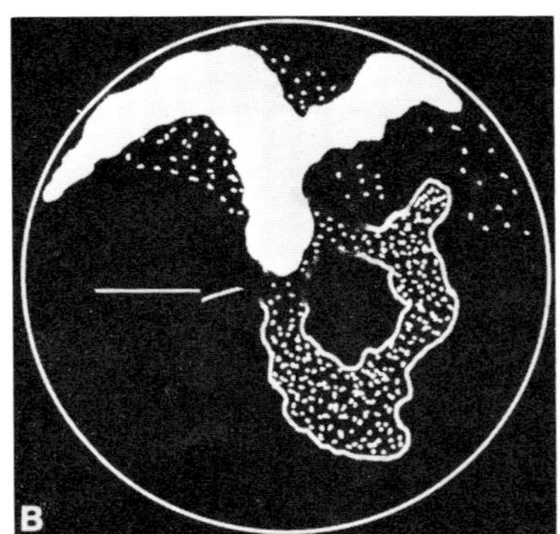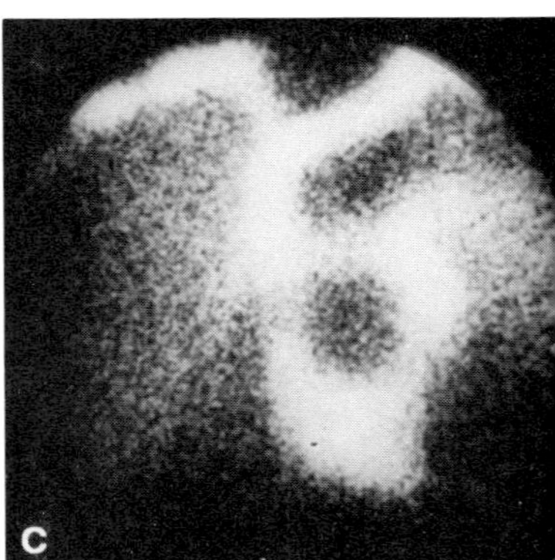
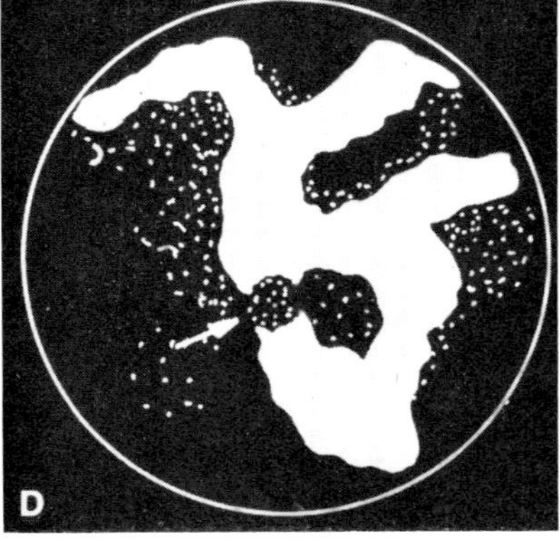

Fig. 1-16. Right pulmonary cross-over sign. Normal superior vena cava—pericardial defect
- **A.** Scan, 6–9 sec. Diminished activity simulating a pinch defect in the lower superior vena cava
- **B.** Line sketch of **A.** Defect identified by arrow
- **C.** Scan, 9–12 sec. The defect is still present but is located below the crossing right pulmonary artery.
- **D.** Line sketch of **C.** Right pulmonary artery cross over is above the pericardial defect.

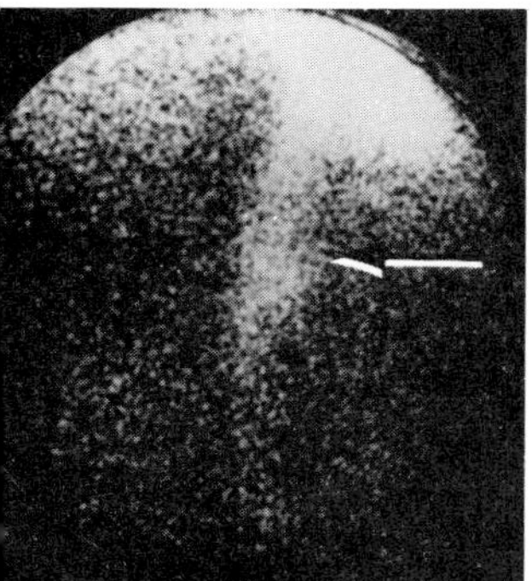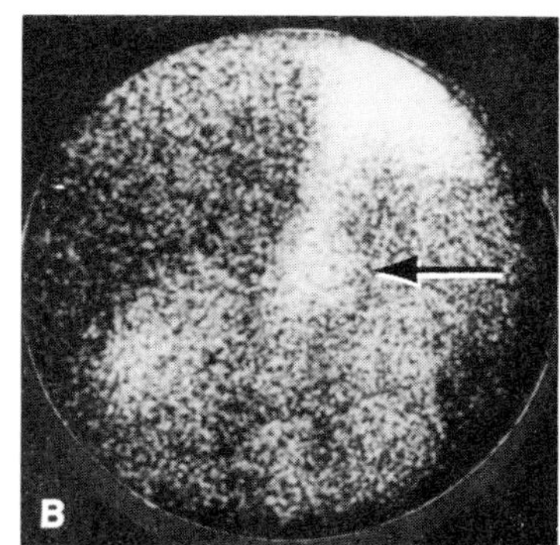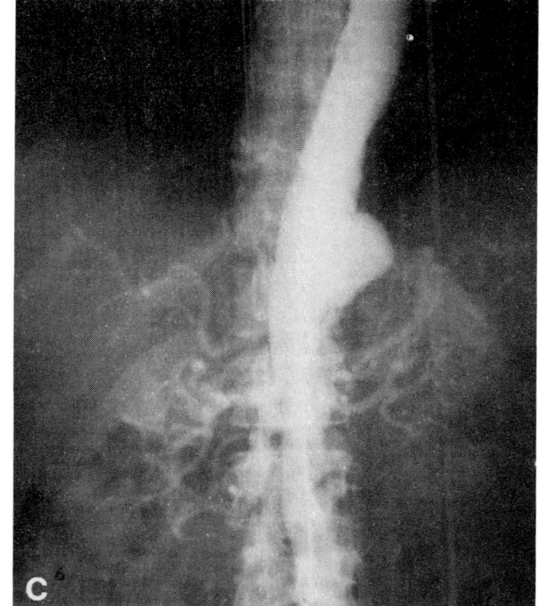

Fig. 1-22. Abdominal aortic aneurysm
A and B. Sequential Scans. On physical examination in a 46-year-old male admitted for elective herniorrhaphy an abdominal bruit was detected. The abdominal aortic image suggests a "bump" just proximal to the kidneys.
    C. Aortography. The small aortic aneurysm is confirmed.

Fig. 1-23. Abdominal aortic aneurysm. An abdominal survey prior to a barium enema identified a questionable aortic calcification.
A. Scan, 15–18 sec. The distal aorta is dilated.
B. Scan, 18–21 sec. The fusiform dilatation is pronounced.
C. Aortography. A large fusiform aortic aneurysm dissects into the iliac arteries.

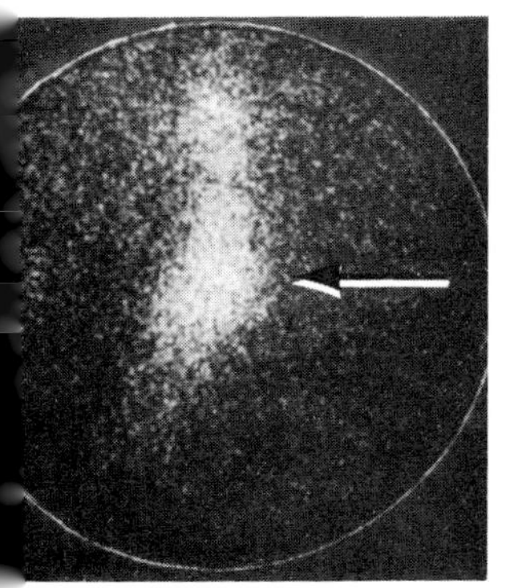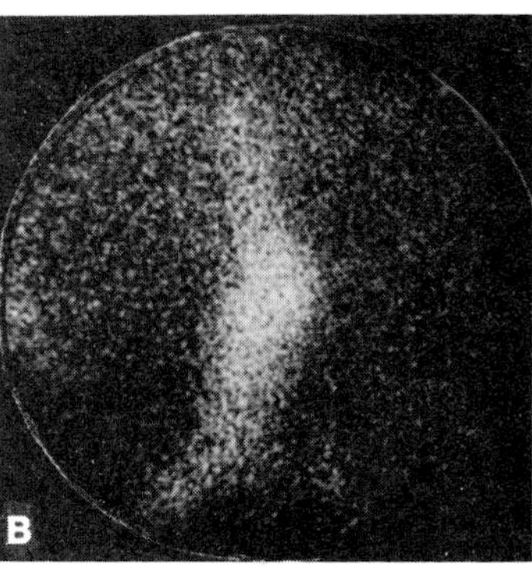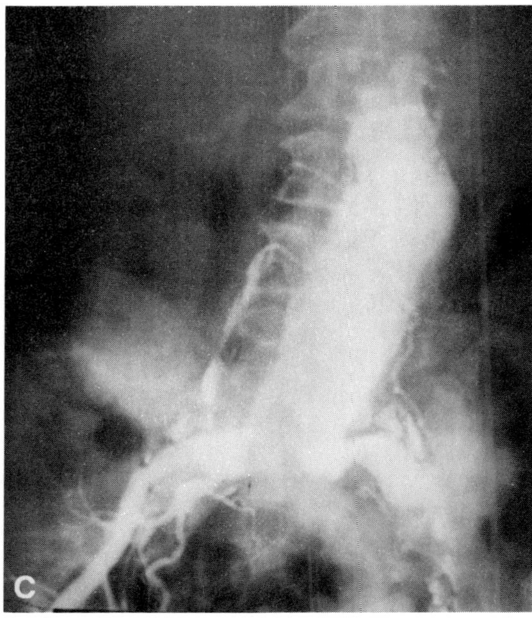

technique. The combination of speed, simplicity, economy, and accuracy make aneurysm detection dependent on only one variable, clinical suspicion, and then clinical action.

Clinical suspicion can be initiated by three general classes of stimuli. The first, and the strongest, is the patient with a full-blown complex of dissecting aneurysm. The second is the inadvertant discovery of changes that "could be consistent with . . ." from an x-ray finding of the chest or abdomen, or of both. The third is physical examination with the unexplained detection of an atypical pulsation or the ascultation of a bruit.

But clinical suspicion is not synonymous with clinical action. The responsible clinician becomes the dialectician and weighs again the age-old conundrum, "does the end justify the means?" In the case of a patient with a full-blown complex of dissecting aneurysm the answer is simple and the catheter crew goes to work. However, in situations two and three the decision is usually no. The age of the patient and the paucity of symptoms must be considered against the rigor of contrast angiography, and the resultant ratio of pluses and minuses is often so disproportionate that further investigation by contrast angiography is usually contraindicated.

And like a TV commercial—"Enter the man from Nuclear!" The type 2 and type 3 situations are his sustenance. Within minutes the nuclear technologist can resolve all clinical doubt. With only an IV anticubital stick the innocuous bruit that did not warrant arteriography becomes or does not become a localized aneurysm on flow study, or the questionable calcification may be seen to be well beyond the aorta and so is safely forgotten. When screening can be done in so simple a manner, the means do justify the ends (Figs. 1-21 to 1-23).

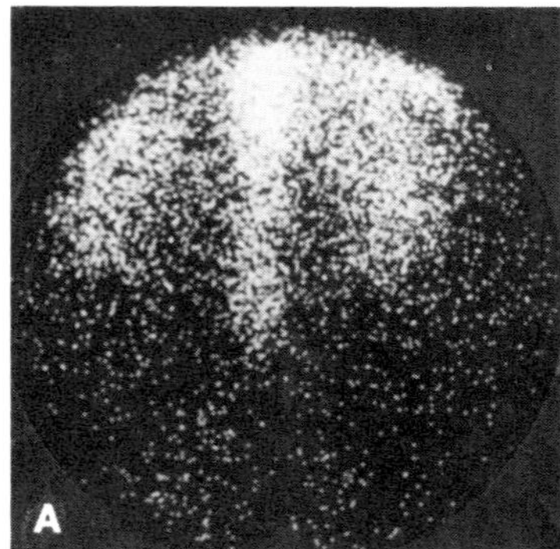

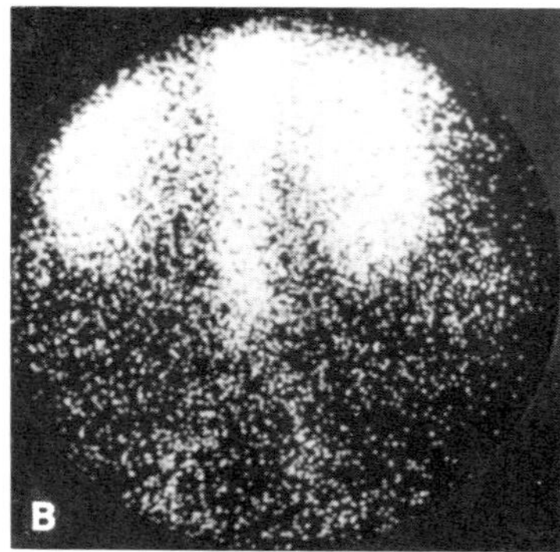

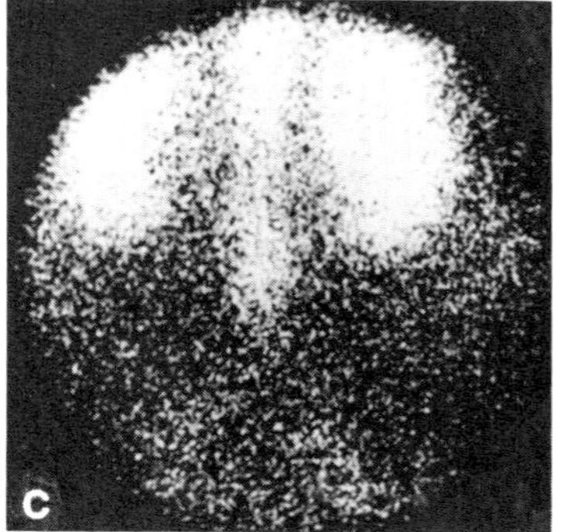

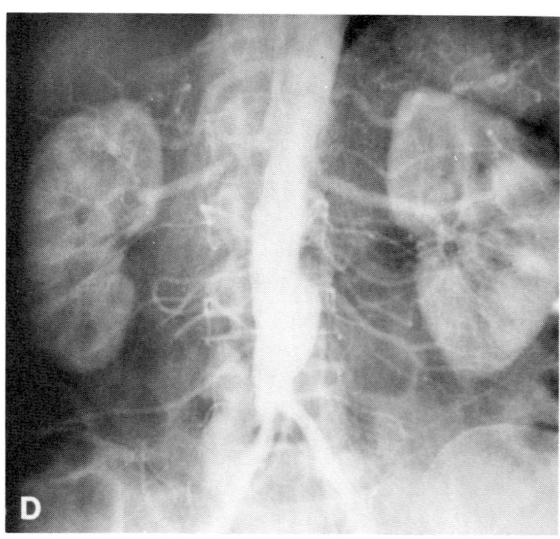

Fig. 1-24. Incomplete iliac artery obstruction
A–C. Sequential scans. The abdominal aorta is well defined to its bifurcation. There is significant delay in transit beyond and poor definition of the iliac arteries.
D. Aortogram. The abdominal aorta is sclerotic. There is a small aneurysm just above the bifurcation. The iliac arteries are markedly narrowed and sclerotic.

Obstruction. If arterial obstruction occurs proximal to the femoral arteries, the diagnosis is possible by isotope angiography. Complete and even partial occlusions of the abdominal aorta and even iliac vessels can be detected (Figs. 1-24 and 1-25). Unfortunately, distal to the iliacs the image quality is too unpredictable for routine reliance. Thus, lesions of the femoral arteries and lower cannot be routinely evaluated by the IV route. Peripheral isotope angiography will be discussed shortly.

PERIPHERAL VASCULAR. Arterial. As has been noted earlier, arterial visualization by the IV flow technique is reliable only to the iliac artery level. More distally, resolution fails primarily as a consequence of bolus dilution. If this did not occur and vascular definition was possible by that technique, it might still prove unsatisfactory in answering certain questions referable to the peripheral perfusion of muscle masses. Definition of the simple presence or absence of occlusive disease is no longer considered sufficient data for surgical decisions, and sophisticated judgment now requires knowledge of the perfusion status distal to the obstruction. Consequently, simple morphologic definition of the arterial tree by contrast angiography (or isotopically, if possible) no longer satisfies the purist. What is the arterial and capillary perfusion distal to the obstruction? What is the collateral status? As with coronary studies the injection of radioactive microspheres into the arterial side at the time of contrast angiography may provide the necessary answers. Preliminary reports suggest the predictable pattern of muscle mass and skin perfusion as a consequence to particular major vessel disease can be obtained by scanning. As with other nuclear techniques,

this preoperative data may both improve prognostic judgment and guide surgical management.

Venous. Radionuclide studies of the peripheral venous structures are assuming two distinct roles: 1) simple isotopic venography or the morphologic depiction of the peripheral venous vasculature and 2) detection of thrombus development.

The first technique is identical to those established for contrast venography. Following the cannulation of a vein on the dorsum of the foot a radionuclide rather than a contrast agent is infused against a tourniquet around the ankle to insure opacification of the deep venous system. Pictures are obtained with a scanning device rather than with an x-ray unit.

Except for those patients who are "allergic" to radiopaque agents it is difficult to become enthusiastic about the study. Isotopic angiography is justifiable when it provides exclusive data, or provides data far more simply, faster, more economically, or with less patient morbidity than comparable contrast studies. Isotopic peripheral vascular venography satisfies none of these criteria, except perhaps a decrease in patient discomfort. It is performed identically to the contrast technique and requires no less time, nor does it offer any sufficient economic advantage. It does, however, provide image detail far inferior to contrast definition. Even so, some justification may exist for its use in other than the special situation of allergy. It has been suggested that in all patients having perfusion lung scans for suspected embolic–infarctive disease the aggregated particles (^{99m}Tc MAA [macroaggregated human serum albumin] or ^{99m}Tc albumin microspheres) be

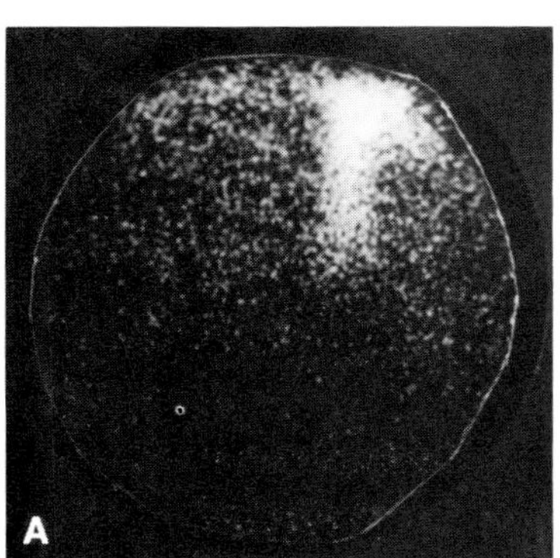
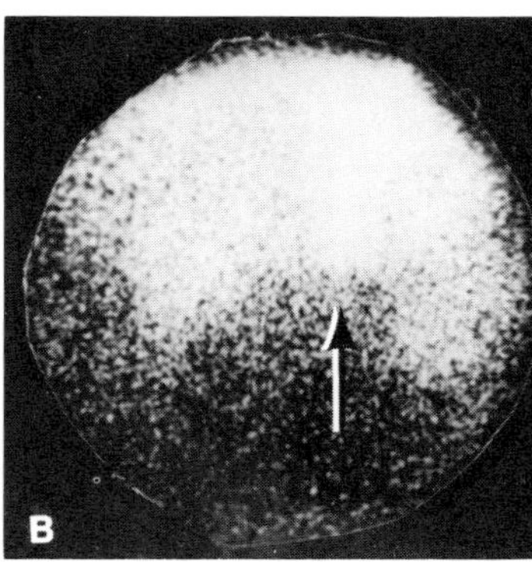

Fig. 1-25. Complete abdominal aortic obstruction
A and B. Sequential scans. Complete occlusion of the aorta immediately below the renal artery take-off (arrow). No contrast angiography was performed prior to surgery.

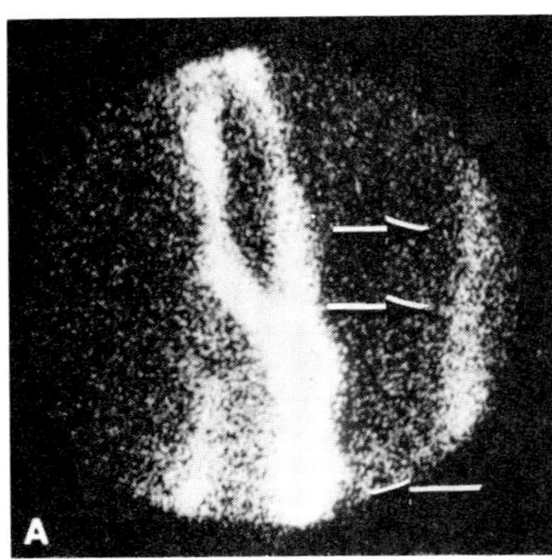
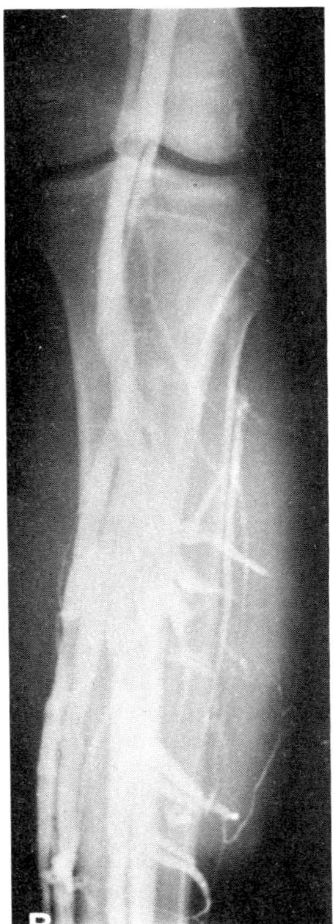

Fig. 1-26. Normal lower leg venography
A. Scan, 15–18 sec. [99mTc] saline infusion on the dorsum of the right foot. The marker (arrow) is at the level of the knee; the stripe of activity (double arrow) is left leg.
B. X ray. Same location during contrast venography

introduced into a foot vein(s). A coincidental lower extremity venogram might be obtained as a screening procedure (Fig. 1-26).

Thrombus detection, on the other hand, holds great promise of being a major diagnostic contribution. As now performed, selected patients are given tagged fibrinogin immediately preoperatively or postoperatively. Imaging is done at the bedside with mobile scanners at regular intervals throughout the immediate recovery. It is hoped that radioactive fibrinogin will incorporate in forming thrombi in sufficiently high concentrations to allow them to be identified and appropriately treated before they become clinically manifest (Fig. 1-27).

However, investigations to date suggest that labeled fibrinogin will not detect preexisting thrombi. Streptokinase labeled with [99mTc] and even similarly labeled urokinase are also being studied. It would seem that these thrombolytic agents, particularly streptokinase, may have certain advantages over fibrinogin since they can detect formed as well as forming thrombi.

Regardless of the agent finally awarded the honor of being "the one," there is every reasonable expectation that the present difficulties in sensitivity and reliability will be mastered and that this technique will assume a position on the menu we call routine procedure.

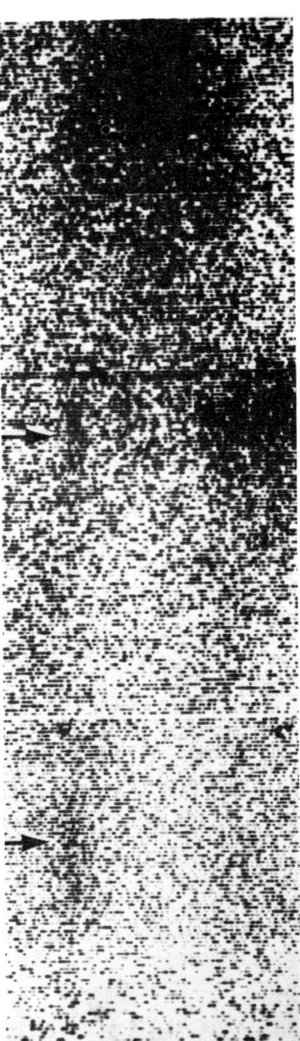

Fig. 1-27. Thrombosis. Two days following the IV administration of [131I] fibrinogen in a patient suffering a left femoral head fracture, a scan of the lower extremities identifies two areas of increased activity (arrows). These foci represent uptake in forming venous thrombi. (Courtesy of N. David Charkes, Temple University Hospital, Philadelphia, Pa.)

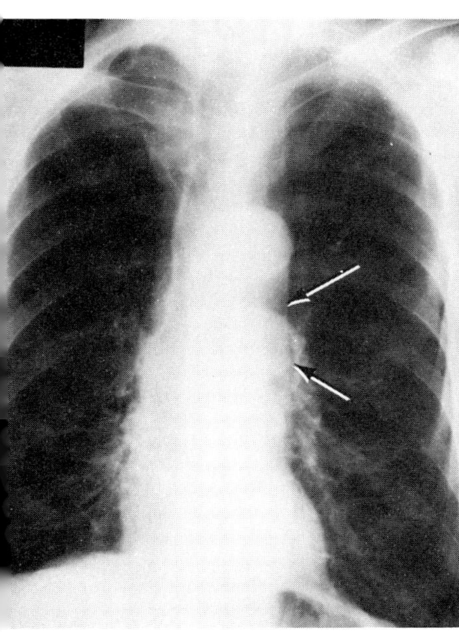

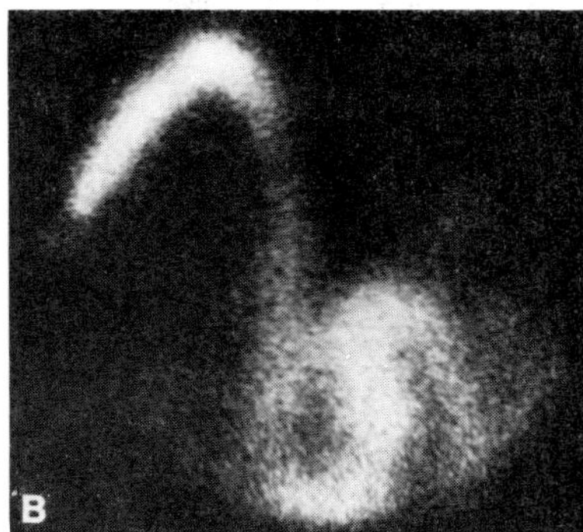

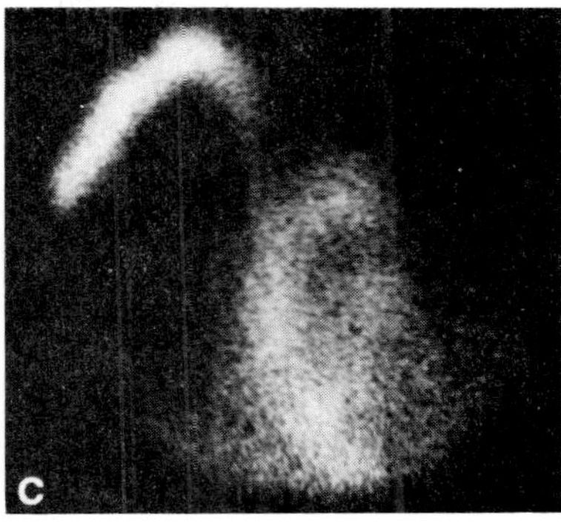

Fig. 1-28. Prominent pulmonary conus—absent right pulmonary artery
A. X ray. Is the prominence (arrows) in the left mediastinum vascular or neoplastic?
B. Scan, 3–6 sec. The pulmonary conus is more prominent than average. The left pulmonary artery is increased in prominence. There is no visualized right pulmonary artery or evidence of right pulmonary perfusion.
C. Scan, 9–12 sec. The pulmonary conus is still seen although the aorta is filling. The left lung perfusion is diminishing. There is still no perfusion of the right lung.

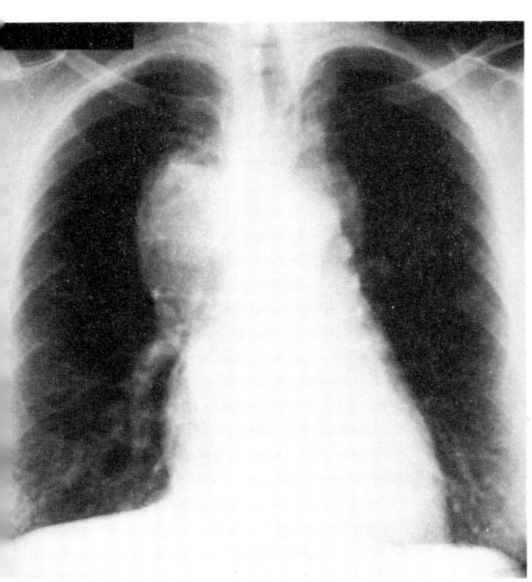

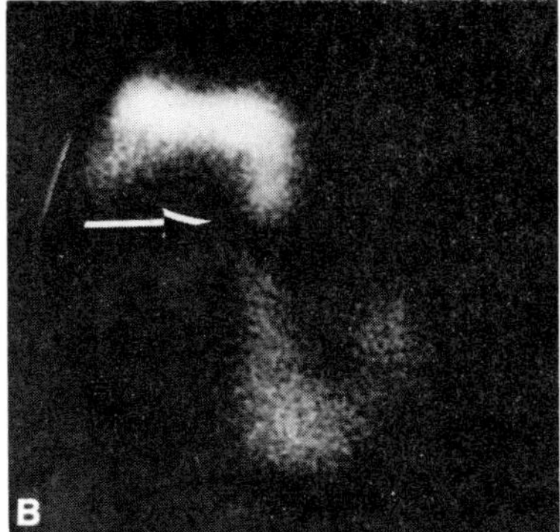

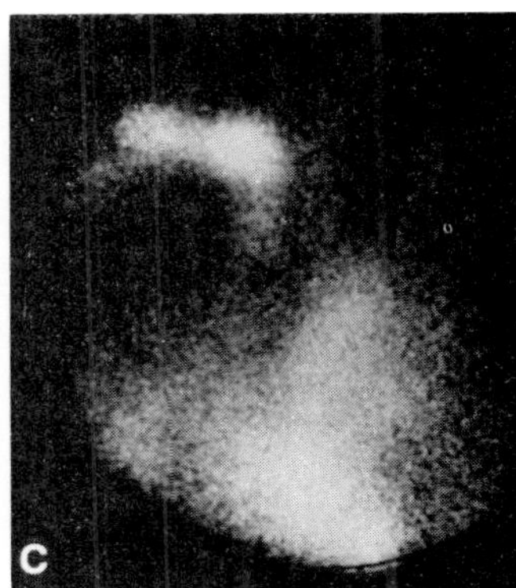

Fig. 1-29. Epidermoid carcinoma of the right lung
A. X ray. Is the widened right superior mediastinal density an aortic aneurysm or pulmonary neoplasm?
B. Scan, 3–6 sec. In the venous phase there is a defect (arrow) in the right innominate vein.
C. Scan, 16–19 sec. The aorta is normal in caliber. There is no perfusion of the right upper lobe.

Others. Others is an ill-defined grab bag of day-to-day problems. Some variation, some changes, some nuisance factor that can't be easily explained or some major defect that is obvious but not readily catalogued, that is noted on physical examination or not uncommonly on x ray—often for some other reason. "Is that a true mass in the hilum?" (Fig. 1-28). "Is that an aneurysm or tumor?" (Fig. 1-29). "Are those really notched ribs?" (Fig. 1-30). "What's displacing the bladder?" (Fig. 1-31). "Where is the catheter?" (Fig. 1-32). Hardly a day passes that some such question does not arise. Don't sweat it! Flow it!

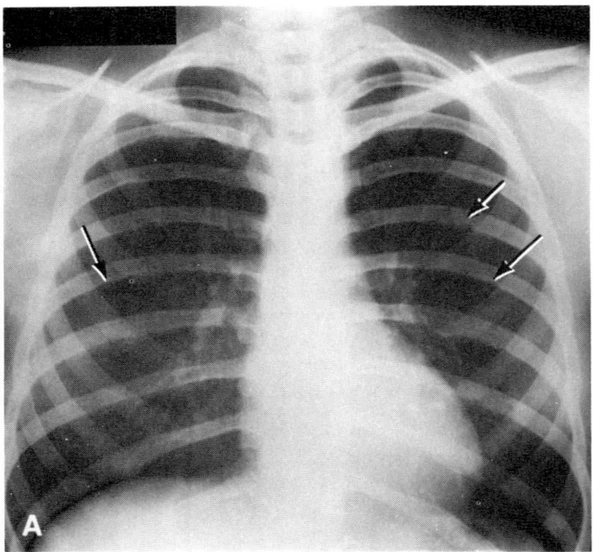

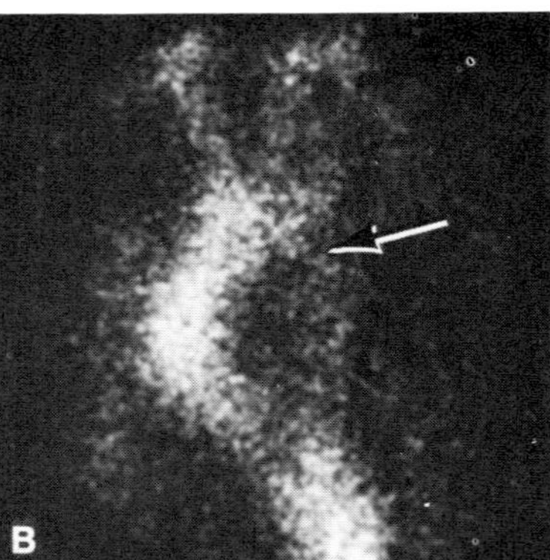

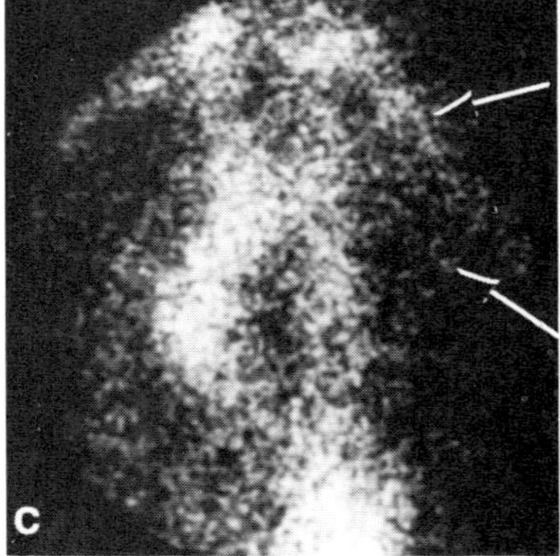

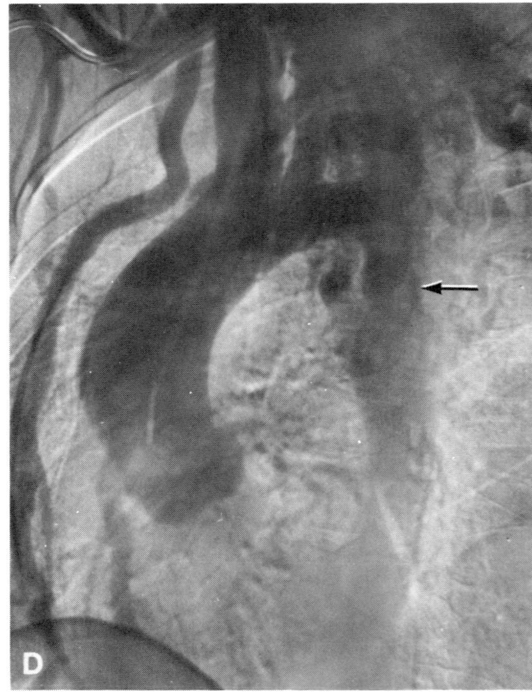

Fig. 1-30. Coarctation of the aorta
A. X ray. Are the ribs really notched (arrows)?
B. Scan, 12–15 sec. The aortic image just distal to
the arch presents a notch defect (arrow).
C. Scan, 15–18 sec. The aorta now is continuous, but
atypical vessels and activity are present (arrows).
D. Aortogram (subtraction mode). The site of
coarctation corresponds with the notch defect in
B (arrow). Collateral vessels are easily identified.

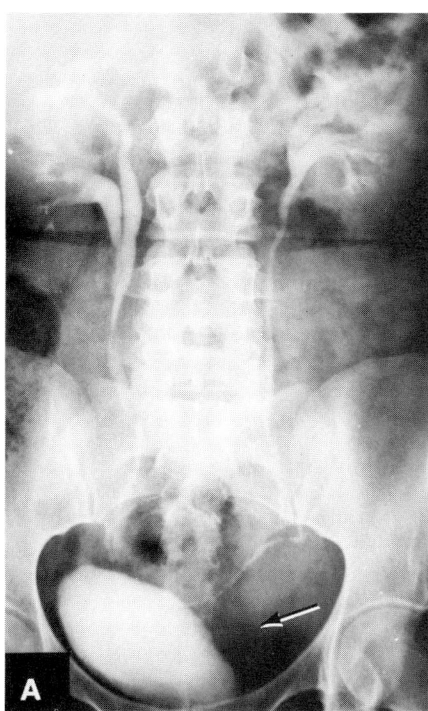

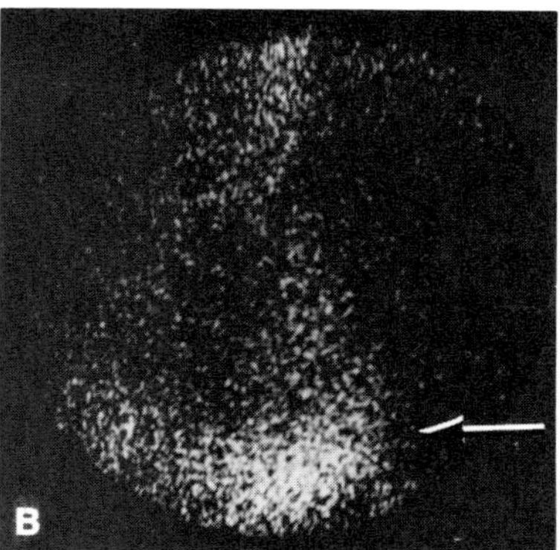

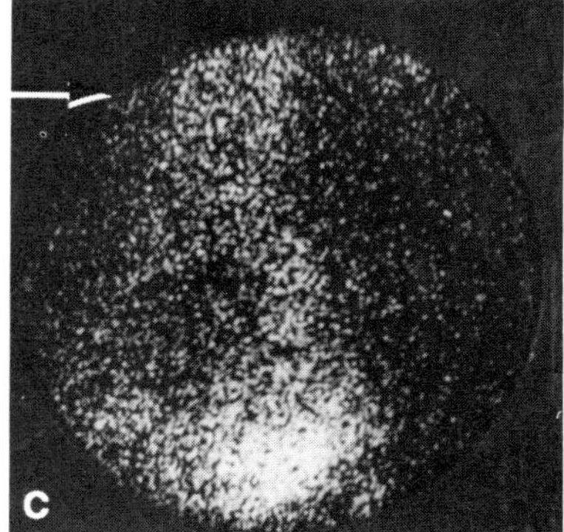

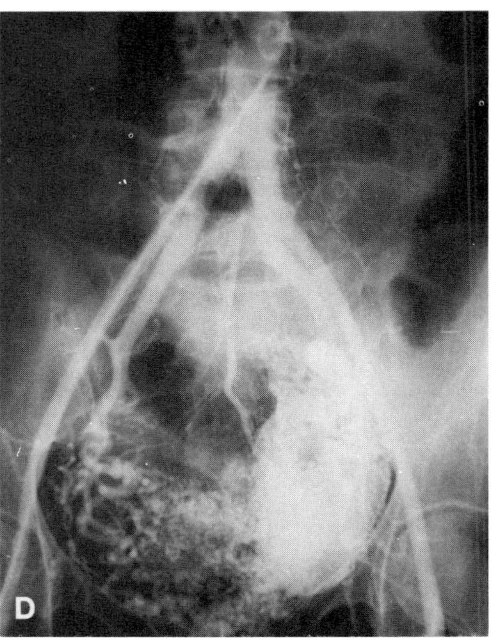

Fig. 1-31. Pelvic arteriovenous malformation

A. X ray. The bladder is displaced to the right (arrow). The distal portion of the left ureter is elevated. Why?

B. Scan, 5–18 sec. A grossly atypical collection of activity (arrow) is present adjacent to the left common iliac artery.

C. Scan, 18–21 sec. A parallel stripe of activity (arrow) appears adjacent to the vertebral band of the abdominal aorta—the inferior vena cava.

D. Arteriogram. A massive arteriovenous malformation

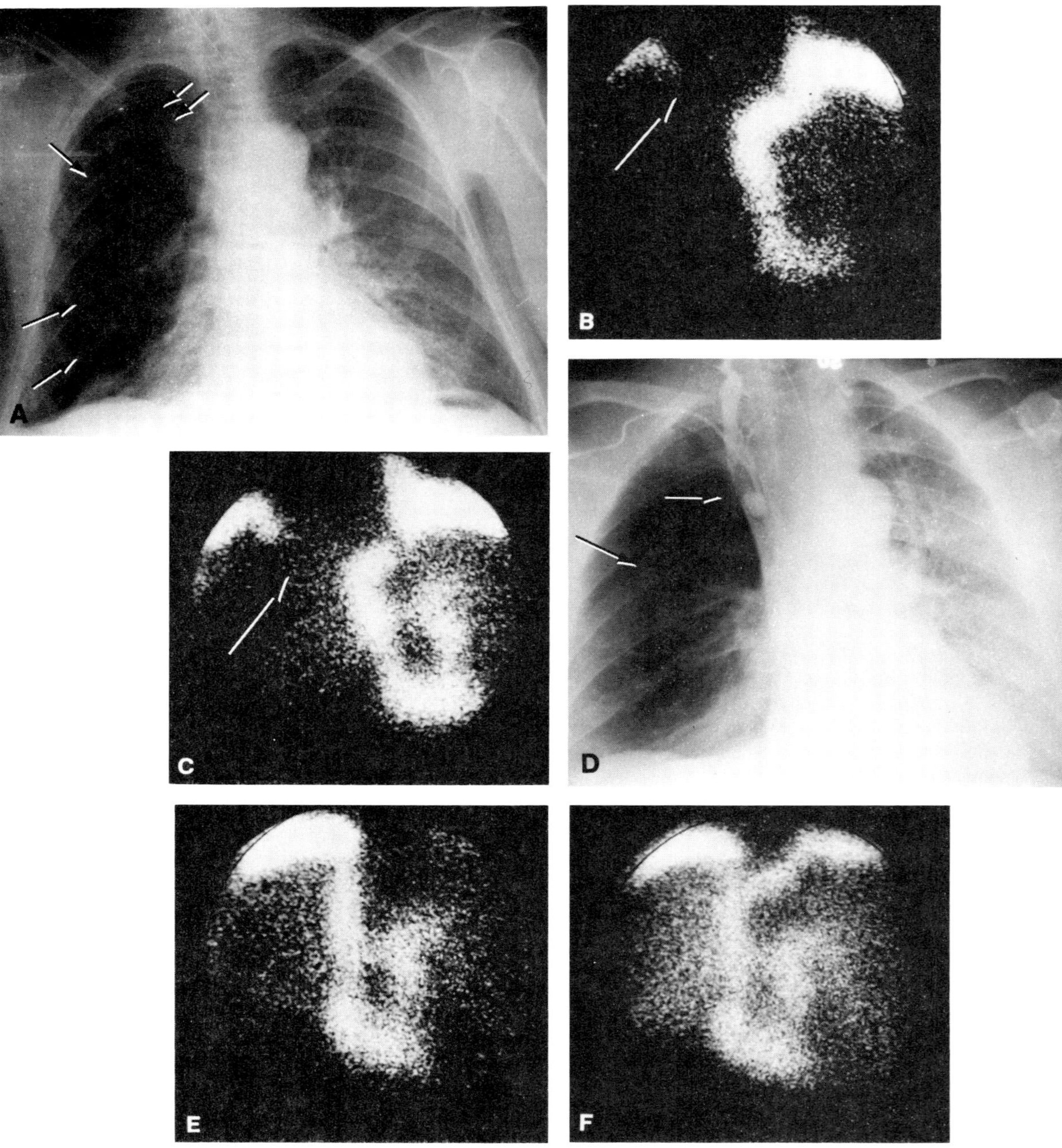

Fig. 1-32. Iatrogenic obstruction and thrombosis of the right innominate vein

A. X ray. Following the placement of a central venous pressure catheter (double arrows) there was no blood flow. A partial right pneumothorax is present (single arrows). Where was the catheter and why no blood return?

B and C. Sequential scans, **B** at 4–6 sec, **C** at 6–8 sec. There is a complete obstruction (arrow) of the right innominate vein.

D. X ray. A new catheter was immediately reintroduced and opaque media injected. A large thrombus (arrow) is present in the innominate vein and it is obstructed. The pneumothorax was increased (arrow).

E and F. Sequential scans, 9 days later. The right innominate vein is completely patent.

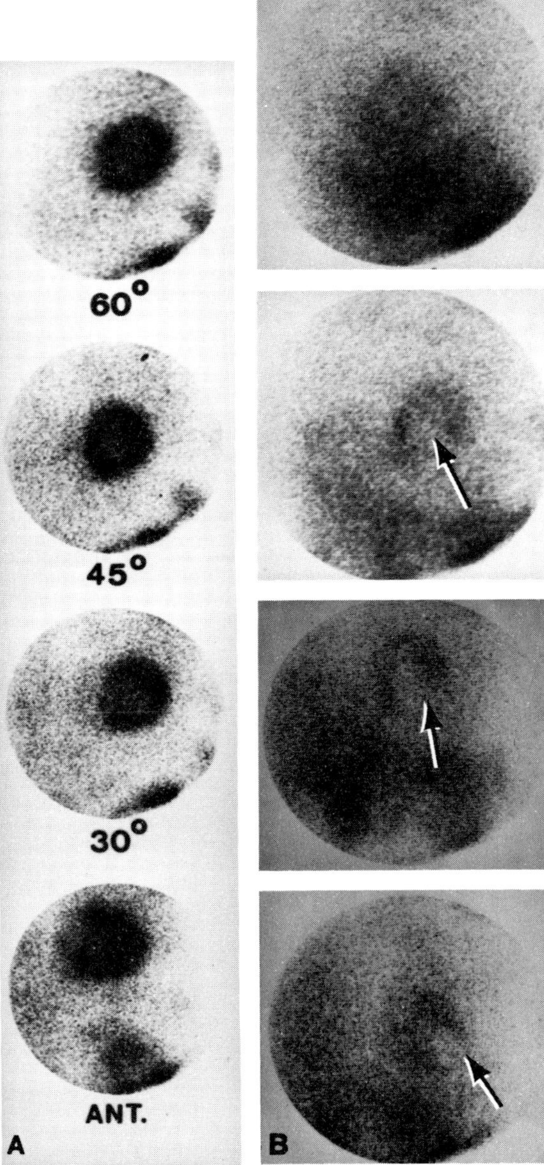

Fig. 1-33. Myocardial infarction (left ventricle)
A. Normal myocardial uptake of [201]Tl. Images are obtained 10 minutes following the IV injection of 2 mCi.
B. Infarction. Large defect (arrow) in myocardial uptake in the region of the anterior inferior segment of the left ventricle
(Courtesy of G. Jackson, Harrisburg Hospital, Harrisburg, Pa.)

Radioisotope Angiocardiography. *CARDIAC.* Although isotopic angiocardiography is a valid, viable, and valuable technique, it has not yet reached broad-based application because the instrumentation required for most problems is beyond that found in the average facility. As with other modalities it will probably be only a matter of time until this area of investigation becomes routine. The work that is being done is exquisite. Initially, investigation was confined to problems of a congenital etiology. Now, acquired lesions are also studied.

As previously discussed istopic angiocardiography can serve as a screening procedure. It is also of value in patients too ill to tolerate catheter studies, in serial evaluation of the efficacy of medical therapy, in the documentation of preoperative and postoperative states, and as a monitoring device to follow the course of disease.

MYOCARDIAL. Despite the well-established diagnostic position of the EKG, despite the reliability of enzyme studies, despite the increasing role of contrast coronary angiography, and despite the acceptance of coronary artery surgery, there is a tremendous concerted effort under way to develop a reliable scanning procedure to evaluate the status and integrity of myocardial perfusion. This extensive effort unquestionably reflects the need for such a technique, and it is well known that necessity is the mother of a new nuclear study.

The established procedures fail to provide needed data in two major areas: 1) the status of myocardial perfusion in the patient with classic angina but with normal or nonspecific EKGs and 2) the status of the capillary and collateral beds distal to a known occlusive lesion. Efforts to delineate these general states result in two general types of study: 1) the IV introduction of a radionuclide with subsequent selective myocardial localization and 2) the intracoronary artery injection of a radionuclide at the time of coronary angiography with hope of delineating perfusion distal to the site of established occlusion.

The study to evaluate areas of reduced coronary blood flow is proving partially successful if the patient has had a previous myocardial infarction. The nuclides currently being investigated, *i.e.,* potassium (^{43}K) and cesium (^{131}Cs and ^{129}Cs) and thallium (^{201}Tl), do localize selectively in the myocardium. Their distribution is a function of vascular integrity so that zones of infarction (and—hopefully—areas of diminished perfusion) will demonstrate diminished uptake and appear cold on scans (Fig. 1-33). The study is performed first with exercise. If positive, it is repeated with the patient at rest. If the stress image is positive and the rest picture negative, some inference of coronary artery disease without infarction is valid. Technical difficulties still persist. Resolution is relatively poor, and lesions in certain locations are far easier to identify than those in others, *i.e.*, anterior wall defects are imaged far better than posterior wall defects.

Prior to experience with ^{99m}Tc phosphates imaging, even when an infarct defect was identified its age was uncertain. Chronic was indistinguishable from acute. Infarction was infarction was infarction. This is no longer true. With pyrophosphate, acute infarcts can be identified as early as 6 hours after the event and images remain positive for approximately 6 days, at which time they begin to fade. Additionally, the technetium bone-scanning agents localize in the infarcted tissue (perhaps in calcified mitochondria) yielding a hot spot as evidence of disease.

Direct nuclide injection into the coronary circulation with immediate imaging will probably become a routine study where coronary angiography and coronary artery surgery are practiced. Contrast angiography, despite its ability to provide exquisite vascular detail, is unable to provide certain critical data that become more important as surgery becomes more commonplace. The angiogram does not delineate capillary flow distal to the site of artery occlusion, nor does it indicate the extent of collateral flow. Consequently, the true status of the infarcted myocardium is not established by this study. However, the addition of a scanning procedure holds promise of improving the prognostic judgment of the efficacy of the contemplated myocardial revascularization and may even aid in identifying the technical procedure of choice.

Table 1–1. Indications, Pharmaceuticals, Methodology and Order of Merit of Radionuclide Study of Heart and Vessels

Why	What	How	Yea–Nay
Blood Pool			
Pericardial effusion	^{99m}Tc pertechnetate or albuminate, ^{113m}In	Static	+++
Placental localization	^{99m}Tc albuminate, ^{113m}In	Static	+++
Cardiac			
Myocardium	^{43}K, ^{129}Cs, ^{201}Tl, ^{99m}Tc pyrophosphate	Static	++
Valvular	^{99m}Tc pertechnetate	Dynamic	++
Vascular			
Central			
Venous			
Occlusion		Dynamic	++++
Displacement		Dynamic	++++
Arterial			
Aneurysm	^{99m}Tc pertechnetate	Dynamic	+++
Obstruction		Dynamic	+++
Congenital		Dynamic	++++
Peripheral			
Venous			
Inflammatory	^{99m}Tc pertechnetate	Dynamic	++
Thrombosis	^{131}I fibrinogen	Static	+++
Arterial	^{99m}Tc microspheres	Dynamic	++

Table 1–2. More About What

Radiopharmaceutical	Dose (mCi)	Physical Half-Life	Energy Peak (keV)
^{99m}Tc pertechnetate	10–15	6 hr	140
^{99m}Tc human serum albumin	1–3	6 hr	140
^{99m}Tc microspheres	10–15	6 hr	140
^{113m}In transferrin	1–2	104 min	393
^{43}K	0.5–1.0	22.4 hr	380
^{129}Cs	2.5–4.0	32 hr	375
^{131}I fibrinogen	0.3–0.4	8.05 days	364

Table 1–3. More About How

Why	Preparation	Administration	Time Between Administration and Exam (min)	Number of Exams	Time for Each Exam (min)	Time for Total Study (min)	Patient's Position	Instrument
Blood Pool								
Pericardial	none	IV	5	1	5–15	5–15	supine	camera or scanner
Placenta	none or skin mark	IV	immed or 5	1	2–15	2–15	supine	camera or scanner or probe
Cardiac	none or exercising	IV	5–120	1 or more	5–15	5–45	recumbent	camera or scanner
Myocardial	cardiac catheter	via catheter	immed	1 or more	1–3	1–10	recumbent	camera
Valvular	none	IV	immed	1	1–2	1–2	supine	camera
Vascular								
Central								
Venous	none	IV	immed	1	1–2	1–2	recumbent	camera
Arterial	none	IV	immed	1	1–2	1–2	recumbent	camera
Peripheral								
Venous								
Infection	none	IV	1–2	1	1–5	1–5	supine	camera
Thrombosis	Lugol's I_2	IV	2–3 days	2–4	15–30	3–4 days	supine	camera or scanner
Arterial	arterial catheter	via catheter	immed	1	15–30	15–30	supine	camera or scanner

BIBLIOGRAPHY

PERICARDIAL

Bonte FJ et al.: Cardiovascular blood pool. In Freeman LM, Johnson PM (eds): Clinical Scintillation Scanning. Hagerstown, Harper & Row, 1969, pp 203–221

Cohen MB: Cardiac blood pool scanning. In Blahd WH (ed): Nuclear Medicine. New York, McGraw-Hill, 1971, pp 513–516

Park CH et al.: Use of simultaneous transmission–emission scanning in the diagnosis of pericardial effusion. J Nucl Med 13(6):347–348, 1972

PLACENTA

Mahon DF et al.: Experimental comparison of radioactive agents for studies of the placenta. J Nucl Med 14(9):651–659, 1973

Nelp WB, Larson SM: The placenta. In Freeman LM, Johnson PM (eds): Clinical Scintillation Scanning. Hagerstown, Harper & Row, 1969, pp 397–413

Sklaroff DM et al.: Measurement of pericardial fluid correlated with I-131 cholografin and IHSA heart scan. J Nucl Med 5:101–111, 1964

RADIOPHARMACEUTICALS

Ansari AN et al.: ^{11}C-norepinephrine as a potential myocardial scanning agent. J Nucl Med 14(8):619, 1973

Chandra R et al.: ^{134m}Cs: A new myocardial imaging agent. J Nucl Med 14(4):243–245, 1973

Go RT et al.: Radionuclide imaging of experimental myocardial contusion. J Nucl Med 15(12):1174–75, 1974

Harper PV et al.: Clinical feasibility of myocardial imaging with ^{13}NH3. J Nucl Med 13(4):278–280, 1972

Holman BL et al.: Detection and localization of experimental myocardial infarction with ^{99m}Tc-tetracycline. J Nucl Med 14(8):595–599, 1973

Lebowitz E et al.: ^{201}Tl for medical use (abstr). J Nucl Med 14(6):421–422, 1973

Metzger JM et al.: Biological clearance and distribution studies of *I-fibrinogen labeled by four methods of iodination (abstr). J Nucl Med 14(6):429, 1973

Parkey RW et al.: Detection of acute myocardial infarction in humans using ^{99m}Tc stannous pyrophosphate (PYP) (abstr). J Nucl Med 15(6):521, 1974

ANGIOGRAPHY–GENERAL

Bonte FJ et al.: Tc-99m pertechnetate angiocardiography in the diagnosis of superior mediastinal masses and pericardial effusions. Am J Roentgenol Radium Ther Nucl Med 107:404–412, 1969

Conway JJ et al.: Evaluation of chest masses in children with early and delayed radionuclide angiography. Am J Roentgenol Radium Ther Nucl Med 108:575–581, 1970

Holmquest DL et al.: Assessment of vascularity in the differential diagnosis of abdominal pathology (abstr). J Nucl Med 13(6):437–438, 1972

Maxfield WS, Meckstroth GR: Technetium-99m superior vena cavography. Radiology 92:913–917, 1969

McIntire FT, Sykes EM: Obstruction of the superior vena cava: a review of the literature and report of two personal cases. Ann Intern Med 925–960, 1949

Miyamae T: Interpretation of ^{99m}Tc superior vena cavograms and results of studies in 92 patients. Radiology 108:339–352, 1973

Nebesar RA et al.: Correlation of angiography and isotope scanning in abdominal diseases of children. Am J Roentgenol Radium Ther Nucl Med 109(2):323–340, 1970

Nelson JP et al.: Rapid bolus injection of radioisotopes (abstr). J Nucl Med 13(6):457, 1972

Ranniger K: Retrograde azygography. Radiology 90:1097–1104, 1968

Rosenthall L: Applications of gamma-ray scintillation camera to dynamic studies in man. Radiology 86:634–639, 1966

Rouviere (Translated by Tobias): Anatomy of Human Lymphatic System. Ann Arbor, Michigan, Edward Bros, 1938

Son YH et al.: ^{99m}Tc pertechnetate scintiphotography as diagnostic and follow-up aids in major vascular obstruction due to malignant neoplasm. Radiology 91:349–357, 1968

Swann SJ et al.: Technique for diagnosing and assessing therapy for degree of superior vena cava obstruction (abstr). J Nucl Med 14(6):477, 1973

Waxman AD et al.: Rapid sequential liver imaging. J Nucl Med 13(7):522–524, 1972

Waxman AD et al.: Sequential liver imaging (abstr). J Nucl Med 13(6):475–476, 1972

Waxman AD et al.: Dynamic imaging of the spleen (abstr). J Nucl Med 14(6):463, 1973

MYOCARDIAL

Ansari AN et al.: ^{11}C-norepinephrine as a potential myocardial scanning agent (abstr). J Nucl Med 14(8):619, 1973

Bennett KR et al.: Correlation of myocardial ^{42}K uptake with coronary arteriography. Radiology 102:117–124, 1972

Bradley-Moore PR et al.: Thallium-201 for medical use. II: Biologic behavior. J Nucl Med 12(2):156–160, 1975

Cannon PJ et al.: Measurement of regional myocardial perfusion in man with ^{133}xenon and a scintillation camera. J Clin Invest 51:964–977, 1972

Chandra R et al.: ^{134m}Cs, a new myocardial imaging agent. J Nucl Med 14(4):243–245, 1973

Grames GM et al.: Safety of the direct coronary injection of radiolabeled particles. J Nucl Med 15(1):2–6, 1974

Holman BL et al.: Detection and localization of experimental myocardial infarction with ^{99m}Tc-tetracycline. J Nucl Med 14(8):595–599, 1973

Lebowitz E et al.: ^{201}Tl for medical use (abstr). J Nucl Med 14(6):421, 1973

Lebowitz E et al.: Thalium-201 for medical use. I. J Nucl Med 16(2):151–155, 1975

Martin LG et al.: Myocardial perfusion imaging with ^{99m}Tc-albumin microspheres. Radiology 107:367–371, 1973

Poe ND: Comparative myocardial uptake and clearance characteristics of potassium and cesium. J Nucl Med 13(7):557–560, 1972

Poe ND et al.: Evaluation of ^{43}K and ^{129}Cs for myocardial imaging. J Nucl Med 14(6):440, 1973

Strauss HW et al.: Noninvasive evaluation of regional myocardial perfusion with potassium 43. Radiology 108:85–90, 1973

CARDIAC–CONGENITAL

Alazraki NP et al.: Detection of left-to-right cardiac shunts with scintillation camera pulmonary dilution curve. J Nucl Med 13(2):142–147, 1972

Freedom RM, Treves S: Splenic scintigraphy and radionuclide venography in the heterotaxy syndrome. Radiology 107:381–386, 1973

Kriss JP et al.: Radioisotopic angiocardiography: findings in congenital heart disease. J Nucl Med 13(1):31–40, 1972

Mishkin F, Prosin MA: Radionuclide angiocardiographic confirmation of tricuspid insufficiency. J Nucl Med 15(3):205–206, 1974

Park HM et al.: Isolated right superior vena cava draining into left atrium diagnosed by radionuclide angiocardiography. J Nucl Med 14(4):240–242, 1973

PERIPHERAL VASCULAR

Charkes ND et al.: Detection of deep-vein thrombosis by photoscanning with ^{131}I-fibrinogen (abstr). J Nucl Med 14(6):385, 1973

Charkes ND et al.: Scintigraphic detection of deep-vein thrombosis with ^{131}I-fibrinogen. J Nucl Med 15(12):1163–1166, 1974

Dugan MA et al.: The use of iodinated fibrinogen for localization of deep venous thrombi by scintiscanning. Radiology 106:445–446, 1973

Giargiana FA et al.: A preliminary report on the complementary roles of arteriography and perfusion scanning in assessment of peripheral vascular disease. Radiology 108:619–627, 1973

Henkin RE et al.: Radionuclide venography (RNV) in lower extremity venous disease. J Nucl Med 15(3):171–175, 1974

McDonald GB et al.: Radionuclide venography. J Nucl Med 14(6):425, 1973

Rhodes BA et al.: Radioactive urokinase for blood clot scanning. J Nucl Med 13(8):646–648, 1972

Siegel ME et al.: Scanning of thromboemboli with ^{131}I-streptokinase. Radiology 103:695–696, 1972

Picture the scene: Prometheus chained to the rock, the vulture swoops down and plucks out his liver, Prometheus writhes in agony, the liver regenerates, the vulture returns and again assaults the liver, the liver regenerates, and on and on each day for over 1000 years. And not one scan to document the course! What an unfortunate waste. His case alone, if followed by an aware clinician, would have been almost sufficient to test all of the wares that the nuclear medicine man has available for problems of the liver. What was the residual function, secondary to the daily pecking? What was the picture pattern of vulture tearing? Were there focal or generalized defects? Did jaundice develop? If so, was it obstructive? Did infection or abscess become a complication? Could it be subdiaphragmatic? If intrahepatic, how could it be differentiated from the focal defects of trauma? Did Zeus ever consider a liver transplant? What would it look like? How could it be monitored?

But for all of these things to have been documented Prometheus's agonies would have had to be extended to the mid-1950s when liver imaging was first successfully accomplished, employing rose bengal tagged with ^{131}I. Several years later, colloidal gold ^{198}Au was introduced, and in the mid-1960s, ^{99m}Tc sulfur colloid became the popular agent.

When the colloids—^{198}Au and then ^{99m}Tc—became standard operational procedure an unanticipated plus was happily accepted. The spleen, also a major site of reticuloendothelial activity, was routinely imaged. Imaging of the spleen prior to the colloids was a tedious chore requiring the tagging of erythrocytes with ^{51}Cr and then damaging the cells, usually with heat, so that they would be sequestered by the organ and thus make the spleen scanable. The resulting images were acceptable but rarely of quality. The combination of prolonged pharmaceutical preparation plus picture paucity plus relatively few specific clinical indications consigned spleen imaging to a sometime thing reserved

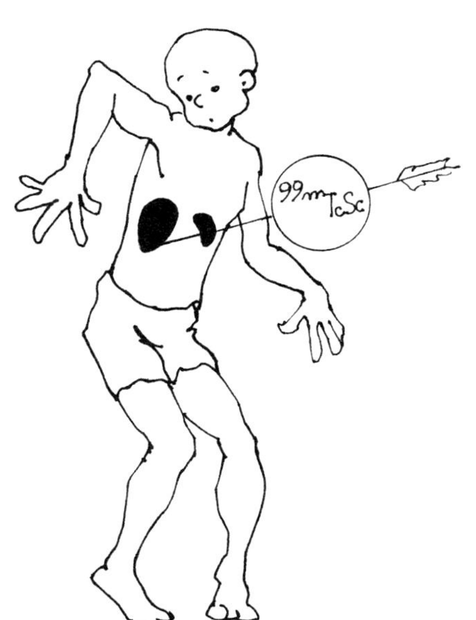
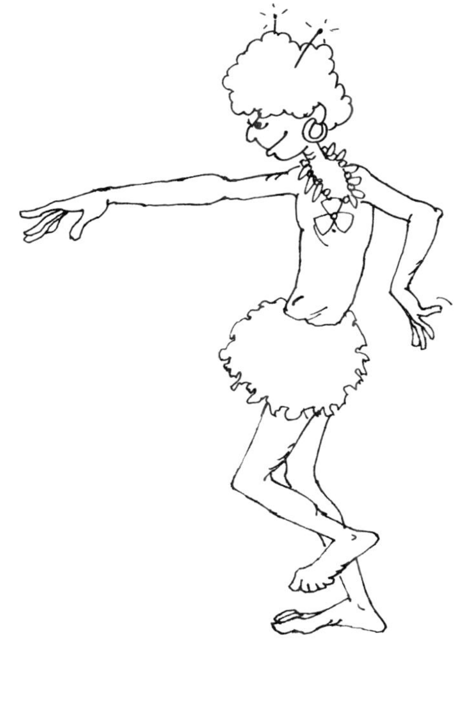

chapter 2

liver and spleen

almost exclusively for some hematologic indication, and most of the older texts discuss it under this heading. However, with the bargain of the "two-fer" liver and spleen at one throw, considerable experience has developed increasing the importance and indications for the study and suggesting that it should be considered in the chapter discussing the liver.

As discussed in chapter 1, the contributions of nuclear capabilities to the investigation of an organ system can usually be considered as functional measurements and structural imaging. Also, mentioned earlier is that, as a rule, the functional determinations usually require a sophistication of instrumentation and personnel that is not "usual and average" to the capabilities of the masses. These generalities obtain again in the isotopic evaluation of the liver and spleen, although as contrasted to some systems, *e.g.,* lung and brain—in which the average department does no functional evaluation— certain measurements of liver function are doable in all departments.

The functional studies of the liver are almost exclusively confined to the measurement of rose bengal clearance from the plasma and its appearance in the GI tract. This information is of value in the jaundiced patient if the mechanism of the jaundice is not clear. There are no routine splenic evaluations of function that do not utilize a scan.

Thus, although of unquestionable merit, the functional contributions are limited. Organ imaging is our main business. The indications are many and varied, and as with the other solid organs, conventional x ray offers little. Laboratory numbers generated as the end points of the measurements of the numerous and complicated functions are of course most valuable, but they ain't no picture. Is the palpated abdominal mass liver? Spleen? Scan it. Is the liver–spleen displaced? Scan it. Is there metastasis? Parenchymal disease? Abscess? Cyst? Scan it. Is the jaundice obstructive? Scan it. Has the known trauma produced rupture? Scan it. And once scanned, the interpretive analysis begins. Each organ presents its own set of peculiar conditions based on its unique anatomy, position, and physiology, which modify the diagnostic analysis. In liver scanning after the first decision of abnormal has been made it is helpful to confine the differential analysis to three major categories: 1) physical characteristics, *e.g.,* size, shape, and position; 2) generalized parenchymal involvement; and 3) focal defects.

WHAT

Any of several excellent nuclide agents may be used to obtain the desired picture. The choice of a particular agent is not capricious, but based on the clinical problem to be solved. It will be remembered that the liver is a most complex organ composed of two major cell types: 1) the polygonal and 2) Kupffer. The polygonal group, which comprises approximately 60% of the liver mass, performs the metabolic and detoxifying functions and also produces and secretes bile. The Kupffer cells represent the major site of the reticuloendothelial system and line the liver sinusoids.

Historically, the first successful scanning agent was rose bengal (a halogenated fluorescein dye) tagged with ^{131}I, which was employed in liver function testing, similar to bromsulphalein (BSP). It is cleared by the polygonal cells and excreted into the intestinal tract with the bile. When an appropriate tag is incorporated, its active transport can be monitored and imaged. Thus, a technique to both evaluate hepatocellular function—*i.e.,* clearance of the dye from the plasma and clearance through the liver with the bile—and image the liver morphology became operational. For years this was the only nuclide available, and we loved it. But, as with our children, love must be tempered with objectivity. Iodine 131 is just not a particularly good nuclide. Because of [131]I's relatively long half-life (approximately 8 days) only relatively low doses can be used, thus diminishing the quality of the image and prolonging the time of the examination. Then, too, a thyroid-blocking agent must be administered to protect that organ. And additionally, the gamma energy is in a range that reduces its efficiency when stationary crystals (cameras) are the scanning instruments. And still more additions, for problems other than possible biliary obstruction the very nature of hepatocellular clearance and biliary discharge of rose bengal works against the creation of an image. The imaging agent is continually leaving the target area. The scan must be obtained almost immediately following introduction of the nuclide since intestinal activity can be identified in nonobstructive problems within 10–20 min. Intestinal activity may interfere or confuse interpretation. Imaging in multiple views or recheck because of a question becomes impossible—it is like scanning uphill. But, despite all of the "additionallys," when the clinical problem is jaundice either in an adult or infant, the hepatocellular clearing agents are the nuclides of choice. Evidence that biliary clearance into the GI tract has occurred clarifies the frequent differential diagnostic problem of obstructive versus nonobstructive jaundice. How then to maximize the profits and diminish the losses? Switch from ^{131}I to [123]I. The latter nuclide has a half-life of 13 hours and a gamma energy range of 159 keV, both of which are ideal. A further switch from rose bengal to BSP, which is also cleared by the hepatocellular system, is also desirable since BSP is tagged with the nuclide more readily (a significant factor when the nuclide's half-life is only hours). Thus, when ^{123}I becomes economically feasible (the high cost and impurity of ^{123}I production at present precludes its routine use) it will probably be the preferred clearance agent.

However, predictions of nuclide ascendancy are about as accurate as guesses of next year's teeny-bopper idol. Interesting reports referring to the superiority of hepatobiliary extraction of thyroxin-glucuronide labeled with ^{131}I may result in the future adoption of these agents rather than the dyes. Also being investigated are agents cleared through the bile which can accept a [99mTc] tag. This has been accomplished with mercaptoisobutyric acid. And the search goes on.

Historically, the first nuclide to successfully image the spleen was [51Cr] tagged to RBCs. The patient's blood was incubated in an acid medium with added [51Cr] and then heat-treated so that crenation occurred. The latter step was important in order that the cells would be "seen" and sequestered in the spleen. But if ^{131}I carries fair credentials, [51Cr]s are for the birds, because a half-life of 27 days is bad news for humans. Additionally, its energy is higher than desirable (323 keV), and its percentage of gamma yield per decay is woefully low. Additionally, the time and nuisance of preparation is only exceeded by the time and nuisance of rescanning when the labeling process is poor and the original study nondiagnostic.

And so it was in the dawn of liver and spleen imaging, there was one choice for each, and each was imaged separately. But during those lean years the persons in the laboratory were cooking and stirring their brews and *voila*—[198Au] as a colloid. Here, finally, was an agent that would be extracted by the reticuloendothelial system component and "stick." The activity did not run away. Thus, scanning could be done at leisure. Multiple views could be obtained. Image

quality and its logical corollary, diagnostic accuracy, were markedly enhanced. And additionally, the spleen, another reticuloendothelial storing organ, was simultaneously imaged. But, [198Au] was not good enough. Its half-life (2.7 days) was far better than that of ^{131}I, but the iodine "ran off" (even in obstructive situations slow clearance through the kidneys occurs with rose bengal) whereas the colloid remained, causing a radiation load to the organ far greater than with the hepatobiliary agents. And lastly, its gamma energy (411 keV) was far from ideal.

So eventually, [99mTc] was tagged to a colloid of sulfur. This satisfied all of the major criteria: half-life was acceptable, gamma energy was acceptable, and the cost was acceptable. Other colloidal agents have their champions, *e.g.,* [113mIn], ^{131}I as aggregated albumin, but except for the exceptions, [99mTc] sulfur colloid is the most commonly employed nuclide.

exceptions

Jaundice. As previously noted, when jaundice is the clinical problem, rose bengal ^{131}I is preferable.

Localized Defects. All localized defects identified by the sulfur colloid scan look the same. Employing other nuclides to specify the nature of the defect is sometimes rewarding (see below, under "Why"). These nuclides include selenium 75 as [75Se] selenomethionine, gallium 67 as [67Ga] gallium citrate, and good old technetium 99m as [99mTc] pertechnetate.

Abscess. Metronidazole (Flagyl) tagged with [99mTc] is being investigated as a possible detector of amebic abscess.

Subdiaphragmatic Abscess. At this time to validate or deny the clinical suspicion of this problem, the lung and liver must be imaged as one continuous unit. This requires two different nuclides, one for each organ. Hopefully, one agent will become available that will do the deed, but with a [99mTc]-tagged pharmaceutical for each, this is hardly a problem.

HOW

The liver–spleen scan ranks high on the list of the easiest diagnostic procedures. The only unpleasantness is the IV introduction of the nuclide. No other preparation is required. Scanning is initiated within minutes of injection. Routinely, four views are obtained. Time per view varies with the instrument and dosage but rarely exceeds 10 min. The standard views are anterior, posterior, right lateral, and left lateral. Occasionally, additional positions are obtained. Thus, instructions are simple and uncomplicated: there is no preparation, one IV injection, and 30–45 min of examination time.

The above refers to the routine liver–spleen scan employing a colloid. As alluded to above, special situations requiring other nuclides change this procedure. In jaundice problems the search centers about detection of radioactivity in the bowel, and this often requires serial scanning. The selected time sequence is not critical, and the number of individual determinations are dependent on whether or not "run off" occurs. Thus, the nonobstructive jaundice problem may require only a single study since bowel activity may be detected within 10–20 min after rose bengal injection. However, a nondetection on initial study demands follow-up; a recheck at 1–6 hours is common. If doubt still exists a 24-hour evaluation is routine. Occasionally, even a 48-hour view may be performed. In these cases it is desirable to inform the patient that several visits may be required and that these repeats are not a result of professional incompetence nor synonymous with dire disease.

In some departments, rose bengal plasma clearance studies are performed in addition to scanning. When this is the style, probes, metal cylinders surrounding a scintillation crystal and attached to some recording device, are placed against the patient (the affluence of a department can be quickly assessed by determining the number of probes possessed). Ideally, this technique is performed with a probe against the side of the head and one over the midabdomen. Although the procedure is absolutely painless, warning the patient helps diminish the feeling of "being surrounded" by hardware. This monitoring may require as long as a half hour and may be repeated at serial intervals.

When the initial colloid scan identifies defects, further investigations to identify the nature of these defects are warranted. If ⁶⁷Ga citrate is employed, there may be a 24- to 48-hour wait from injection to scan. Bowel preparation is usually performed, but the actual scanning is similar to the colloid techniques. If ⁹⁹ᵐTc as a perfusion or flow technique is selected, then a simple 2- to 3-min study under the camera is all that is required.

Of all the major organs accessible to the scanning eye perhaps none provide a wider range of normal configurations. Whereas paired structures provide symmetry as a simple guide to normalcy, and the brain provides a confined constancy of size and contour, the liver provides only variations. No one ventures into liver land without a handy guide to identify the friendly natives from the foe. At least 12 general contours are recognized as normal. Figure 2-1, often referred to as the triangular type, is by far the most common. However, there is also the square, globular, Riedel's lobe, *en chapeau de gendarme,* and many, many more.

WHY

liver

Focal Defects. In the analysis of liver scan abnormalities the changes are initially classified as reflecting focal or diffuse disease. Space-occupying lesions produce focal defects. In scan parlance a focal defect is defined as a discrete zone of nonactivity. Unfortunately, there is no unique or distinguishing characteristic that permits differentiation of the nature of one focal defect from another. Therefore, all of these lesions will be considered together.

The search for metastasis probably initiates more liver scans than any other single differential consideration. Typically, a patient is sent for imaging because a known primary exists and therapy planning must identify the presence or absence of liver invasion. In many of these situations there is clear evidence of metastatic invasion and the scan findings simply confirm the obvious clinical state (Fig. 2-2), but in other situations there are no physical findings to bias the interpretation. A ⁹⁹ᵐTc sulfur colloid scan is done and a focal defect (or defects) is found. Although statistically the lesion is probably a metastasis, it can also be a nonspecific granuloma, a hamartoma, a cyst, an abscess, a hemangioma, a primary malignant neoplasm, a defect secondary to trauma, Hodgkin's disease, or even cirrhosis (Fig. 2-3). Few clues exist except historic review, which will assist the sorting out. Recent surgery, unexplained temperature elevation, right upper quadrant pain, and a focal defect may imply abscess (?). Known polycystic kidney disease and a focal

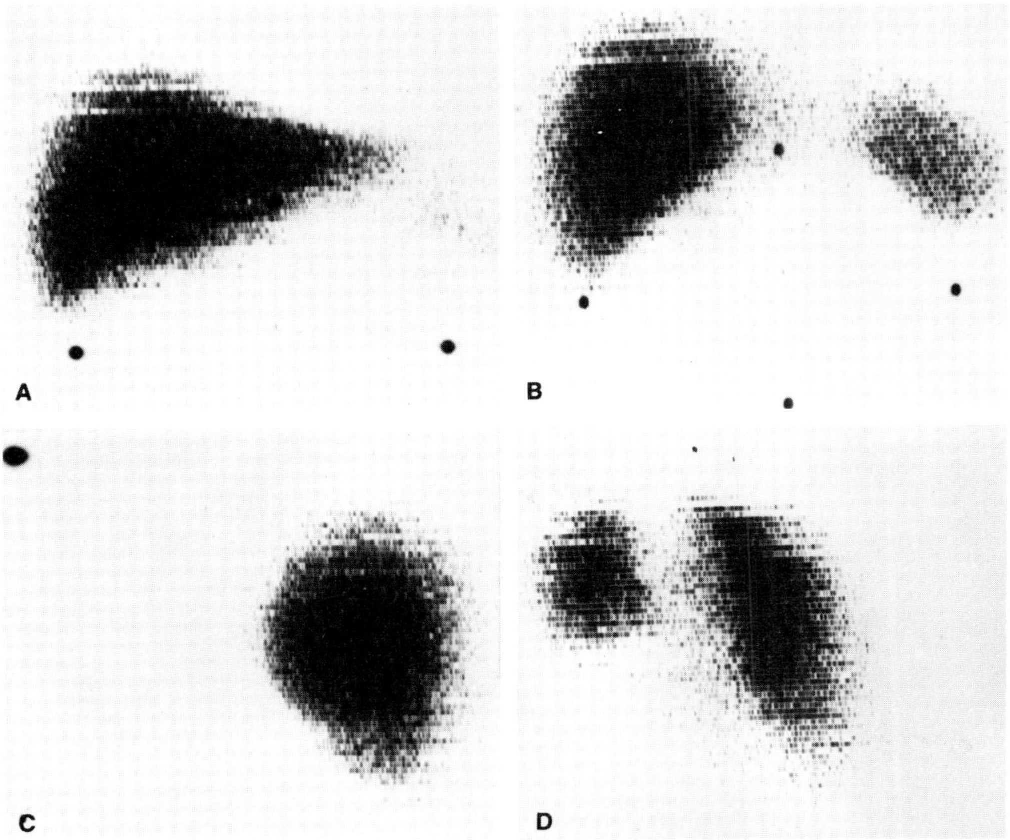

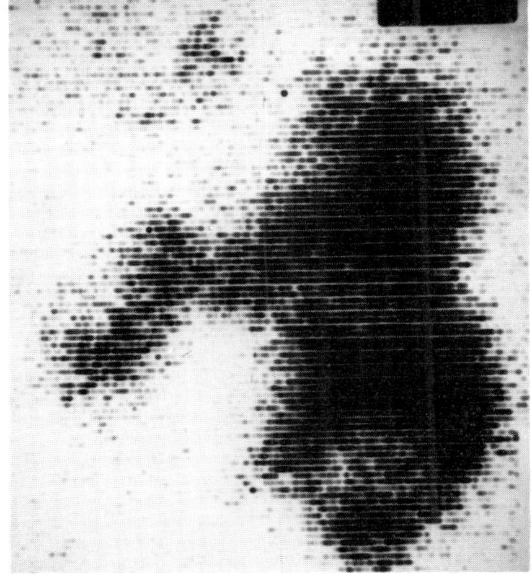

Fig. 2-1. The conventional liver scan consists of four views
A. Anterior. Black dots identify the zyphoid notch, the right and left costal margins, and umbilicus. The liver margins are smooth and the distribution of activity uniform. The spleen may not be identified on this view.
B. Posterior. The spleen is always seen, and its activity may equal that of the liver.
C. Right lateral. The spleen is obscured by the liver.
D. Left lateral. The liver is anterior and the spleen posterior.

Fig. 2-2. Focal defects: metastasis from colon carcinoma. Massive hepatomegaly and massive invasion. The right lobe is almost completely replaced. The left lobe extends into the pelvis and is focally replaced.

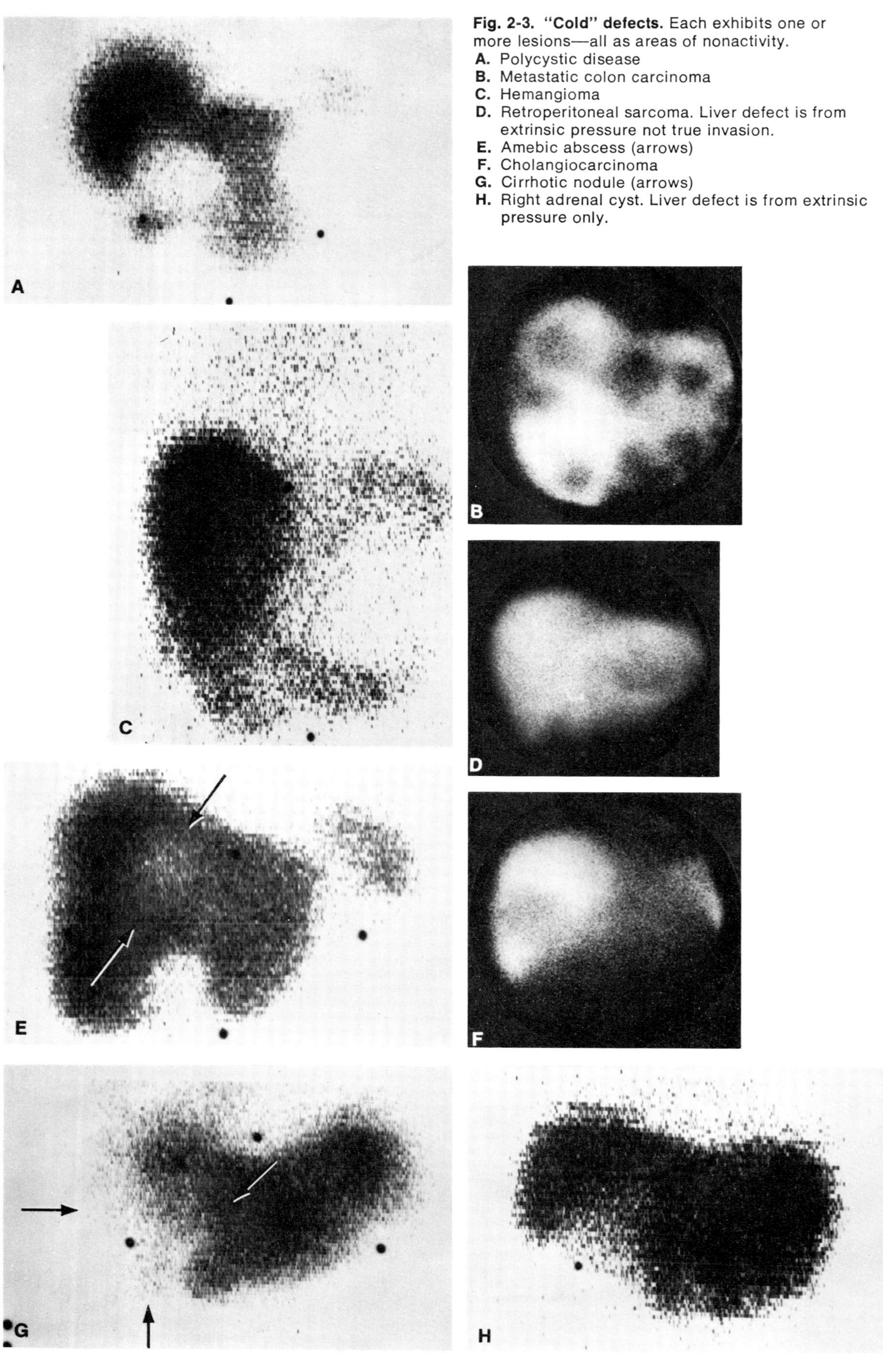

Fig. 2-3. "Cold" defects. Each exhibits one or more lesions—all as areas of nonactivity.
A. Polycystic disease
B. Metastatic colon carcinoma
C. Hemangioma
D. Retroperitoneal sarcoma. Liver defect is from extrinsic pressure not true invasion.
E. Amebic abscess (arrows)
F. Cholangiocarcinoma
G. Cirrhotic nodule (arrows)
H. Right adrenal cyst. Liver defect is from extrinsic pressure only.

Fig. 2-4. "Hot" defect: lesion as area of increased activity. Diagnosis: Metastatic bronchogenic carcinoma

A. Posteroanterior chest x ray. Large bronchogenic carcinoma right upper lobe

B–E. Flow study. Superior vena cava (see chapter 1) sequential images of mediastinal region following injection of ^{99m}Tc. There is complete obstruction at right innominate vein and massive collateralization. **B,** 5–8 sec; **C,** 8–11 sec; **D,** 11–14 sec; **E,** 14–17 sec

F and G. Anteroposterior **(F)** and lateral oblique **(G)** liver scan. Focal area of increased activity (hot spot) (arrow 1), probably secondary to caval obstruction adjacent to a focal defect (arrow 2), probably metastatic disease

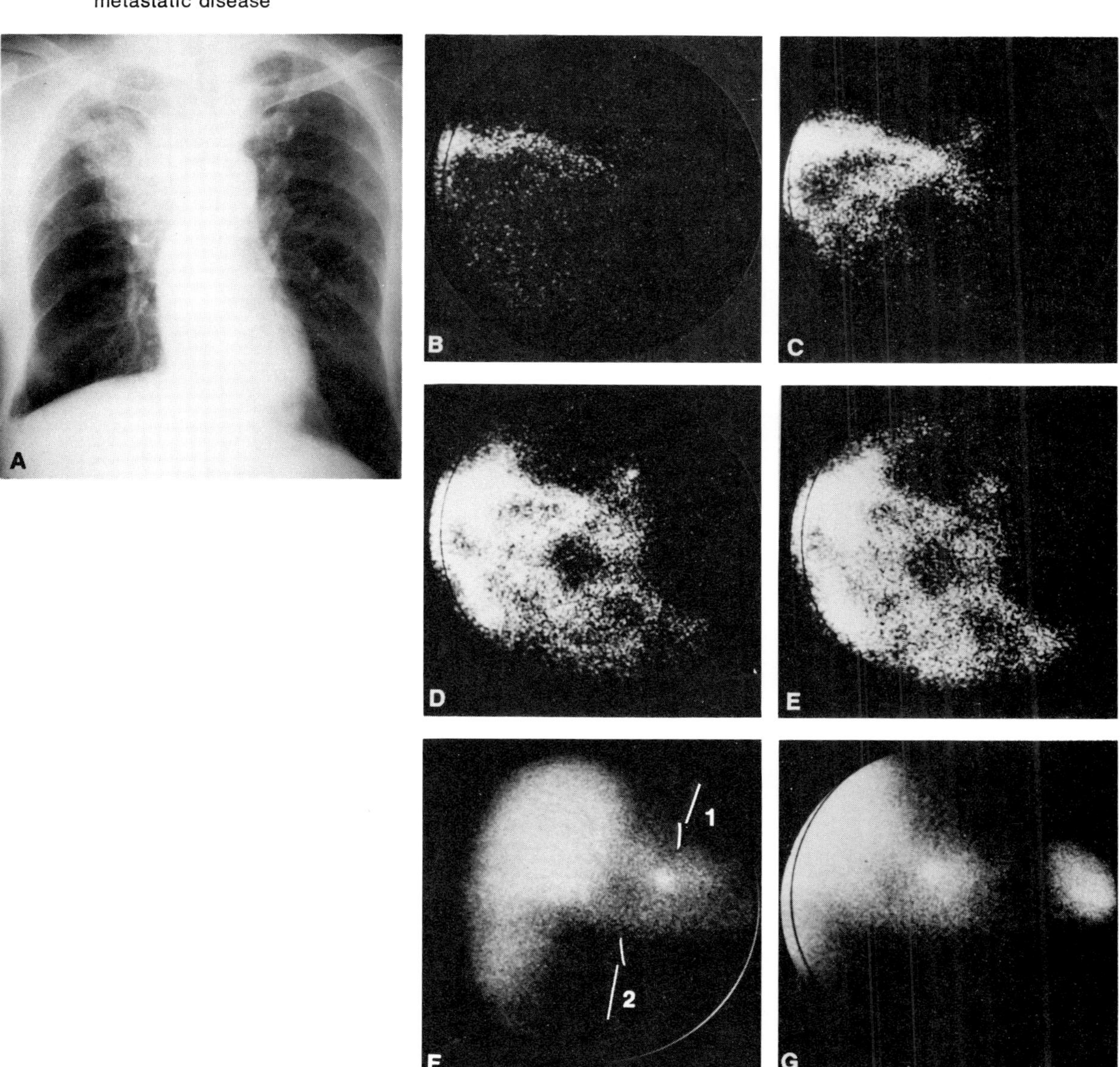

defect or defects may imply polycystic liver disease (?). A positive diagnosis of Hodgkin's disease and a focal defect may imply Hodgkin's disease of the liver (?) (?). A history of trauma to the abdomen, laboratory evidence of blood loss, right upper quadrant pain, and a focal defect may imply liver rupture (?). It's not the picture alone that makes it.

There is one exception to all of the above. Those focal defects are all cold. Occasionally, a focal defect will be hot, *i.e.,* its activity will exceed that of the surrounding parenchyma (Fig. 2-4). Almost without exception these have been observed in cases of superior vena caval obstruction and have been localized to the region of the porta hepatis. It is felt that the increased collection reflects systemic venous bypass secondary to the caval obstruction, with the resultant high specific activity of colloid in the portal branches appearing as a hot spot in the region of the porta.

Until recently, after eliminating some of the differential considerations by obvious historic and laboratory review and citing the statistical probabilities of the causes of the focal defect, all that was left for the nuclear medicine man was to punt. Further sophistication of the judgment became someone else's responsibility. Today, before giving up the ball, there are a few

more plays that can be run. The focal lesion can be studied further with nuclear techniques that attempt to determine whether or not the defect is vascular or exhibits any functional integrity. The vascular versus nonvascular parameter is evaluated by a "flow" or perfusion scan employing ^{99m}Tc as pertechnetate. Indium 113m may also be used in this technique. The study is similar to all other organ flows. Following the IV injection of 10–15 mCi of tracer, rapid sequential images are obtained over the liver. The patient is usually supine. Perfusion is usually identified 5–10 sec after activity is seen in the kidneys or spleen. The images are evaluated for any evidence of activity in the previously identified focal defect. If any increase is present, it is safe to exclude cysts, abscesses, and cirrhotic nodules from consideration. If the defect "fills in" so that its activity is equal to the surrounding parenchyma or even becomes hot, *i.e.,* its activity exceeds that of the surrounding parenchyma, then primary hepatoma and hemangioma becomes the chief considerations (Fig. 2-5). Metastatic defects can be found somewhere between the hot and cold (Fig. 2-6). Their pattern, unfortunately, is variable. They may be "warm," "warmish" (a little more active than cold) or even cold, depending on their cell type. Thus, if the focal defect demonstrates any

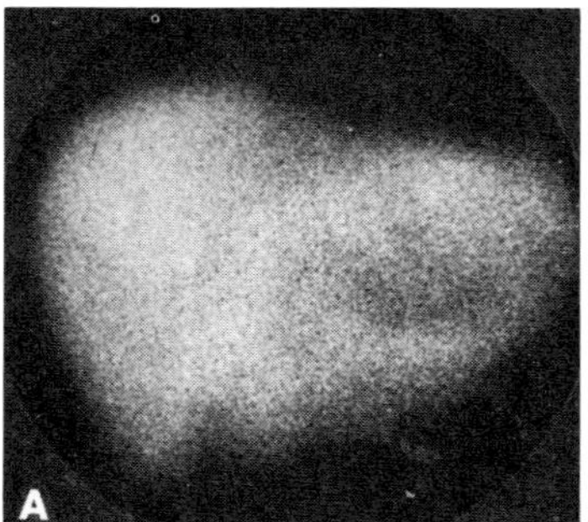
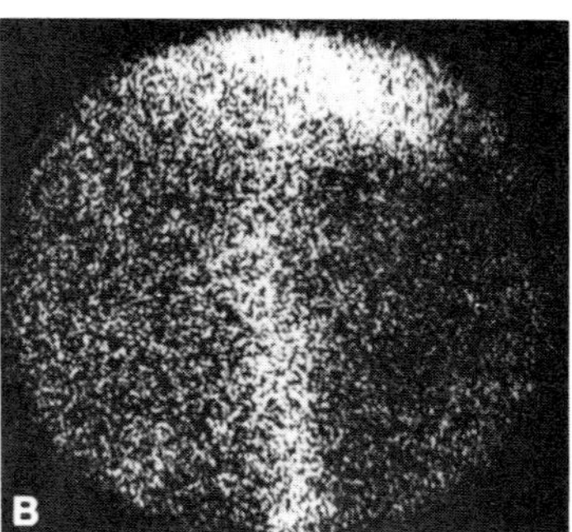
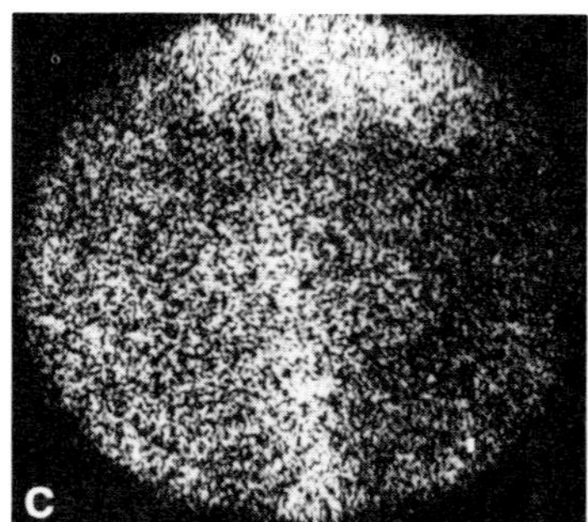
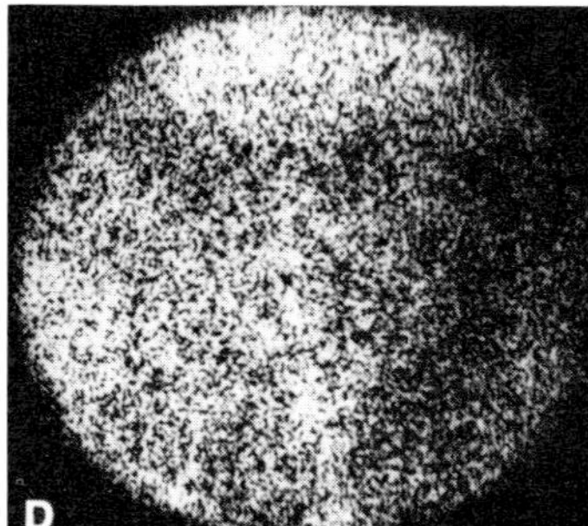

Fig. 2-5. Focal defect with perfusion study. Diagnosis: Retroperitoneal sarcoma with extrinsic pressure but no true invasion
    A. Sulfur colloid static scan. Large focal defect replacing a major portion of the enlarged left lobe
B–D. Technetium flow. Sequential images
        B. Activity primarily in cardiac blood pool and abdominal aorta
      C and D. Perfusion throughout the liver including the site of defect, which is to the left of the aorta

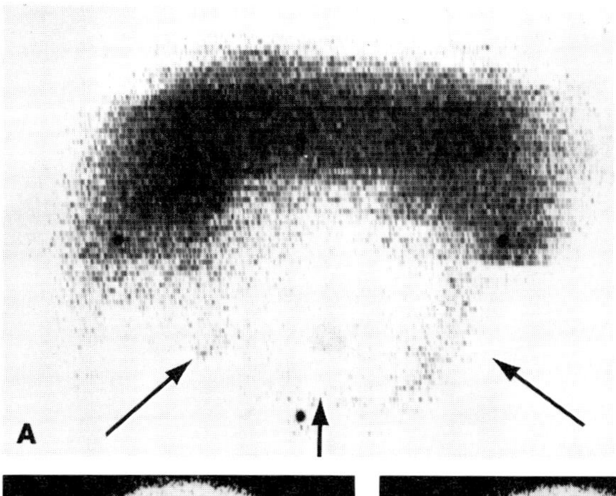

Fig. 2-6. Focal defects with perfusion study. Diagnosis: Metastatic breast carcinoma
  A. Conventional sulfur colloid scan identifies a huge focal defect (arrows).
  B–D. Sequential images with ^{99m}Tc suggest some perfusion, particularly at the periphery of the lesion (arrows).

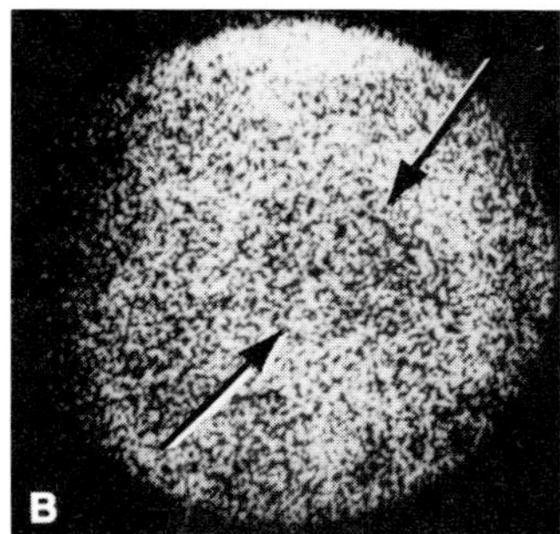

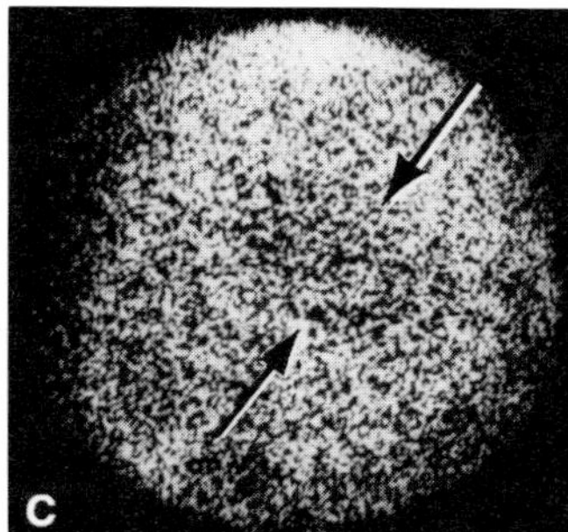

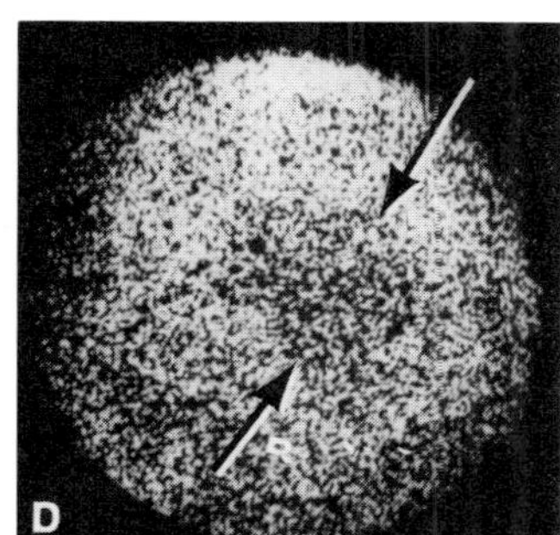

evidence of perfusion, benign lesions are usually excluded. If the perfusion exceeds surrounding parenchyma, metastasis is unlikely. Unfortunately, these are only generalities. Primary neoplasms may not perfuse (Fig. 2-7), and metastatic lesions may exhibit excellent perfusion (Fig. 2-8). Thus, as with many other techniques, only sufficient experience on the part of the examiner will decide their ultimate worth.

Other nuclides may be employed in the differential sorting. Selenium 75 selenomethionine surfaces in the literature with predictable regularity as an agent to be considered. Conceptually, the defects, if neoplastic, will incorporate the methionine and cause the lesion to light up. Advocates of ^{75}Se cite higher yields in the detection of hepatomas, but detection requires initial suspicion, and hepatomas, when unassociated with cirrhosis, are rarely suspected. They may present as a single large lesion or as multiple small defects and are found predominantly in the right lobe. However, if there is an established diagnosis of cirrhosis and the scan identifies a focal defect associated with the typical diffuse cirrhotic pattern, the

nerve endings that heighten concern should tingle. Statistically, probability states that the vast majority of these focal lesions are cirrhotic nodules, but if one should shine with ^{99m}Tc perfusion or ^{75}Se incorporation, the nuclear man deserves the courtesy of a hello the next time you pass him in the corridor.

Gallium 67 citrate has also been employed in these problems. This agent resembles the proverbial little girl in the poem in that when it is good . . . , but when it is bad it is not very good. Unfortunately, ^{67}Ga citrate is totally unpredictable. Suffice it to say that it may be helpful, and its help is similar to the results of the other agents. If the defect takes up the material, it is not cystic (Fig. 2-9), but if it does not, there is no change in the previous consideration.

Although the above modalities are not described with ebullience, they should not be ignored. Experience has certainly shown that experience improves with experience. The continued use of these investigative techniques, particularly the perfusion scanning, if history is repeated, will hopefully improve their diagnostic accuracy. This has already occurred with flow studies of the brain and kidney, which were

This pathophysiologic state is reasonably captured in a scan image. When effective liver flow is uniform, the Kupffer cell extraction efficiency of more than 95% for the injected colloid results in an image of uniform distribution of activity. When shunting exists as a consequence of hepatocellular disease, the pattern becomes nonuniform, and the extent of this aberration is proportional to the severity of the process. Additionally, as the intravascular liver bed undergoes change, pressure gradients throughout the portal system are affected, often resulting in portal hypertension. This in turn, and in association with the reduced extraction efficiency, results in increased colloid uptake at other reticuloendothelial sites, notably the spleen and marrow.

Of the general group of diseases that produce diffuse defects, cirrhosis is the most common. Other causes of diffuse changes to be considered and differentiated are: congestive heart failure; infections; metabolic disturbances that result in fatty infiltration or amyloidosis; granulomatous diseases, *e.g.,* sarcoidosis, histoplasmosis, brucellosis, and tuberculosis; a miscellaneous category that includes the infiltrative changes of leukemia; diffusely invasive metastases; and chemical poisons (Fig. 2-10).

The sensitivity of detection of diffuse involvement is not as good as that of focal defects, particularly if the involvement is early or mild. However, in each case of diffuse involvement the responsible condition invariably produces some degree of hepatomegaly, and it is often this change in size that alerts the viewer to possible changes in the homogeneity of the trapping pattern. The notable exception in this size rule is advanced cirrhosis, which may be first imaged when contraction has already occurred. Occasionally, and also more commonly

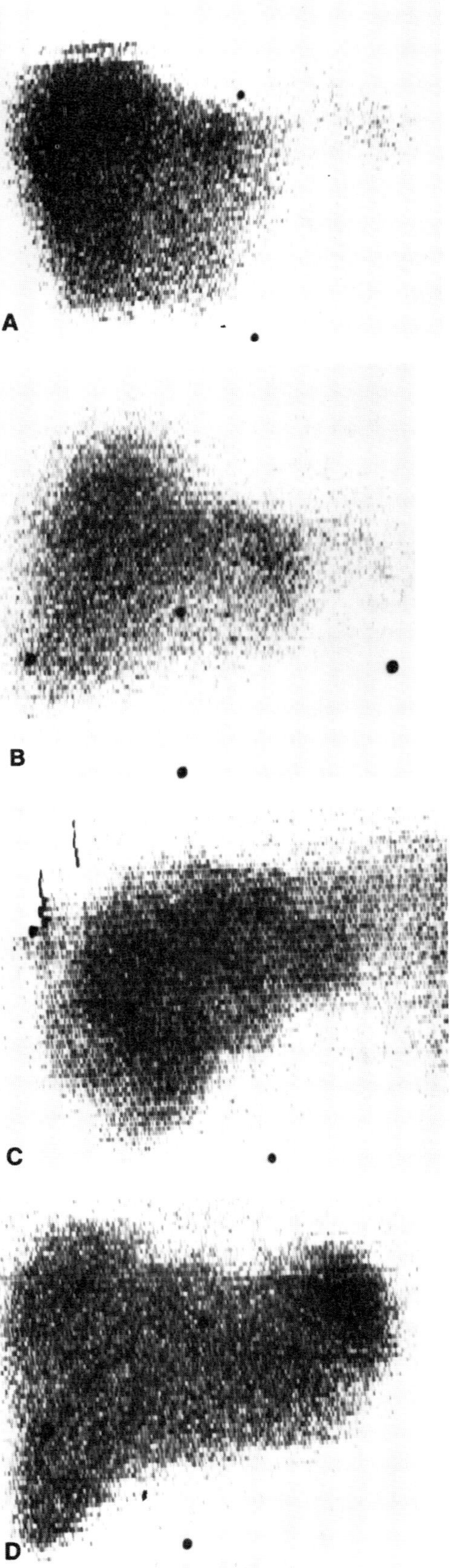

Fig. 2-10. Diffuse defects. The liver is usually enlarged. Activity is nonhomogenous. The changes are generalized, not focal.
A. Miliary tuberculosis
B. Sarcoidosis
C. Diffuse metastatic colon disease
D. Congestive heart failure

Fig. 2-11. Diffuse defects. Diagnosis: Cirrhosis (early). Only left lobe hypertrophy is noted although nonhomogenous trapping is present throughout the organ.

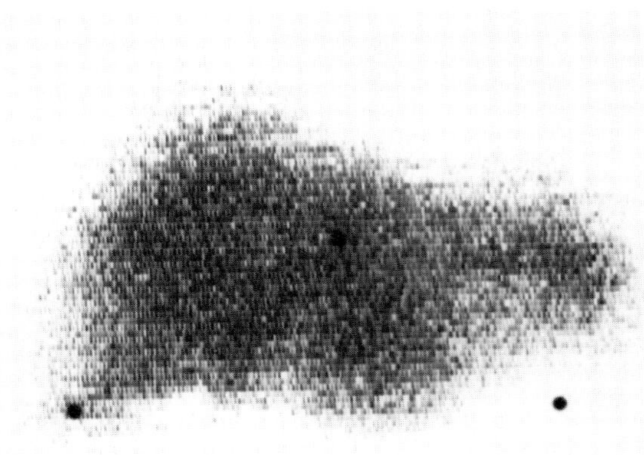

Fig. 2-12. Diffuse defects. Diagnosis: Cirrhosis (moderately advanced) **A and B.** Hepatomegaly and nonhomogenous trapping associated with diminished liver activity, increased splenic size and activity and uptake in the vertebral marrow. **A,** anteroposterior; **B,** posteroanterior

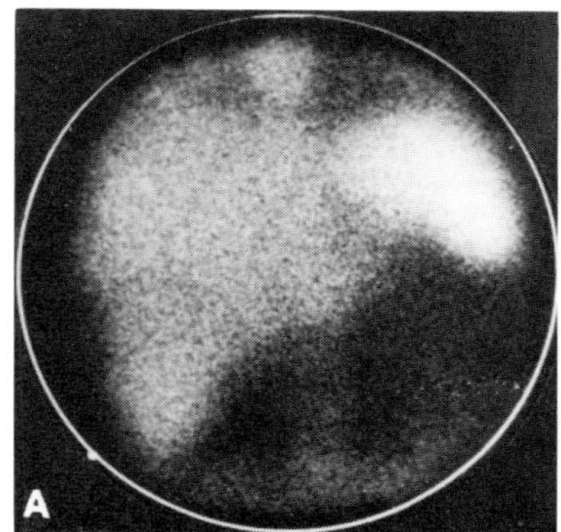
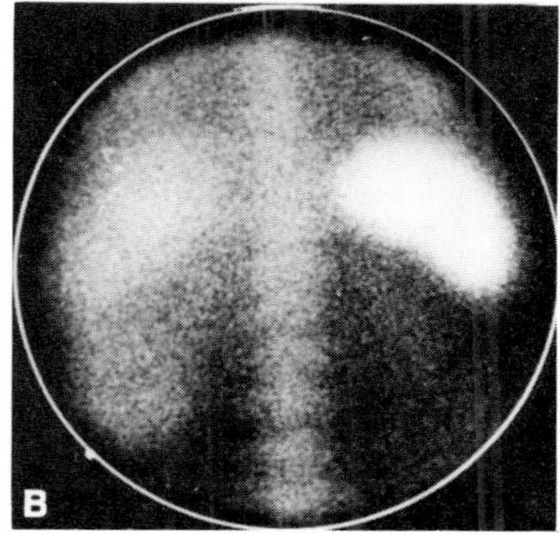

in cirrhosis, the enlargement may be confined only to the left lobe (Fig. 2-11). More-advanced changes are easily identified and have been characterized as "mottled" or "salt and pepper" patterns. Normally, the activity and thus the intensity of the liver image is five times that of the spleen in the anterior view and essentially equal in the posterior view. Frequently associated with nonuniformity, however, there is a shift in intensity of trapping away from the liver, with a reversal of the liver:spleen ratio. Initially, the spleen reflects this shift and its intensity begins to exceed that of the liver. It may also enlarge. As the pathologic process worsens, the liver extracts less and less colloid as a consequence of a shrinking hepatic vascular bed, and the reticuloendothelial components in the marrow begin to extract more colloid. It is not uncommon in advanced cirrhosis to see a small, poorly trapping liver, a large bright spleen, and activity throughout the marrow, so that the study almost suggests a bone scan (Figs. 2-12 and 2-13).

Occasionally, trapping is identified in the lungs (Fig. 2-14). There is at this historic moment a raging controversy as to the significance of this finding. Obviously, the first possibility that must be ruled out is pulmonary deposition secondary to a poorly prepared batch of colloid. If colloid size is not carefully controlled, pulmonary vascular trapping can occur (the mechanism of the conventional lung scan), and lung activity is identified. If this then is the mechanism, all other patients examined with that particular batch of reagent will also exhibit pulmonary uptake. When colloid size is not the answer, what is responsible and what is its significance?

It has been observed that when faulty colloid has been ruled out as the cause, lung trapping, although infrequent, always occurs in severely ill patients, more than half of whom suffer from malignancy and the others from cirrhosis and abscess. It was also observed that approximately half of the group expired within 3 months of the scan finding. Therefore, the existence of lung trapping on a conventional colloid liver scan

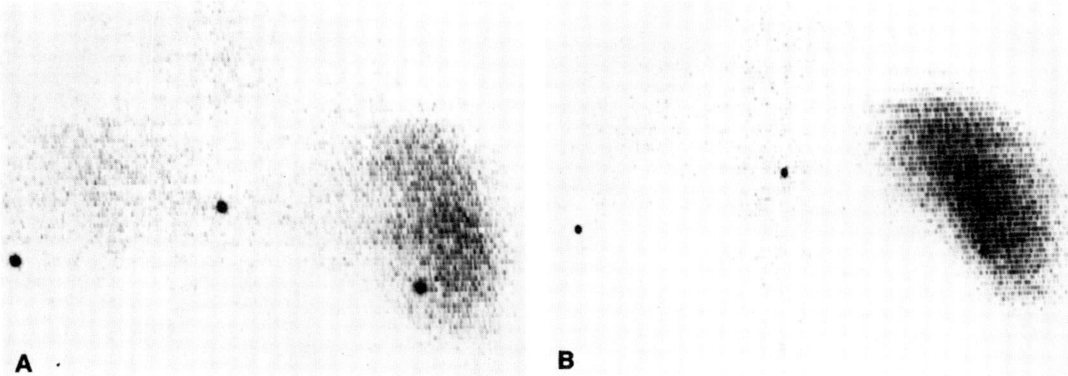

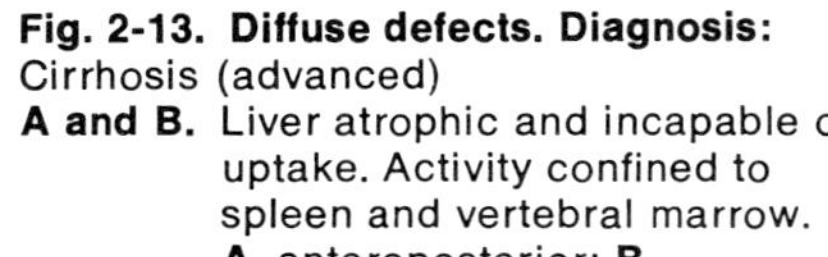

A   B

Fig. 2-13. Diffuse defects. Diagnosis:
Cirrhosis (advanced)
A and B. Liver atrophic and incapable of
uptake. Activity confined to
spleen and vertebral marrow.
A, anteroposterior; **B,**
posteroanterior

may have dire prognostic significance, but the
mechanism of uptake still resists unanimous
agreement. Although some evidence suggests
enhanced reticuloendothelial system (RES)
stimulation in the lung secondary to the
underlying illness, the current prevailing
hypothesis seems to favor some mechanism that
alters the physiologic pattern of intravascular
foreign colloid clearance triggered by the other
physiologic changes associated with the severe
or terminal illness.

Jaundice. When there is clinical indecision as to
the mechanism of jaundice and extrahepatic
obstruction is a distinct differential consideration,
nuclear techniques can be helpful. As previously
discussed, this problem is best attacked with a
hepatocellular clearing agent. Of these, the most
popular is still ^{131}I rose bengal. The procedure
consists of starting at A, the IV injection of the
nuclide, and proving that the nuclide gets to B,
the GI tract (Fig. 2-15). If this is accomplished,
the extrahepatic obstruction is ruled out since
the path from A to B is the extrahepatic biliary
tract. But, and a most important but, if A does
not reach B, if there is no GI activity, this does
not necessarily mean extrahepatic obstruction.
Intrahepatic obstruction secondary to severe
chronic disease states or acute viral or drug-
induced hepatitis will simulate the same rose

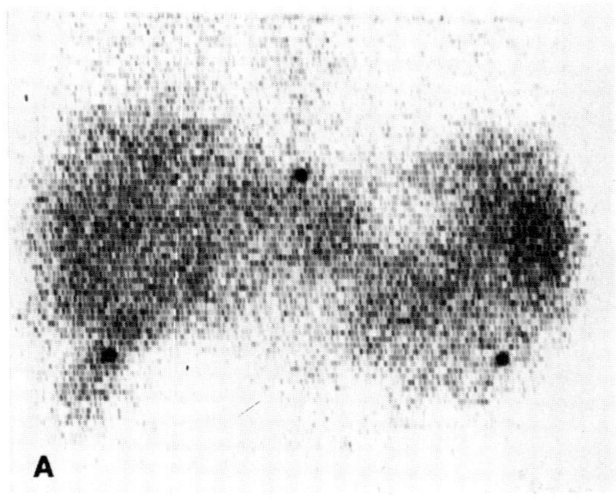

A

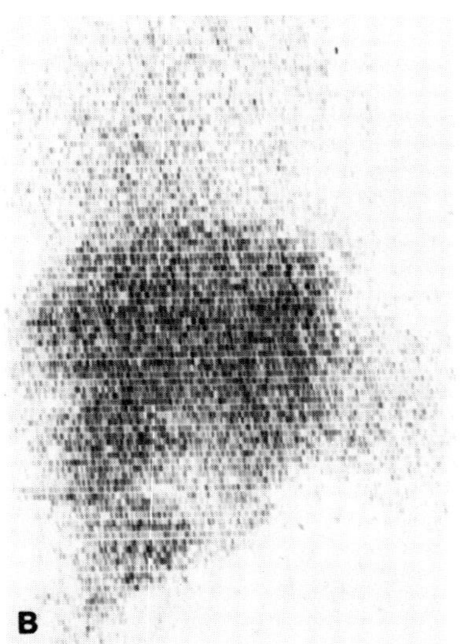

B

Fig. 2-14. Focal defects with lung trapping.
Diagnosis: Metastatic carcinoma—gall bladder
A and B. Focal defects are present in the liver.
Splenic and marrow uptake is increased.
Significant trapping present in the lungs is
best appreciated on the lateral view **(B).**
A, anteroposterior

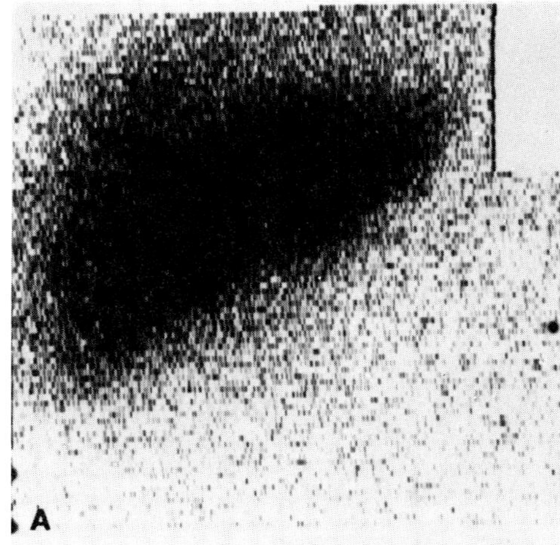

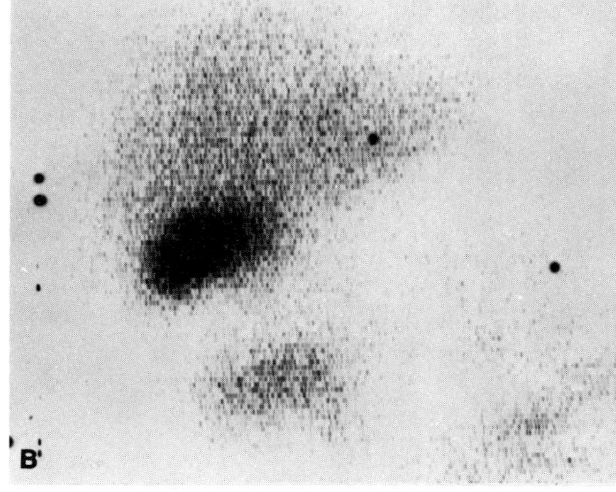

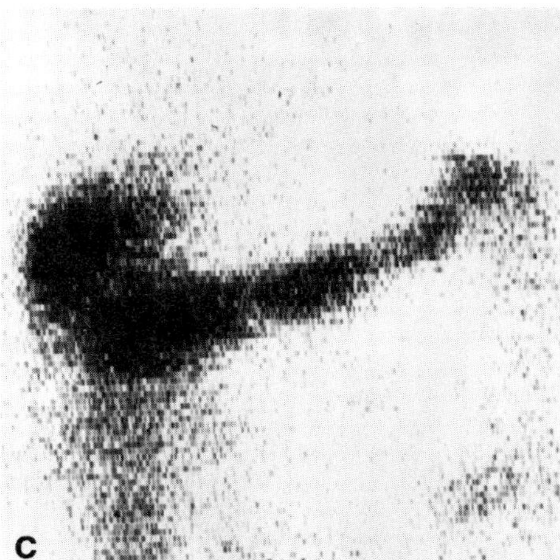

Fig. 2-15. Jaundice without obstruction. Rose bengal
[131]I is employed. Scans are made at intervals to confirm
or deny clearance of nuclide into the GI tract.
A. 15 min. Activity is confined to the liver.
B. 6 hours. The liver is almost cleared; activity is
localized to the gall bladder and small bowel.
C. 24 hours. The liver is cleared, activity still present in
gall bladder and colon.

Fig. 2-16. Jaundice with obstruction
A. Anterior, 24 hours. Liver activity is prominent. Activity is present beyond the
liver, but not in the bowel. Clearance is occurring through the kidneys. This
may be confused with GI activity unless a posteroanterior view is obtained.
B. Posterior, 24 hours. Obvious activity in the kidneys, as well as retention in
the liver

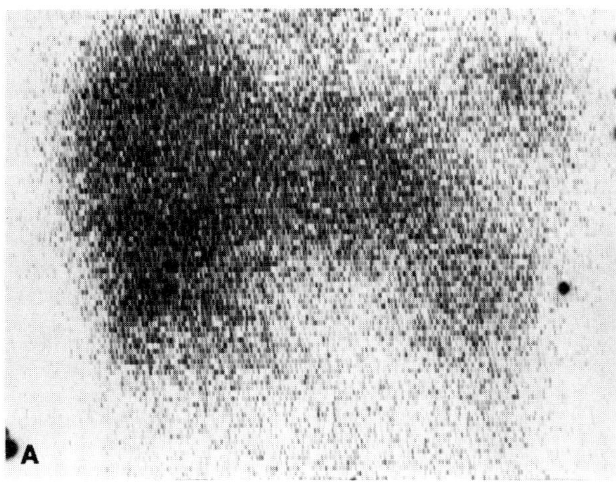

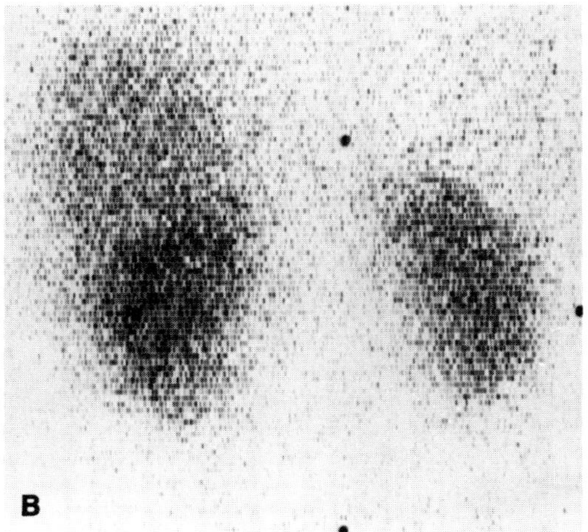

bengal pattern. The absence of "run off," a term frequently used to indicate that there is activity in the bowel is not synonymous with a surgical problem, although some suggest that the total absence of bowel activity through 48 hours is diagnostic of extrahepatic obstruction (Fig. 2-16).

Occasionally, obstruction can be deduced from the conventional colloid image. The occluding mechanism produces dilatation of the intrahepatic biliary ducts which may be identified as linear or band lucencies throughout the liver or even as a focal trapping defect in the region of the porta hepatis. Thus, a history of long-standing jaundice with scan changes as above noted would suggest an obstructive etiology.

The differential diagnosis of neonatal biliary atresia from cholestasis is also resolvable with rose bengal run-off techniques. Monitoring is carried out through 72 hours. Failure to detect the nuclide within the GI tract during this interval establishes the diagnosis of atresia.

The compulsion to touch all bases requires the inclusion of techniques that monitor plasma clearance, liver retention, and bowel activity levels. Clearance curves and ratios of clearance are established, and diagnoses are deduced from their patterns. Adherents, by definition, claim excellent correlative scores. To date, the adherents of external monitoring probes are far outnumbered by scanners. This is not to impugn the technique, but simply to suggest that imaging techniques provide the same basic data in far simpler fashion.

Size, Shape, Position. It is somewhat embarrassing to state that after the more than 10×10^{10} numbers of livers that have been scanned since the world began, no absolutely accepted criteria exist as to what constitutes hepatomegaly. This does not refer to obvious significant enlargement, but to minor changes. Much of this uncertainty is due to the inordinately high number of normal variants in contour and size. Rather than resorting to the complicated and time-consuming exercises in solid geometry that have been offered to triangulate, equilibrate, and titrate a standard "normal" most examiners simply "eye ball" the image and, based on individual experience, decide whether or not the liver is normal.

It is not infrequent that abdominal palpation raises questions as to "what is that?" Often the question is initiated by the x-ray report of extrinsic pressure on or displacement of the barium-filled stomach or flexures of the bowel.

Nothing is debated with greater vigor than whether or not a palpable structure was lower pole of spleen or muscle guarding, or whether there is hepatomegaly or habitus variation.

The liver-spleen image satisfies many of the questions raised on physical examination and x rays:

Yes, the mass is liver—the next question is why is it enlarged?

No, the mass is not liver—look to the kidneys, pancreas or adrenals as the cause.

No, there is no evidence of splenomegaly.

Yes, the impression on the stomach is liver but it is secondary to displacement rather than enlargement. The malposition being explained by a low right diaphragm, an interposition of bowel, ascites, or a subdiaphragmatic abscess (Fig. 2-17).

Trauma. More and more the rapid screening of abdominal trauma includes liver and spleen imaging. Information can be obtained in minutes by flow or perfusion techniques. If time is not that critical, the perfusion study can be followed by conventional static imaging. Evidence of ruptures, tears, infarcts, displacements secondary to bleeding, and functional variation as a consequence of vascular impairment are reasonable expectations. A positive or questionable change validates the initiation of definitive contrast angiography (Fig. 2-18).

External radiation therapy may be considered as trauma to the liver. When dosages approximate 3500 rads to the organ reticuloendothelial incorporation of colloid is suppressed, and defects may be identified that clearly mirror the configuration of the skin portal. Full "scan recovery" may be anticipated if the dosage does not exceed 5500 rads.

Subdiaphragmatic Abscess. The close proximity of the right-sided subdiaphragmatic abscess to the liver results in changes that are often scan-detectable. The right lobe of the liver is in intimate contact with the base of the right lung, separated only by the right leaf of the diaphragm. Potential spaces are created by various ligamentous attachments of the liver to the diaphragm. When abscess collection is loculated in one of these recesses, there is a separation of the liver from the lung equivalent to the volume of the collection and—frequently—a displacement of the liver. If the abscess is either in the posthepatic recess created by the

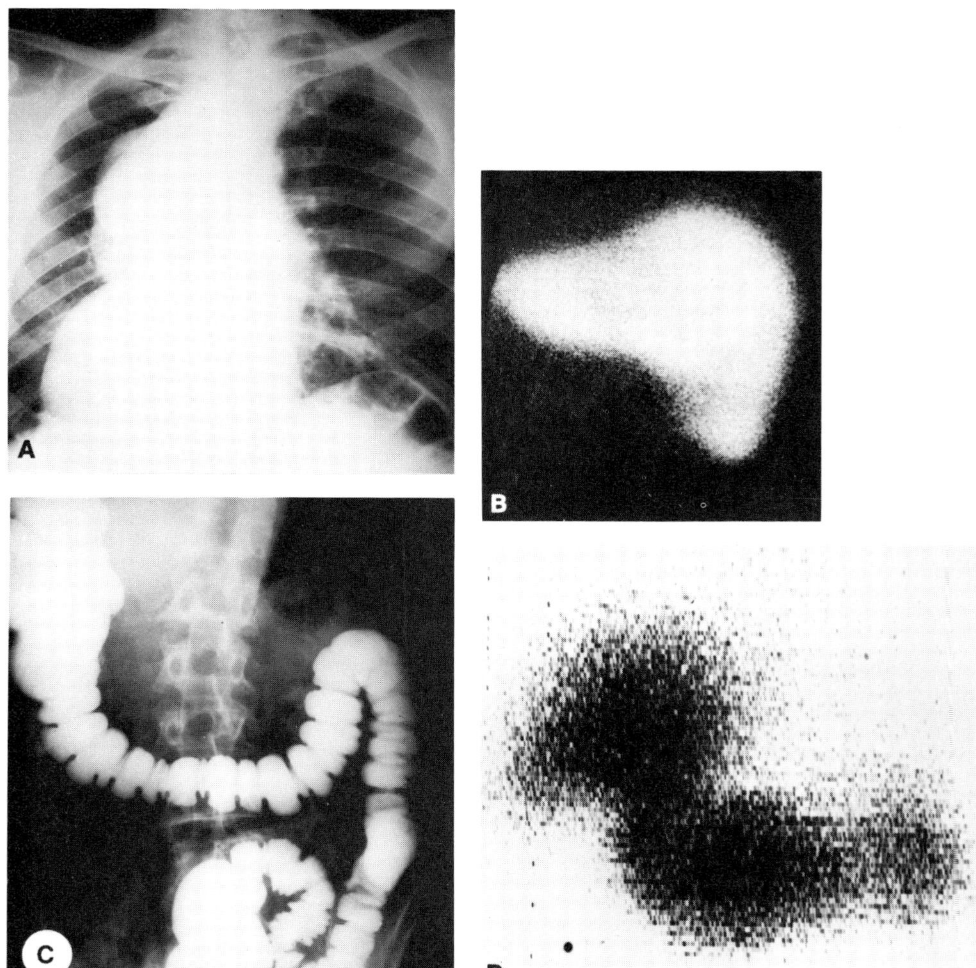

Fig. 2-17. Size, contour, position
Diagnosis: situs inversus
A. Posteroanterior chest x ray. Dextracardia
B. Anterior liver scan. Left-sided liver
Diagnosis: Anomalous position of the hepatic flexure
(palpation suggested an epigastric mass)
C. Barium enema. Position of the hepatic flexure is
atypically high.
D. Anterior liver scan. Palpated epigastric mass is
obviously the left liver lobe. The atypical liver
contour is secondary to the anomalous position of
the colon.

posterior attachment of right triangular ligament or in the right subphrenic space created by the falciform ligament, the liver will be displaced either caudad or medially, or both. Thus, when abscess is suspected (and this is one disease that requires clinician input), a combination liver–lung scan is performed. The right lung and liver must be imaged simultaneously so that any separation or displacement can be detected. Commonly, this is accomplished with ^{99m}Tc sulfur colloid for the liver and ^{99m}Tc albuminate macroaggregates for the lungs. Since the radionuclide is common to both areas the mechanics of imaging are simple. The abscess will be represented as a cold or clear zone separating the hot or active lung and liver (Fig. 2-19). Gallium 67 citrate may localize in the

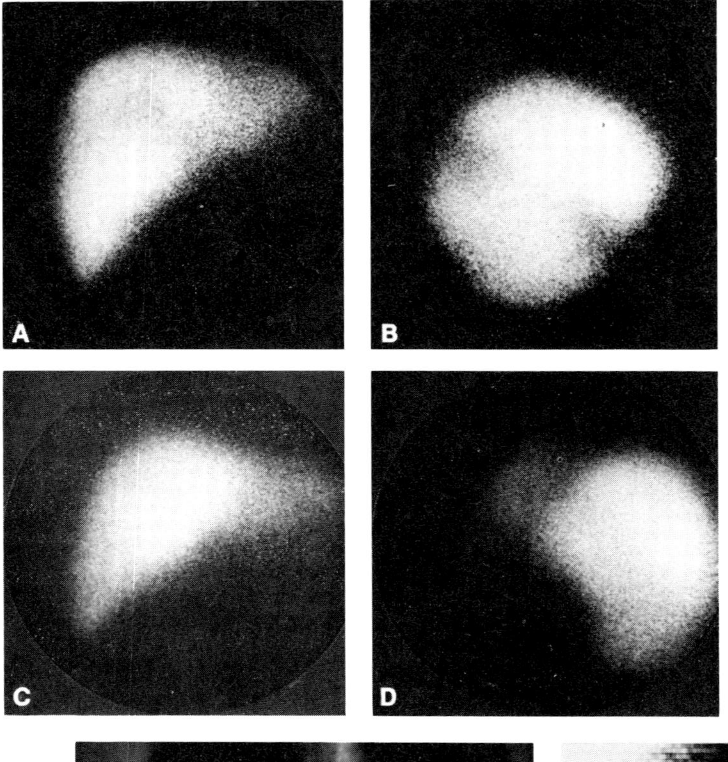

Fig. 2-18. Trauma. Diagnosis: Liver laceration with healing

A and B. Anterior **(A)** and right lateral **(B)** views. An ill-defined bandlike defect (decreased uptake) crosses the liver horizontally **(A).** Defects at both the anterior and posterior margins are more apparent in **B.** The patient had fallen from a scaffold and received blunt trauma to his upper right quadrant.

C and D. Anterior **(C)** and right lateral **(D)** views. 6 weeks later—no evidence of liver defect

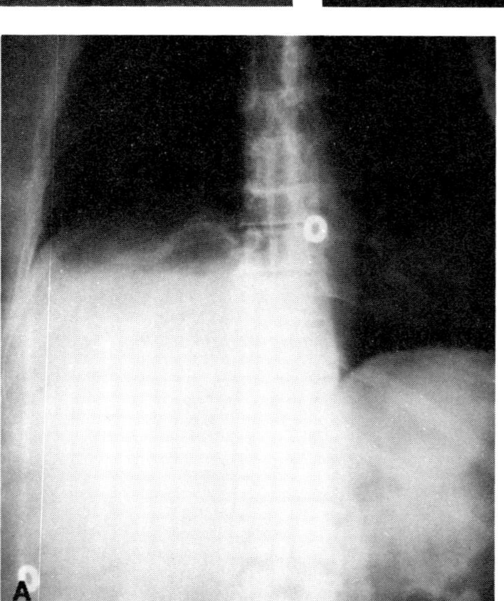

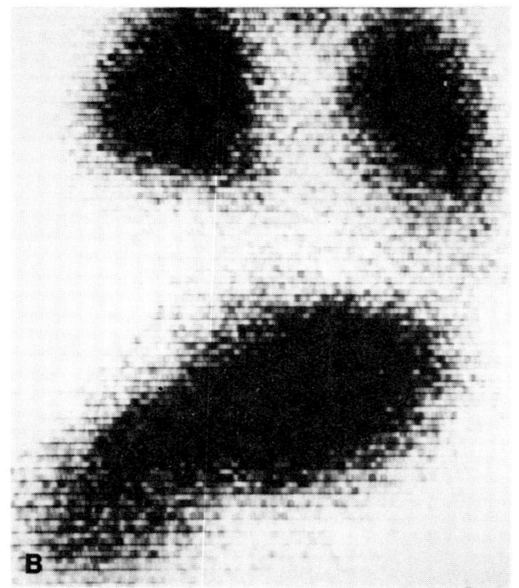

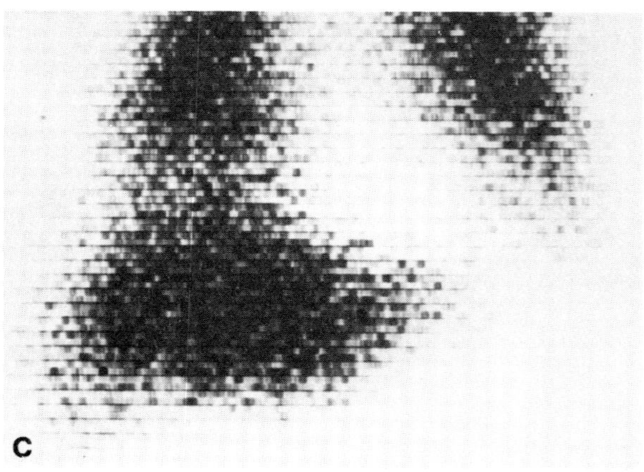

Fig. 2-19. Right subdiaphragmatic abscess.
Simultaneous imaging of the liver and lungs with ^{99m}Tc sulfur colloid and ^{99m}Tc MAA or ^{131}I MAA.

A. X ray (supine). High right diaphragm and subsegmental atelectasis in right lung base

B. Anterior liver-lung scan. Marked separation between base of right lung and dome of liver

C. Anterior liver-lung scan. Normal relationship of liver to right lung one week following drainage of abscess

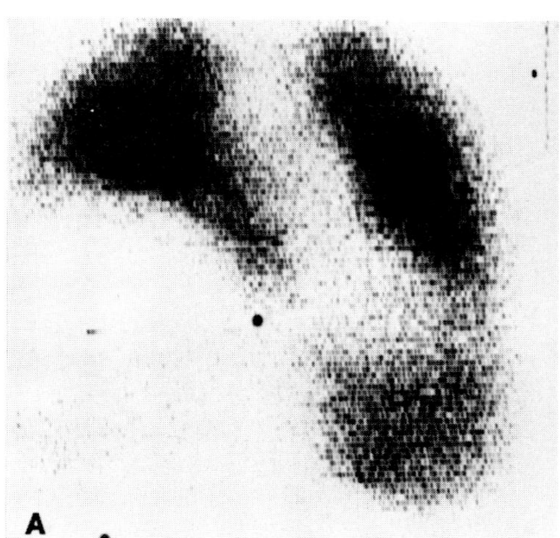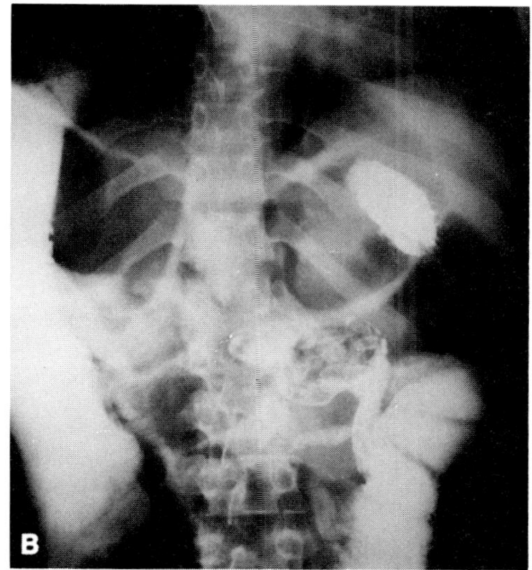

Fig. 2-20. Subdiaphragmatic abscess. Diagnosis: Granulomatous colitis associated with interposition of the hepatic flexure
A. Liver-lung scan. Gross depression of liver trapping. Marked separation of liver and right lung and atypical contour of right lung base. Splenic uptake is preserved.
B. Barium enema. Gross dilatation and interposition of hepatic flexure of the colon between the liver and right diaphragm. Patient also had granulomatous colitis.

abscess and has been advocated as another possible method of detecting this pathology.

The use of imaging is extremely valuable in right-sided problems. Care must be exercised not to misinterpret ascites or bowel interposition for abscess since these also cause displacement of the liver (Fig. 2-20). Unfortunately, left subphrenic space collections are poorly appreciated, although the same criteria are applicable. The relationship of the left lung base to the spleen can be evaluated. When left-sided problems are suspected, imaging with the patient prone is recommended. Also to be recommended is ^{67}Ga whose abnormal accumulation may be detected more easily on the left than on the right side.

Infection. Inflammatory involvement of the liver is either of the focal or diffuse type. If focal, the problem is usually an abscess, although isolated cases of focal change in acute viral hepatitis have been described. As previously discussed under focal defects, without clinical guidance the defects are indistinguishable, one cause from the other. When the problem is hepatitis from any source, the scan changes are of the diffuse type and again require clinical input to be recognized.

Infections of the gallbladder are again receiving investigative interest. Early in liver-imaging history, it was quickly discovered that the hepatocellular clearing agents being used would at some point localize in the gallbladder. For a short period Cholografin tagged with ^{131}I was even used to improve the predictability of this localization. The absence of a tracer in the gallbladder in clinically correlated situations suggested a cystic duct obstructive problem. Since the exact moment of accumulation was an unpredictable variable, the study never achieved a lasting position in the diagnostic menu. However, scattered reports in the literature suggest a possible renaissance attributable to newer, more-specific pharmacologic agents and to the addition of nonradioactive pharmaceuticals, such as cholecystokinin, which improve the normal predictable range of nuclide accumulation. Also reported is the ability to identify acute cholecystitis with ^{67}Ga citrate,

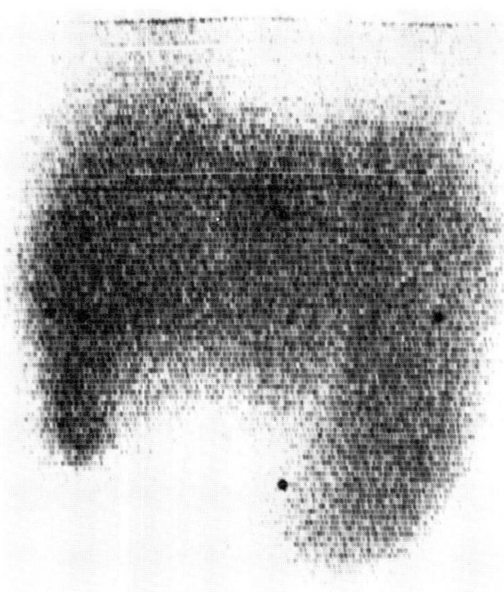

Fig. 2-21. **Acute lymphatic leukemia.** Anterior liver-spleen scan with ^{99m}Tc sulfur colloid. The spleen (which is usually not seen on this view) is grossly enlarged and extends below the umbilicus. The liver is also enlarged. Activity is minimally nonhomogenous.

Fig. 2-22. **Reticulum cell sarcoma**
A. Barium enema. The proximal descending colon is markedly displaced medially.
B. Posteroanterior liver-spleen scan. The splenic trapping is diffusely decreased although the organ appears enlarged.

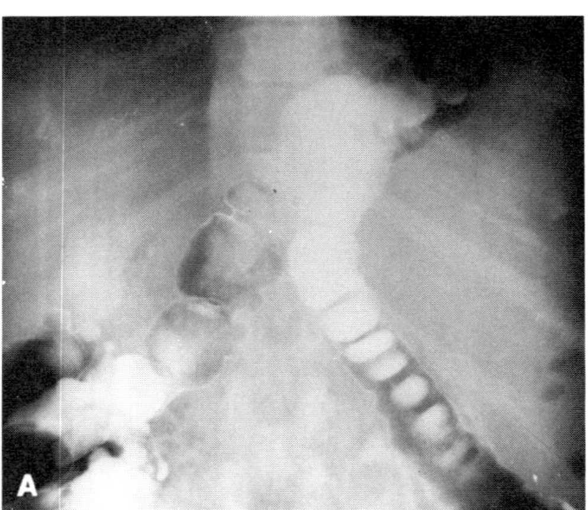

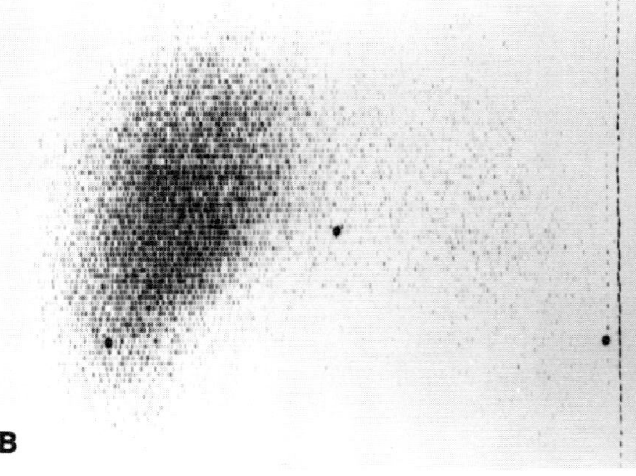

particularly in patients in whom the conventional x rays fail to visualize the gall bladder.

spleen

Size and Position. The single commonest indication for a definitive spleen scan is suspected organ enlargement. Is the upper left abdominal mass splenomegaly? That's what turns it on. This question is answerable (Fig. 2-21). When enlargement is established its etiology may also be suggested by a variation in the scan pattern. Normally, the tracer activity is homogeneously distributed throughout the spleen. Diffuse defects may be secondary to leukemia or lymphomatous processes or granulomatous diseases, such as sarcoidosis (Fig. 2-22).

Trauma. The growing appreciation of the value of screening the spleen in cases of blunt trauma to the abdomen is moving this indication up on the "Why" popularity charts (Fig. 2-23). Few false negative results are obtained, particularly if serial studies are performed when the initial examination is negative but symptoms and

Fig. 2-23. Splenic rupture
A and B. Posterior **(A)** and left lateral **(B)** spleen scans. During automobile accident patient was thrown against door handle with resultant pain in left upper quadrant. An obvious trapping defect appears in the lower pole of the spleen. The liver is normal. (Courtesy of P. Chase, John F. Kennedy Memorial Hospital, Stratford, N.J.)

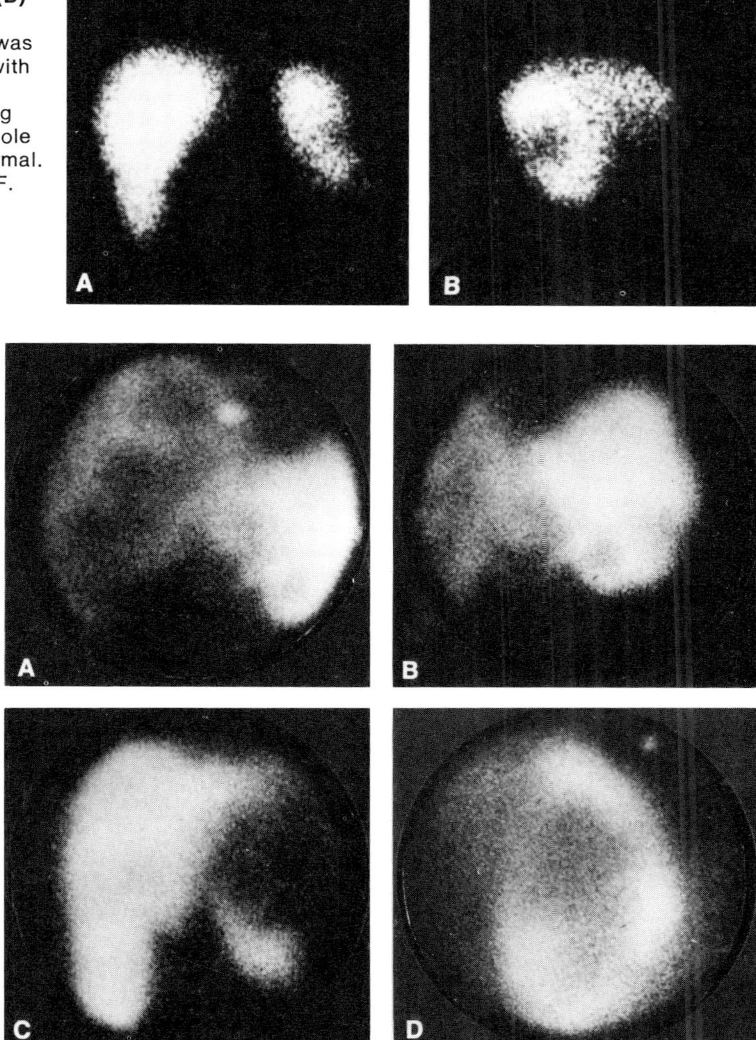

Fig. 2-24. Masses
Diagnosis: Metastatic colon carcinoma
A and B. Anterior **(A)** and oblique **(B)** views. Focal defects in spleen and liver
Diagnosis: Lymphosarcoma
C and D. Anterior **(C)** and left lateral **(D)** views. Focal defects in spleen

clinical suspicions persist. Although delayed ruptures occurring months after trauma have been documented, the vast majority are manifest within the first 2 weeks. Rupture is identified as a zone of absent activity. Complete transection is not uncommon. If a camera is available, multiple views can be obtained without changing the patient's position. Angiography is obviated in many instances.

Masses. Only rarely does clinical concern of a splenic mass (not splenomegaly) initiate the study. Metastatic invasion does occur. Focal defects secondary to lymphosarcoma, abscess, infarct, cyst, and hemangioma are all known, however, these are usually identified on the "two-fer" end of a liver scan and except for additional clinical data are indistinguishable one from the other (Fig. 2-24).

Hematologic Problems. When splenectomy has been performed in the therapeutic management of certain anemias without the anticipated response, the possibility of accessory spleens must be ruled out. Although far from an everyday demand, when indicated, the identification of an accessory spleen is most helpful. In these cases the study is probably best done with an erythrocyte-tagged agent, *e.g.,* ^{51}Cr, ^{99m}Tc stannous glucoheptonate, or ^{203}Pb. These agents avoid the confusion of liver activity and diminish the concern that a small functioning splenic unit will be obscured by the left hepatic lobe, as with the more conventional colloidal nuclides.

Table 2-1. Indications, Pharmaceuticals, Methodology, and Order of Merit of Radionuclide Study of Liver and Spleen

Why	What	How	Yea–Nay
Liver			
Mass lesions (focal)			
Primary	^{99m}Tc sulfur colloid	Static	+++
Metastatic	^{99m}Tc sulfur colloid	Static	++++
Other	^{99m}Tc sulfur colloid	Static	+++
Parenchymal disease (diffuse)			
Cirrhosis	^{99m}Tc sulfur colloid	Static	++++
Congestive heart failure	^{99m}Tc sulfur colloid	Static	++
Other	^{99m}Tc sulfur colloid	Static	++
Jaundice	^{131}I rose bengal	Static	+++
Size, shape, position	^{99m}Tc sulfur colloid	Static	++++
Trauma	^{99m}Tc sulfur colloid	Static	+++
Subdiaphragmatic abscess	^{99m}Tc sulfur colloid	Static	+++
Infection	^{99m}Tc sulfur colloid	Static	+++
Spleen			
Mass lesions	^{99m}Tc sulfur colloid	Static	+++
Size, shape, position	^{99m}Tc sulfur colloid	Static	++++
Trauma	^{99m}Tc sulfur colloid	Static	+++
Accessory	^{51}Cr heat-treated erythrocytes	Static	++

Table 2-2. More About What

Radiopharmaceutical	Dose (mCi)	Physical Half-Life	Energy Peak (keV)
Liver			
^{99m}Tc sulfur colloid	1–3	6 hr	140
^{131}I rose bengal	0.15–0.30	8.4 days	364
^{113m}In colloid	1–3	104 min	393
^{131}I microaggregated albumin	0.15–0.30	8.05 days	364
^{67}Ga citrate	2–4	79 hr	93,184,296
^{75}Se methionine	0.25	120 days	136,265,280
Spleen			
^{99m}Tc sulfur colloid	1–3	6 hr	140
^{51}Cr heat-treated erythrocytes	0.1–0.3	27.8 days	320

Table 2-3. More About How

Why	Preparation	Administration	Time Between Administration and Exam (min)	Number of Exams	Time for Each Exam (min)	Time for Total Study (min)	Patient's Position	Instrument
Liver								
Mass lesions	none	IV	5–15	1	20–30	20–30	recumbent	camera or scanner
Parenchymal disease	none	IV	5–15	1	20–30	20–30	recumbent	camera or scanner
Jaundice	none	IV	15	2 or more	10–20	20 min–48 hr	supine	camera or scanner
Size, shape, position	none	IV	5–15	1	20–30	20–30	recumbent	camera or scanner
Trauma	none	IV	5–15	1	20–30	20–30	recumbent	camera or scanner
Subdiaphragmatic abscess	combined with lung scan	IV	5–15	1	1–2 hr	1–2 hr	supine and rt. lateral	camera or scanner
Spleen								
Mass lesions	none	IV	5–15	1	20–30	20–30	recumbent	camera or scanner
Size, shape, position	none	IV	5–15	1	20–30	20–30	recumbent	camera or scanner
Trauma	none	IV	5–15	1 or several	5–15	15 min to days	recumbent	camera or scanner
Accessory	^{51}Cr heat-treated erythrocytes	IV	4 hr	1 or more	1–2 hr	2–24 hr	prone	camera or scanner

BIBLIOGRAPHY

LIVER

General

Christie JH, Chaudhuri TK: Measurement of hepatic blood flow. Semin Nucl Med 2:97–107, 1972

DeLand FH, Wagner HN: Liver. In Reticuloendothelial System, Liver, Spleen and Thyroid. Philadelphia, WB Saunders, 1972, pp 65–202

Johnson PM: The liver. In Freeman LM, Johnson PM (eds): Clinical Scintillation Scanning. Hagerstown, Harper & Row, 1969, pp 260–303

Mangum JF, Powell MR: Liver scintiphotography as an index of liver abnormality. J Nucl Med 14(7):484–489, 1973

Shingleton WW: Liver scanning-gastrointestinal tract function and disease. In Blahd WH (ed): Nuclear Medicine. New York, McGraw-Hill, 1971, pp 366–374

Silberstein EB: Efficacy of technetium-99m sulfur colloid, angiography, and liver function tests in the diagnosis of hepatic disease (abstr). J Nucl Med 15(6):533, 1974

Wagner HN Jr, Mishkin F: The liver. In Wagner HN Jr (ed): Principles of Nuclear Medicine. Philadelphia, WB Saunders, 1968, pp 599–620

Pharmacology

Bastomsky CH et al.: Gamma-study of the hepato-biliary excretion of ^{131}I-thyroxine-glucuronide and ^{131}I-rose bengal in the rat. J Nucl Med 14(1):34–39, 1973

Chaudhuri TK et al.: A new radiopharmaceutical for combined lung-liver scan—preliminary experiment in animals. J Nucl Med 14(6):346–347, 1973

Goris ML: ^{123}I-iodo-bromsulphalein as a liver and biliary scanning agent. J Nucl Med 14(11):820–825, 1973

Jacksen RA et al.: Technetium-mercaptide complexes and their potential application as a liver specific agent (abstr). J Nucl Med 14(6):411–412, 1973

Lin TH et al.: A ^{99m}Tc-labeled replacement for ^{131}I-rose bengal in liver and biliary tract studies. J Nucl Med 15(7):613–615, 1974

Subramanian JG: ^{99m}Tc-stannous phytate: A new in vivo colloid for imaging the reticuloendothelial system (abstr). J Nucl Med 14(6):459, 1973

Space-Occupying Lesions

Chaudhuri TK et al.: Uptake of [87mSr] by liver metastasis from carcinoma of colon. J Nucl Med 14(5):293–294, 1973

Freeman LM, Mandell CH: Dynamic vascular scintiphotography of the liver. Semin Nucl Med 2:133–138, 1972

Geslien GE et al.: Gallium scanning in acute hepatic amebic abscess. J Nucl Med 15(7):561–563, 1974

Kaplan E, Domingo M: [75Se]-selenomethionine in hepatic focal lesions. Semin Nucl Med 2:139–149, 1972

Kew MC et al.: False–Negative [75Se]-selenomethionine scans in primary liver cancer. J Nucl Med 15(4):234–236, 1974

Lee GC et al.: Correlation of scintigraphic and sonographic findings in focal liver disease (abstr). J Nucl Med 15(6):511, 1974

Levin J et al.: Radionuclide scanning of the liver in primary hepatic cancer: an analysis of 202 cases. J Nucl Med 15(4):296–299, 1974

Lubin E, Lewitus Z: Blood pool scanning in investigating hepatic mass lesions. Semin Nucl Med 2:128–132, 1972

McCartney WH et al.: Use of the CEA titer as an adjunct to the liver scan in the diagnosis of hepatic metastases (abstr). J Nucl Med 15(6):514–515, 1974

McCready VR: Scintigraphic studies of space-occupying liver disease. Semin Nucl Med 2:108–127, 1972

Siemsen JK et al.: Scintigraphic differentiation of focal hepatic disease (abstr). J Nucl Med 14(6):452–453, 1973

Tubis M et al.: Development of [131I] and [99mT]-labeled metronidazoles as new agents for amebic hepatic abscess imaging (abstr). J Nucl Med 14(6):461, 1973

Yeh S–H et al.: Intravenous radionuclide hepatography in the differential diagnosis of intrahepatic mass lesions. J Nucl Med 14(8):565–567, 1973

Jaundice

Christy B et al.: Preparation of iodine-123 labeled rose–bengal and its distribution in animals (abstr). J Nucl Med 15(6):484, 1974

Czerniak P et al.: Parenchymal and obstructive jaundice—radionuclide differential diagnosis (abstr). J Nucl Med 14(6):388, 1973

Nordyke RA: Metabolic and physiologic aspects of [131I] rose bengal in studying liver function. Semin Nucl Med 2:157–166, 1972

Winston MA, Blahd WH: [131I] rose bengal imaging techniques in differential diagnosis of jaundiced patients. Semin Nucl Med 2:167–175, 1972

Subdiaphragmatic Abscess

Alter AJ, Farrer PA: The perihepatic halo in liver scintiangiographic perfusion studies: a sign of ascites. J Nucl Med 15(6):396–398, 1974

Beihn RM et al.: Subtraction technique for the detection of subphrenic abscesses using [67Ga] and [99mTc]. J Nucl Med 15(5):371–373, 1974

Briggs RC: Combined liver-lung scanning in detecting subdiaphragmatic abscess. Semin Nucl Med 2:150–156, 1972

Pinsky SM et al.: Lung overlap sign in combined liver-lung scanning (abstr). J Nucl Med 14(6):438, 1973

Hot Spots

Chayes Z et al.: The "hot" hepatic abscess. J Nucl Med 15(4):305–307, 1974

Holmquest DL, Burdine JA: Caval–Portal shunting as a cause of focal increase in radiocolloid uptake in normal livers. J Nucl Med 14(6):348–351, 1973

Mikolajkow A, Janinski WK: Increased focal uptake of radiocolloid by the liver. J Nucl Med 14(3):175, 1973

Morita ET et al.: Further information on a "hot spot" in the liver. J Nucl Med 14(8):606–608, 1975

Pasquier J, Dorta T: Letter: Focal hyperfixation of radiocolloid by the liver. J Nucl Med 15(8):725, 1974

SPLEEN

DeLand FH, Wagner HW: Spleen. In Reticuloendothelial System, Liver, Spleen and Thyroid. Philadelphia, WB Saunders, 1972, pp 206–233

Gilday DL, Alderson PO: Scintigraphic evaluation of liver and spleen injury. Semin Nucl Med 4(4):357–370, 1974

Goswitz F: Radiocolloid spleen scanning in lymphoma and chronic lymphocytic leukemia (abstr). J Nucl Med 15(6):496, 1974

Gutkowski RF, Dworkin HJ: A new kit for RBC labeling and spleen scanning: Tc-99m stannous glucoheptonate (abstr). J Nucl Med 15(6):498, 1974

Habibian MR, Abernathy EM: Splenomegaly with uniformly decreased splenic uptake of [99mTc]-sulfur colloid: a new observation in childhood sarcoidosis. J Nucl Med 15(1):45–46, 1974

Handmaker H, Freedman GS: Preoperative diagnosis of splenic abscess using scintigraphic techniques (abstr). J Nucl Med 15(6):499, 1974

Johnson PM: The spleen. In Freeman LM, Johnson PM (eds): Clinical Scintillation Scanning. Hagerstown, Harper & Row, 1969, pp 414–446

McIntyre PA: Diagnostic significance of the spleen scan. Semin Nucl Med 2(3):278–287, 1972

Slavin JD et al.: Scan demonstration of delayed splenic rupture. J Nucl Med 15(7):632–633, 1974

Spencer RP: "Healing" of a splenic infarct. J Nucl Med 15(4):303–304, 1974

Surprenant E, Steffens J: Diagnosis of space occupying lesions of the abdomen. J Nucl Med 15(6):536, 1974

Uchida T et al.: Survival and sequestration of [51Cr]- and [99mTcO4]-labeled platelets. J Nucl Med 15(9):801–807, 1974

Wilson GA, Keyes JW Jr: The significance of the liver-spleen uptake ratio in liver scanning. J Nucl Med 15(7):593–597, 1974

The application and usefulness of radionuclide investigations varies considerably from one organ system to the next. In some there just ain't no magic. In others, all systems are Go! The kidneys are ideally suited to radioisotopic investigation. Their paired anatomy is an obvious initial advantage that permits visual and measured comparison of one to the other as well as against a standardized norm. Additional advantages derive from the fortuitous availability of acceptable nuclides and instrumentation to monitor their unique physiologic functions.

Despite these natural advantages it was not until relatively recently that isotopic investigation of the kidney developed the enthusiasm we believe it deserves. Perhaps its relatively late acceptance stemmed from the existence of other well-established techniques for study. Although the tracer studies of the thyroid, brain, liver, and even lung provided data not obtained by other "routine" techniques, the dutiful duo of x ray and laboratory was considered adequate to attack renal problems and the urgency for other parameters of view was not compelling. Coupled with this lack of urgency was the unfortunate early experience with the renogram. This technique was introduced in 1955 as a method to recognize renal vascular disease and diagnose correctable renal artery hypertension. Initial

excitement, even to the extent of development of instrumentation specifically designed for this study, was quickly dampened. Experience proved that interpretations were less than satisfactory because the parameters of the measurement were far more complex than originally perceived. It could be said without fear of contradiction that this study was "an idea born before its time." More on the renogram later.

Renal incorporation is accomplished by the binding of the sulfhydril radicals of chlormerodrin in the cystoplasm of the proximal convoluted tubules. Thus, images could be obtained of the cortical elements of the kidney using existing rectilinear instrumentation. (The camera was still just "a gleam" and as yet unavailable commercially.) This ability to image the cortex "kosherized" scanning since the x-ray studies with opaque were primarily keyed to visualization of the medullary elements (the collecting systems). Remember that way back then IVPs did not look the way they do now. Infusion techniques did not exist and routine tomography

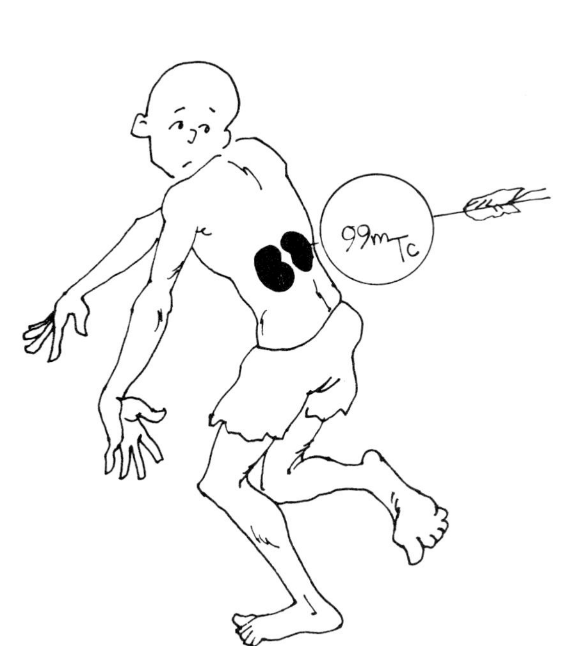

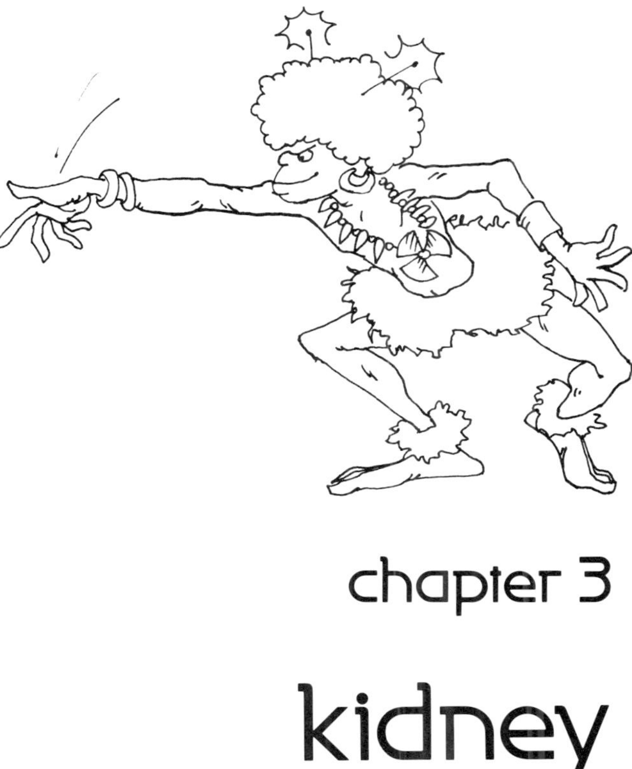

chapter 3

kidney

was unheard of. Yet, it was hard to buck the common misconception that the mercury scan and the standard IVP were essentially competitive techniques. Indeed, an alternative was present if such contraindications as allergy to opaques or obscuring abdominal densities existed, but common practice did not suggest that complementary benefits were obtainable in many situations by employing both methods. Not until the advent of the camera imaging system allowed dynamic events to be viewed and the development of suitable nuclides capable of identifying these events did general acceptance occur. In this time span the original agents ^{131}I acetrizoate sodium (Urokon) and ^{131}I-iodopyracet (Diodrast) were discarded in favor of the more-specific ^{131}I-orthoiodohippurate (Hippuran). This latter material, like paraaminohippuric acid, is handled by a combination of glomerular filtration (20%) and tubular secretion (80%), so that approximately 92% of the unbound material is cleared from the plasma in a single passage through the normal kidney. Technetium 99m in the pertechnetate form was found to supply reliable data on the vascular perfusion pattern. Finally, the coupling of ^{99m}Tc to both Fe ascorbate DTPA and Sn-DTPA chelates and to glucoheptonate achieved the ultimate (at least for now) of imaging both the perfusion and excretion pattern with a single agent in a single study.

Tables 3-1 and 3-2 under What summarize the agents now in popular usage. Each contributes specific information, and in combination they often more sharply define differential distinctions. As with any rapidly changing body of data the four or five standard agents identified herein may and probably will become obsolete in the future. In the past 2 years, 13 additional materials have been noted in the literature, each with an appropriately positive descriptive glow: [113m]In-DTPA, [169]Yb-DTPA, ^{131}I-fibrinogen, ^{123}I-sodium iodohippurate, ^{99m}Tc-gelatin, ^{99m}Tc-mannitol, ^{133}Xe, ^{99m}Tc-penicillamine acetazolamide complex (TPAC), ^{99m}Tc-inulin, ^{99m}Tc-labeled tetracyline, ^{51}Cr-EDTA, and even ^{99m}Tc-polyphosphate. This tabulation is simply appended to indicate the continuing investigational search for superior agents. It in no way affects that which has already been established.

With respect to the *how* (Tables 3-1 and 3-3) the only pain to be anticipated is the "ouch" of the IV injection. All studies start from that common origin, with later variations depending on the problem. If the study is for hypertensive screening the total time commitment is 1–2 min —no one ever misses lunch for this one. The evaluation of the integrity of a renal transplant, on the other hand, may require daily monitoring throughout several weeks. However, in none is discomfort to be anticipated. The position of examination is usually prone or supine. In most situations no preparations are necessary. Occasionally, hydration may be requested in the renogram. Except for the renogram in which

Table 3-1. Indications, Pharmaceuticals, Methodology and Order of Merit of Radionuclide Study of Kidney

Why	What	How	Yea–Nay
Mass lesion	[197]Hg chlormerodrin	static	++++
	[99m]Tc pertechnetate	dynamic	
Vascular			
Hypertension	[99m]Tc pertechnetate	dynamic	+++
	[131]I sodium iodohippurate	renogram	++
Infarction	[197]Hg chlormerodrin	static	+++
Acute tubular necrosis	[99m]Tc pertechnetate	dynamic	+
Mechanical obstruction	[99m]Tc diethylenetriaminepentaacetic acid (DTPA)	dynamic	++++
	[99m]Tc glucoheptonate	static	
Trauma	[197]Hg chlormerodrin	static	+++
	[99m]Tc glucoheptonate	static	
Congenital	[197]Hg chlormerodrin		++++
	[99m]Tc glucoheptonate	static	
Inflammatory			
Nephritis	[99m]Tc glucoheptonate	static	++
Abscess		static	+++
Transplant	[99m]Tc pertechnetate	dynamic	+++

Radiopharmaceutical	Dose (mCi)	Physical Half-life (hr)	Energy Peak (keV)
[197]Hg chlormerodrin	0.2	64.8	77
[131]I iodohippurate	0.3	201.6	364
[99m]Tc pertechnetate	10–20	6	140
[99m]Tc Sn-Diethylene-triaminepentaacetic acid (Sn-DTPA)	10–20	6	140
[99m]Tc glucoheptonate	10–20	6	140
[99m]Tc dimercapto-succinic acid	1–5	6	140

Table 3-3. More About How

Why	Preparation	Administration	Time Between Administration and Exam (hr)	Number of Exams	Time for Each Exam (min)	Time for Total Study (min)	Patient's Position	Instrument
Mass	none	IV	static: 1–2	1	30	30	prone	camera or scanner
			dynamic: immed.	1	1–2	1–2	prone	camera
Vascular Hypertension	renogram: hydration	IV	immediate	1	20–45	30–45	sitting	probes and strip chart or camera
	dynamic: none	IV	immediate	1	1–2	1–2	prone	camera
Infarction	none	IV	1–2	1	30	30	prone	camera or scanner
Acute tubular	none	IV	immediate	1 or more	1–10	1 min–24 hr	prone	camera or scanner
Mechanical Obs.	none	IV	immediate	2 or more	1–10	6–24 hr	prone	camera or scanner
Trauma	none	IV	immediate	1	1–10	1–10	prone	camera or scanner
Congenital	none	IV	immediate	1	1–10	1–10	prone or supine	camera or scanner
Inflammatory Nephritis	none	IV	1–2	1	30	30	prone	camera or scanner
Abscess	none	IV	static: 1–2	1	30	30	prone	camera or scanner
			dynamic: immed.	1	1–2	1–2	prone	camera
Transplant	none	IV	immediate	1 or more	1–2	min to days	prone or supine	camera

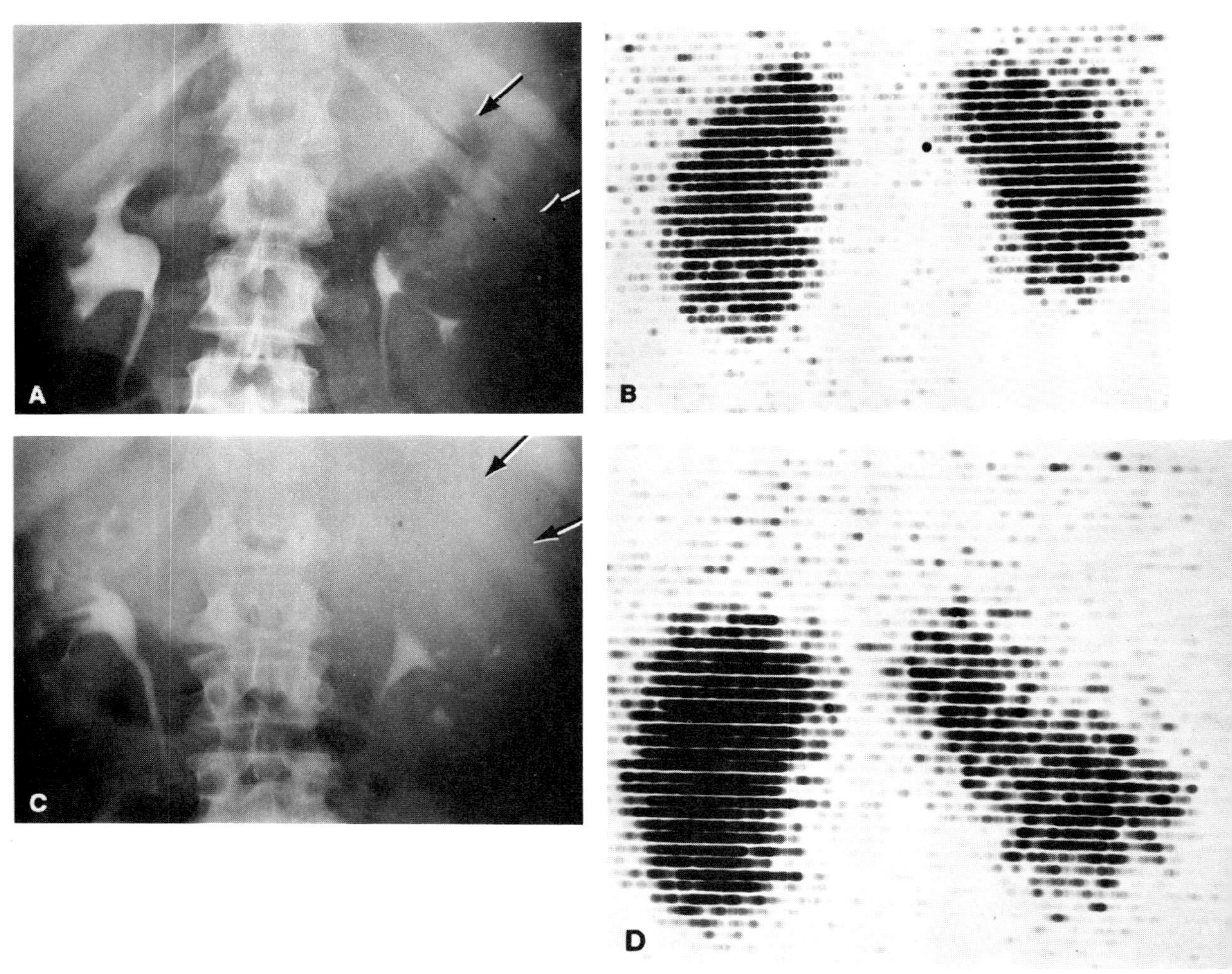

strip chart recorders are employed to graph the results, almost all of the other examinations have images as their record.

WHY

mass

Except in isolated situations, the average patient suspected of harboring a space-taking lesion in either or both kidneys is initially investigated by x ray. The prime exception is the contraindication to the use of iodinated radiopaque contrast agents. When the contrast study is definitely positive, the need for radionuclide investigation is debatable. When the contrast study is suggestive, questionable, or unsatisfactory for

reasons of poor film quality or from any other cause, then further investigation with nuclides is almost mandatory.

Review of the usual sequential diagnostic pathways with editorial order of merit comments may prove helpful in establishing a different and hopefully more-productive sequence.

When for any number of clinical reasons an IVP is obtained and the findings are suspicious of a mass lesion one of two possibilities exists: 1) definitely positive; 2) questionable.

There is also that small group of patients in whom suspicion of an intrarenal disease exists but who cannot be studied with contrast agents. This group can be considered in the questionable category and managed similarly. In both, further qualification is necessary. In 1 the definite

Fig. 3-1. Mass lesion?
Diagnosis: Normal kidneys
  A. X ray. Left kidney suggests a possible space-occupying lesion. The superior and middle calyceal groups are ill-defined and questionably stretched (arrows).
  B. Scan. Static scan employing ^{197}Hg. Trapping pattern is homogeneous. There is no evidence of a space-occupying lesion. Study was performed with a rectilinear scanner.
Diagnosis: Hypernephroma (right kidney)
  C. X ray. Right kidney (reversed for ease of comparison with **(A)** also suggests a possible space-occupying lesion. The superior and middle calyceal groups are ill-defined. The renal margin is obscured (arrows).
  D. Scan. Static image confirms a defect in the superolateral half of the right kidney. Trapping is defective. The renal contour is distorted.

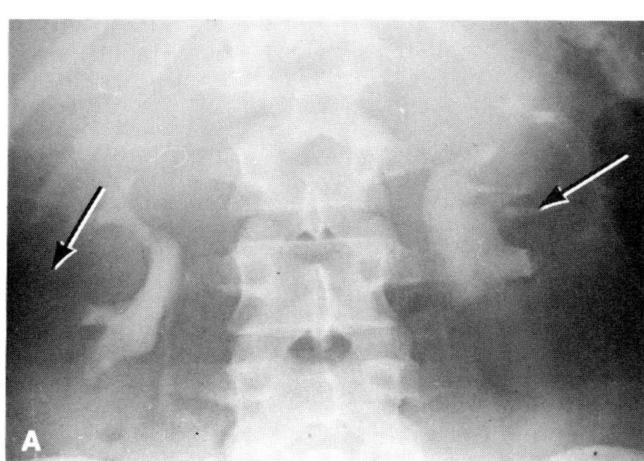

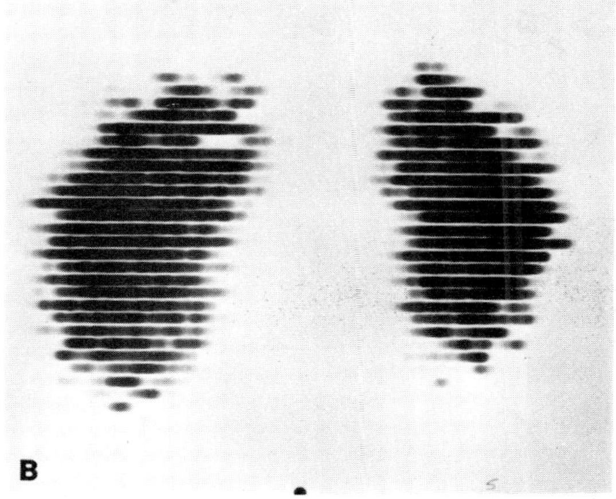

Fig. 3-2. Mass lesion?
Diagnosis: Normal kidneys
  A. X ray (IV urogram).
    Right kidney—possible spreading of superior and middle calyx (arrow)
    Left kidney—possible stretching of superior and middle calyces (arrow)
  B. Scan. The image is normal. Size, contour, position, and trapping integrity are preserved.
Diagnosis: Benign cyst (right kidney)
  C. X ray (IV urogram)
    Right kidney—possible spreading of superior and middle calyx (arrow)
    Left kidney—normal
  D. Scan. Large focal defect midright kidney. Left is normal.

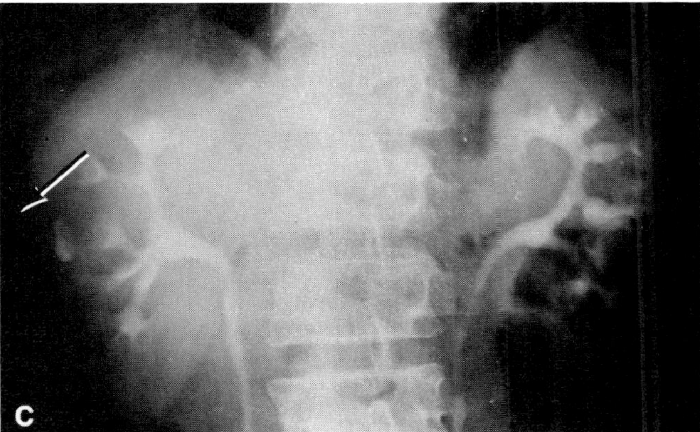

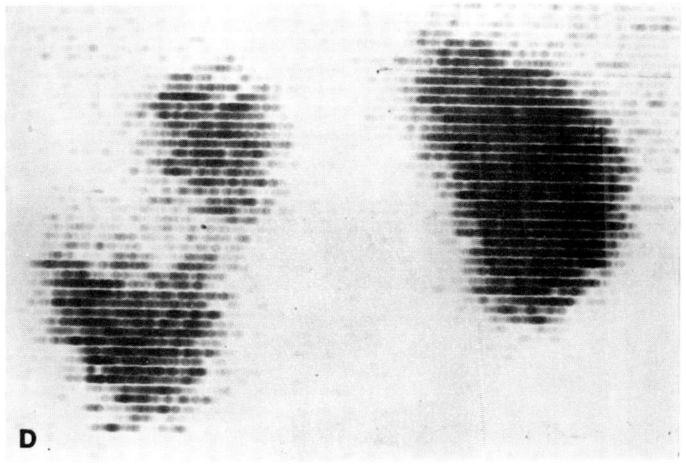

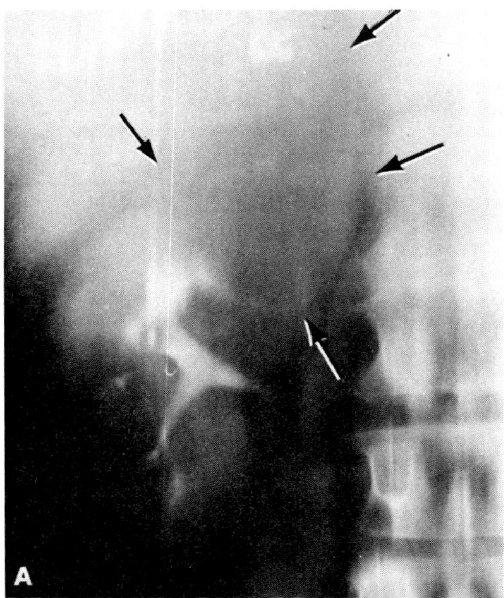

**Fig. 3-3. Avascular defect upper pole right kidney: Benign
renal cyst**
A. X ray. An apparent defect (arrows) of the upper pole of the
right kidney extending cephalad
B. Scan. ^{197}Hg image of the right kidney does not confirm an
upper pole lesion. Image is normal. Examination is made
with gamma camera.
C. Renal flow, 22–25 sec. Superior pole of right kidney is
ill-defined (arrow) and activity is diminished.
D. Renal flow, 25–28 sec. The superior pole fails to perfuse
(arrow). Activity is uniform throughout the remainder of the
kidney.

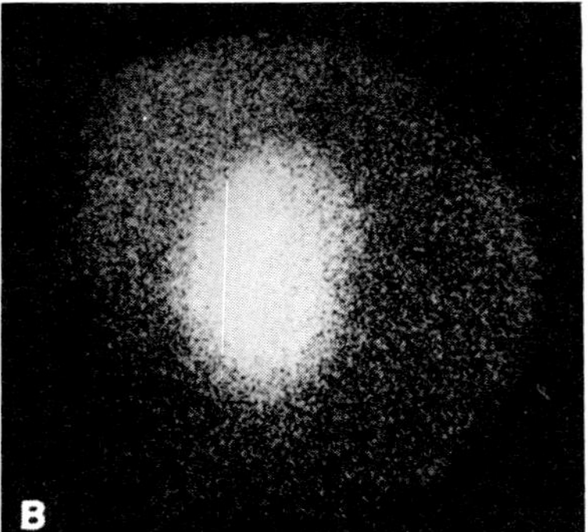

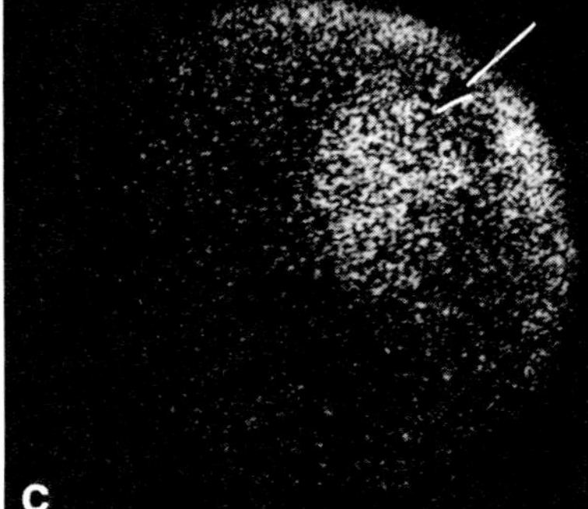

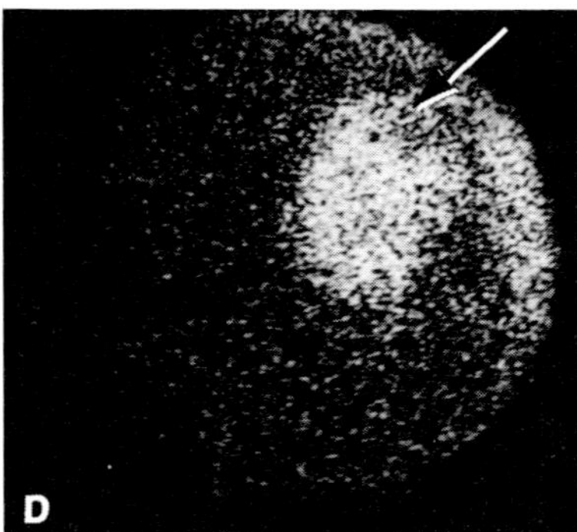

intrarenal mass must be further defined as to
type so that appropriate management can be
initiated. Situation 2's status (questionable) must
be upgraded to 1 and studied accordingly or
demoted to normal and the search discontinued.

The questionable group is our *raison d'etre,*
so let's discuss it first. The urogram is neither
definitely negative nor positive. There is a
questionable alteration in renal contour, and
nephrotomography has not, can not, or should not
be performed; there is a possible displacement
of a calyx; the kidney is obscured by superimposed gas shadows. The presence or absence
of an intrarenal mass of cortical origin can be
established by scanning in most cases if that
lesion is 2.5 cm or more in size and is not situated
on a renal margin and extending outward. Any
of the nuclides listed which are capable of
defining cortical integrity are satisfactory. Any
space-taking lesion, regardless of histology or
morphology will affect tubular integrity such that
the isotope cannot be trapped or stored, and a

negative defect will be noted. The defect may be
single or multiple, but is characteristically
discrete. Thus, the recognition of a negative
defect establishes a space-taking lesion (Figs.
3-1 and 3-2).

Although the reliability of this approach is
excellent, there are certain known exceptions in
which this search-and-destroy technique may
fail. As noted above, lesions less than 2.5 cm
may not be discernable and a false negative
opinion rendered. More commonly missed is the
lesion that originates at the periphery and
extends outward. If this type of problem is
suggested on the questionable urogram, a
negative static or cortical trapping scan is
insufficient and further imaging is required.
Dynamic or perfusion images may be helpful.
The scans obtained may identify the peripheral
or extrarenal component (Fig. 3-3), but these
scans, too, may fail to confirm the presence of
pathology (Fig. 3-4). Lastly, any space-taking
lesion that is confined to the medullary portion of

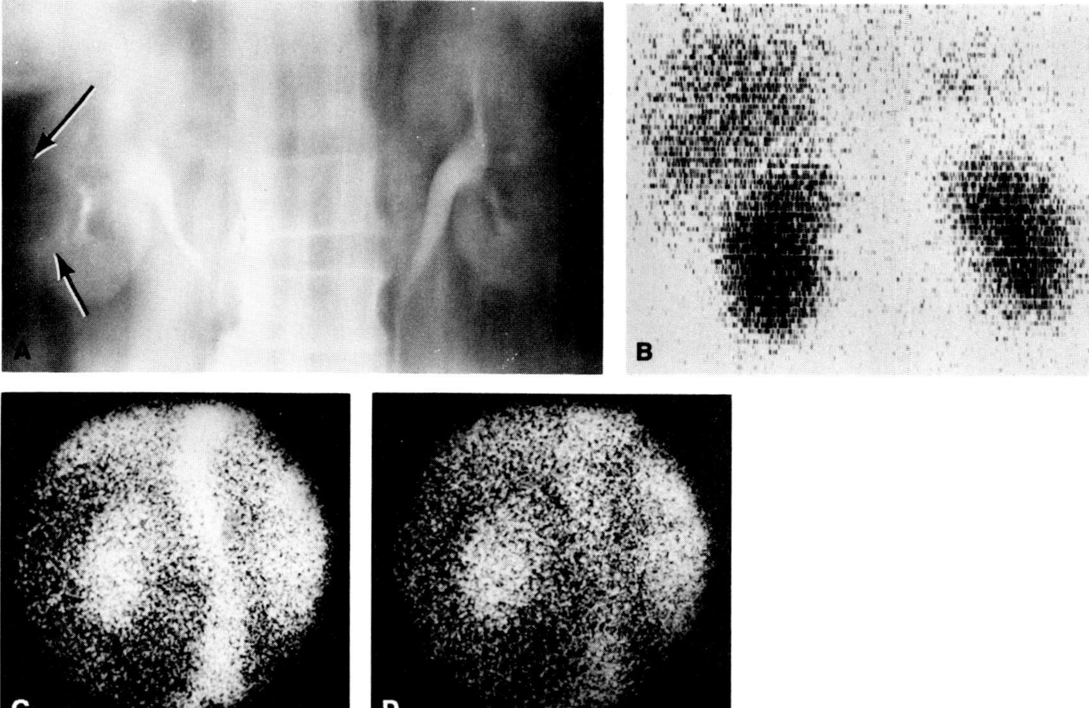

Fig. 3-4. Benign renal cyst
- **A.** X ray. A circumscribed defect appears at the lateral margin of the right kidney (arrows).
- **B.** ^{197}Hg image is normal. Activity above the right kidney is within the liver.
- **C and D.** Renal flow. Sequential images 3 sec apart suggest a normally perfusing right kidney. The marginal defect is not appreciated. The vertical band of activity is ^{99m}Tc in the abdominal aorta. A portion of the left kidney and spleen is visible.

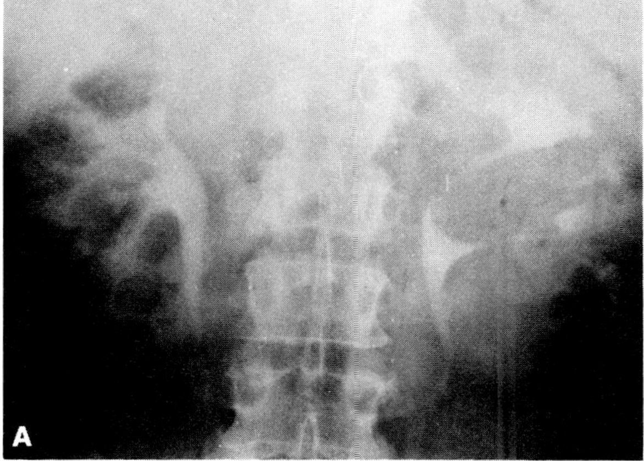

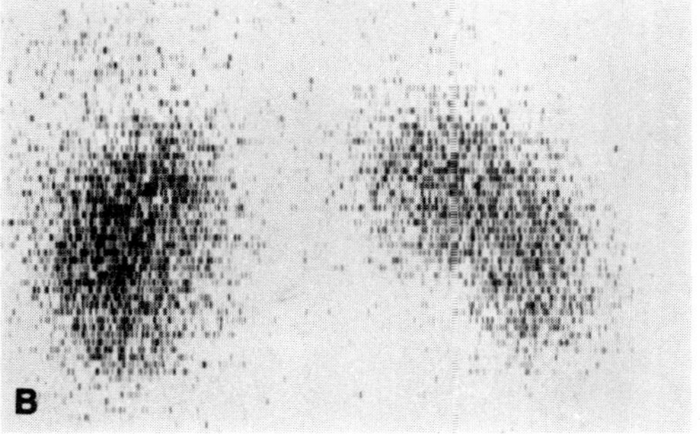

Fig. 3-5. Peripelvic cyst (left kidney)
- **A.** X ray. A large defect distorting the contour of the left kidney and stretching the calyces
- **B.** Scan. The left kidney's axis is minimally altered, but no trapping defect is present.

the kidney or assumes a peripelvic location may also be missed on both the static and dynamic studies, but this combination of an obvious urographic lesion with negative static and dynamic scans is pathogenic of a peripelvic cyst (Fig. 3-5).

Fortunately, these exceptions are numerically small, and although exact figures are unavailable, our clinical experience utilizing this approach to the "is there or ain't there" problem suggests an accuracy yield in excess of 90%.

This leaves only the 1 type situation: the IVP defines an intrarenal mass. Where do we go from there? Differentiation between benign and malignant is essential. Three approaches are generally recognized:

1. Further x ray: retrograde pyelography, nephrotomography, angiography
2. Radionuclide imaging
3. Ultrasound

Further analysis is complicated by multiple considerations, including many as yet unsettled opinions. Perhaps a major decision to be established is whether or not angiography is necessary regardless of clear-cut evidence of either benignancy or malignancy. If the answer is yes, the arterial or venous supply, or both, must be visualized prior to surgical intervention; then definitive angiography becomes the obvious next and only follow-up examination. If, however, contrast angiography is "nyet" because of age, allergy, medical contraindications, or a surgeon content to know only if the lesion is benign or malignant, additional evaluation with isotopes and ultrasonics becomes invaluable (Fig. 3-6).

On the other hand, the vascular lesion may appear normal on the perfusion examination. The "negative defect" on the static image "fills in" on the perfusion study and may be indistinguishable from the surrounding tissue. Occasionally, the vascular lesion may hyperperfuse and appear as a "blush" or hot spot against the adjacent structures (Figs. 3-7 to 3-9). Thus, the combination of a defect on the static and a "normal" or hot-spot perfusion scan warrants a diagnosis of malignant neoplasm. Some rare benign renal tumors, *e.g.*, renal cell adenomas and xantho-granulomatous pyelonephritis are often misdiagnosed by this combination scanning

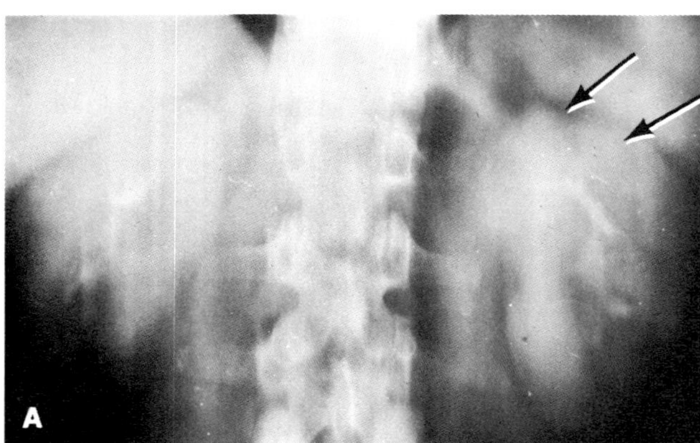

Fig. 3-6. Avascular intrarenal lesion (benign cyst)
A. X ray. There is a questionable flatting of the left superior minor calyces and a questionable lobulated left renal margin (arrows).
B. Renal scan. The static image confirms the suspicious defect on the IV urogram. A circular zone of nonactivity is present in the upper portion of the left kidney (arrows).
C. Renal flow, 24–27 sec. The defect seen on static imaging is identified on the perfusion study employing ^{99m}Tc Sn-DTPA (arrows).
D. Renal flow, 1 min. Defect is still visible.

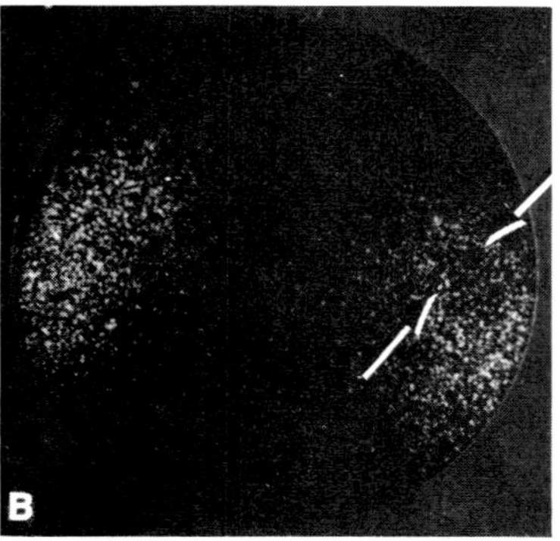

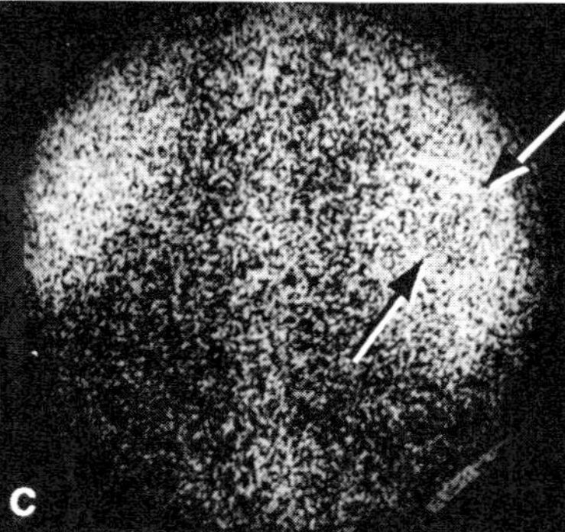

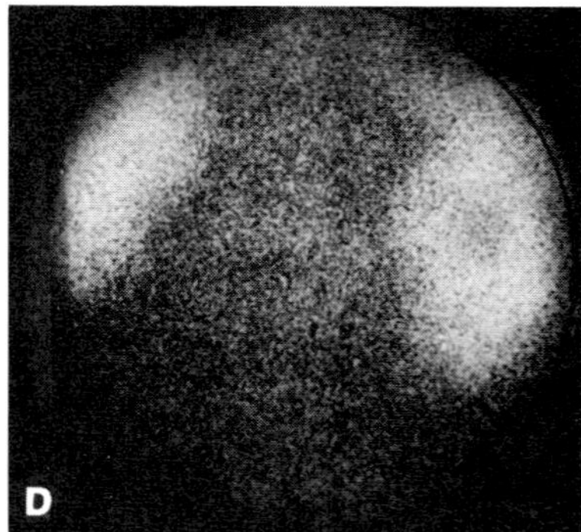

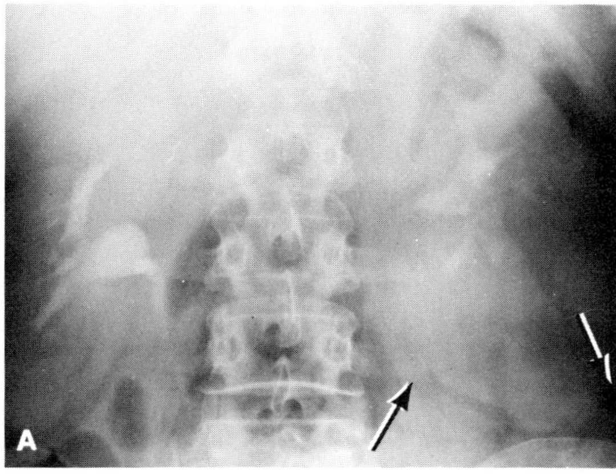

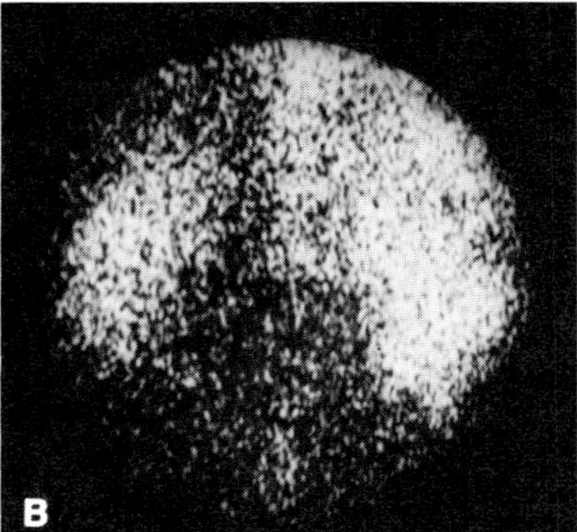

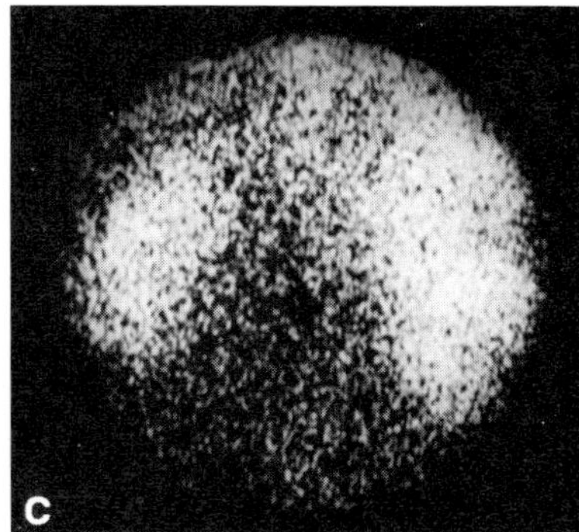

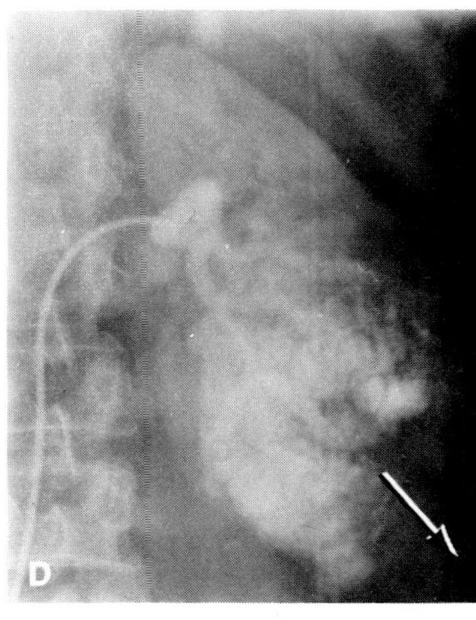

Fig. 3-7. Hypernephroma
A. X ray. There is a large left lower pole mass (arrows).
B and C. Renal flow. Sequential images suggest the lesion (confirmed on static imaging) perfuses completely.
D. Renal arteriogram. The lower pole lesion is hypervascular with typical tumor vessels (arrow).

approach. Unfortunately, they are usually misdiagnosed with equal frequency when studied angiographically.

Unfortunately, a small but not insignificant percentage of renal neoplasms undergo some degree of necrosis by the time they are studied (Fig. 3-10). Additionally, it is becoming recognized that contrary to original opinion about 4%–12% of primary renal tumors are poorly vascularized. These situations, when encountered, may result in the combination typical of benign cystic defects, namely, a defect on static imaging which persists as a defect on the perfusion study (Fig. 3-11). When this combination is encountered, further investigation is unfortunately still necessary since the fundamental question (benign versus malignant) has not been resolved. Review of the entire clinical picture along with the conventional x rays and scans frequently permits recognition of the true nature of the lesion, but we strongly recommend, in contra-distinction to the dictates of teachers of English, the adoption here of the double negative rule:

if the defect is negative by both static and dynamic imaging, there is a "stand off" and no opinion is permissible until further studies clarify the process. Classically, these cases were all examined by contrast angiography. However, coming up fast on the outside is ultrasound. In sophisticated hands, this is becoming the most impressive noninvasive tool. In this situation, the differential diagnosis of avascular or necrosing neoplasm versus the cystic is resolvable by sonography. The echo pattern distinguishes solid from cystic lesions. If the lesion is solid, a strong presumption of malignancy is valid, and contrast angiography or definitive management becomes the next procedure. If the lesion is cystic, certain questions remain to be resolved. Is it benign, or a necrotic neoplasm, or a neoplasm arising in a cyst? This is not an infrequent diagnostic dilemma. A recent study identified asymptomatic space-occupying lesions

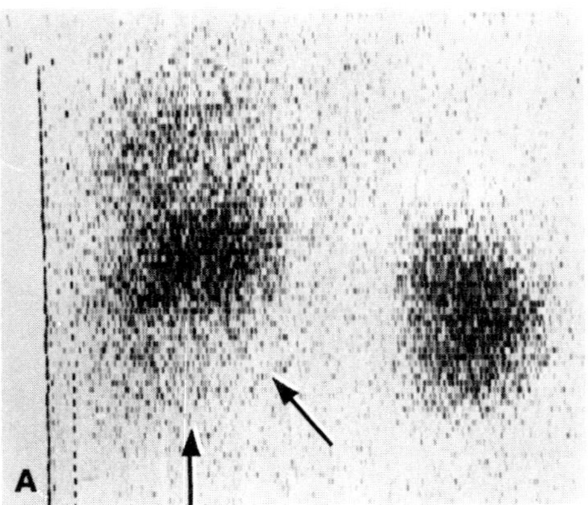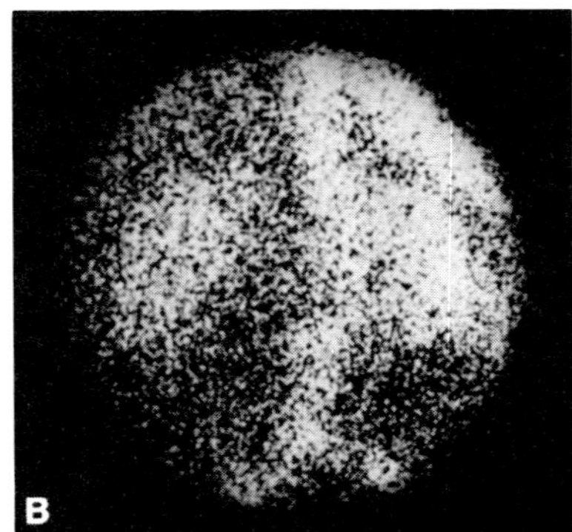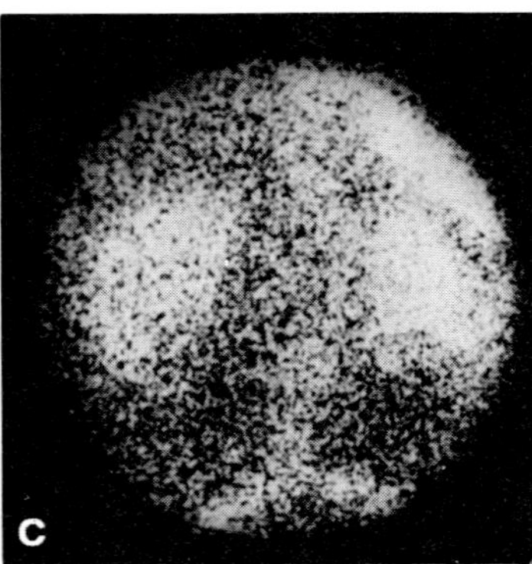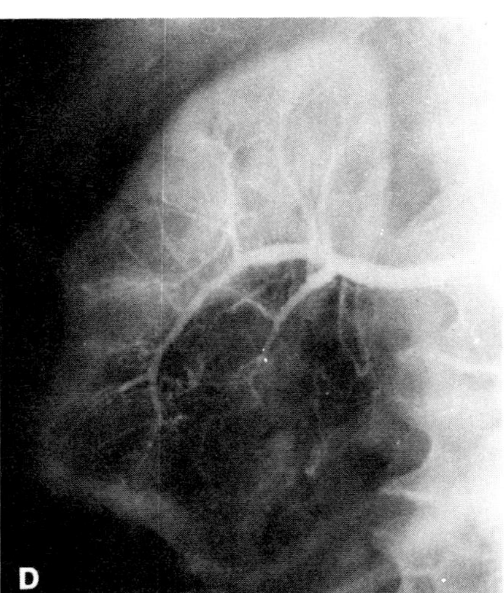

Fig. 3-8. Clear cell carcinoma (right kidney)

A. Static renal scan. The IV urogram suggested a lesion in the lower pole of the right kidney. The ^{197}Hg scan confirms a defect by a nontrapping deficit in the lower pole (arrows).

B and C. Renal flow. The sequential perfusion images indicate that the lower pole of the right kidney is equal in vascular integrity with all other portions of the right and left kidney.

D. Renal arteriogram. The arterial phase of the right arteriogram. Vascular stretching is associated with neovascular puddling.

of the kidney in the general hospital population to be 5%; when only elderly males were considered, the incidence was 15%—and of these, 5%–6% were malignant.

Cyst puncture and aspiration techniques have been recommended to resolve this problem in differential diagnosis. Either under fluoroscopic or ultrasound control the cystic lesion is punctured through a translumbar approach. Its contents are aspirated and studied visually, histochemically, and histocytologically. Additionally, both air and contrast media are instilled and roentgen renal cystography performed. If this combination says "benign," the problem has been resolved by a series of relatively benign techniques. If the combination precipitates out as "malignant" or "highly suspicious," the investigation continues with angiography and possibly surgery.

Thus, in the search for intrarenal mass lesions radioisotopic investigation is excellent for establishing the presence of most lesions and highly effective in defining their character. Whether or not contrast angiography is indicated for every intrarenal lesion is as yet unsettled. It is this decision, established in each case on its own merits, which regulates sequential diagnostic patterns.

hypertension

Perhaps more has been written about the isotope renogram employing ^{131}I sodium iodohippurate than about any other single examination. The pros and cons of this technique have waxed and waned in the literature over the past 20 years. Conceptually, the study is faultless. It is

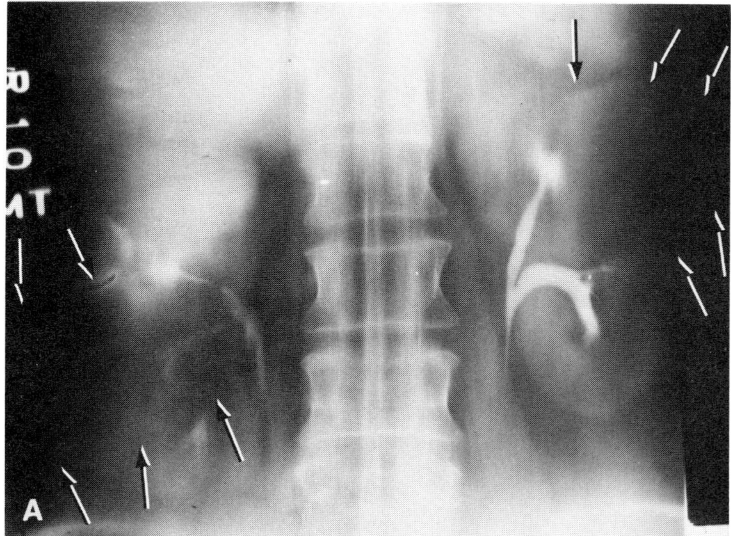

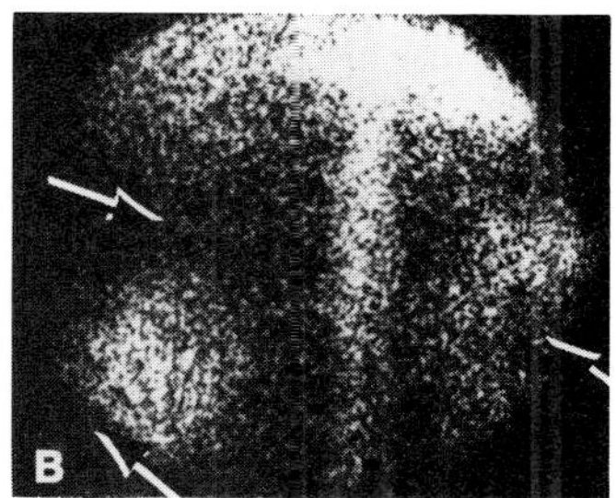

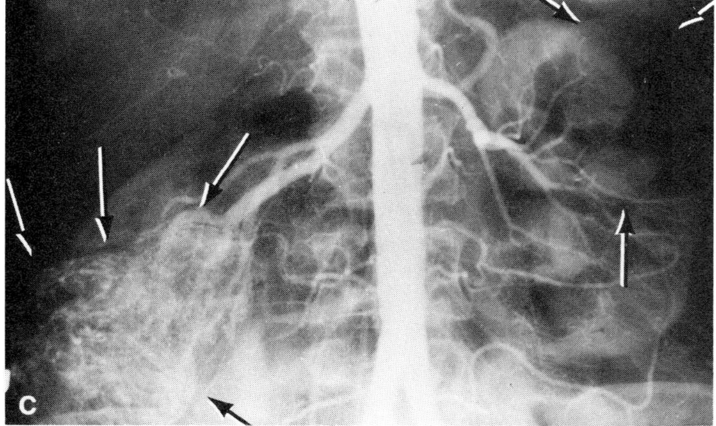

Fig. 3-9. Benign cyst (left kidney); hypernephroma (right kidney)

A. Nephrotomogram. Space-occupying lesion appears in the upper pole of the left kidney and lower pole of the right (arrows).

B. Renal flow. The lesion on the left kidney does not perfuse (arrow). The right lower pole lesion perfuses excessively (arrows) with resultant under perfusion of the superior half of the kidney.

C. Renal arteriogram. The left renal lesion is decreased in vascularity. The vessels are stretched (arrows). There is no evidence of malignancy. The right renal lesion is obviously malignant (arrows).

predicated on the direct intercomparison of the uptake and excretion pattern of each kidney of a tracer compound delivered to it from its own renal artery. Therefore, if a suitable detector is placed over each organ and a suitable radio-nuclide injected into the vascular system, the measurement of the passage of that nuclide through each kidney should readily identify asymmetry whether the problem is a unilateral or bilateral abnormality when compared against a set of norms. Unfortunately, the resulting measurements which were initially and are still obtained by many in graphic form, are far more complicated than a simple pass-through. Numerous modifications in both procedure and interpretation have occurred. It is now common

to obtain an image record in addition to or instead of the graphic representation. The camera is necessary for these and sequential pictures are obtained over an average of 20–30 min. Experience has established that nonvascular disease can also be recognized. In particular, urinary tract obstruction is readily depicted and parenchymal disease is detectable. These uses, however, by strict nomenclature, are not what is meant by the renogram. It is interesting to note that a great deal of renewed interest in this technique has developed as a result of the application of computer analysis to renogram curves. By adequate corrections, extrapolations, manipulations, and the like, proponents indicate that unilateral artery disease is now accurately

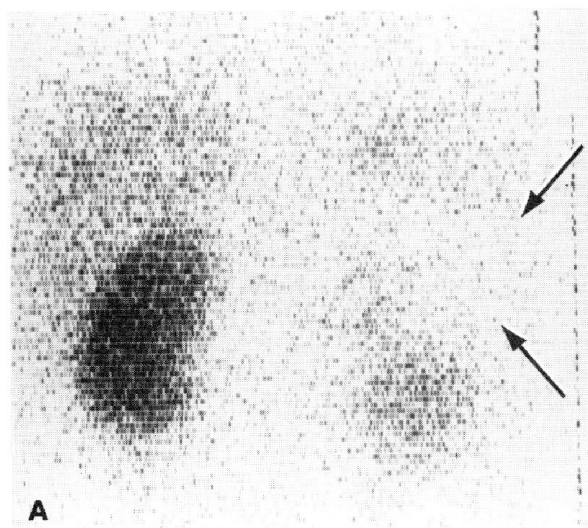

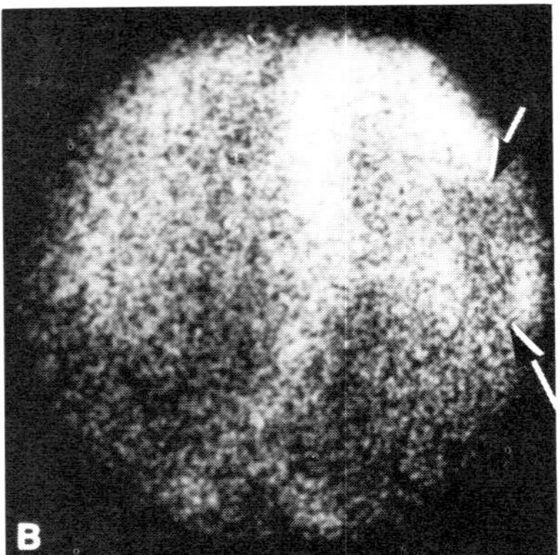

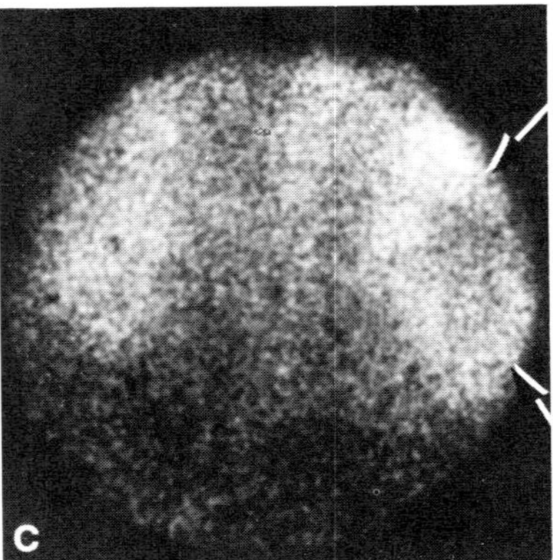

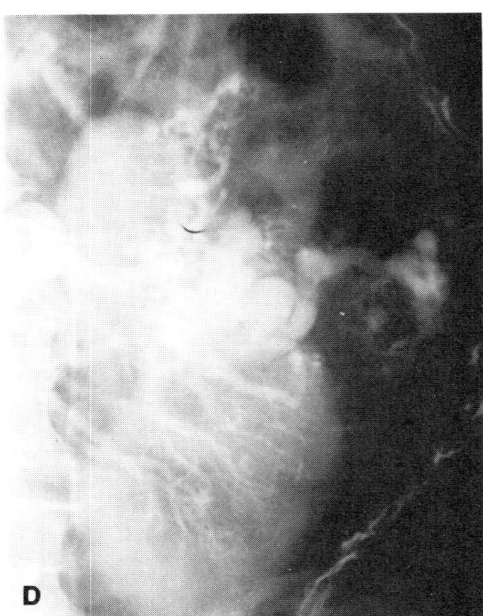

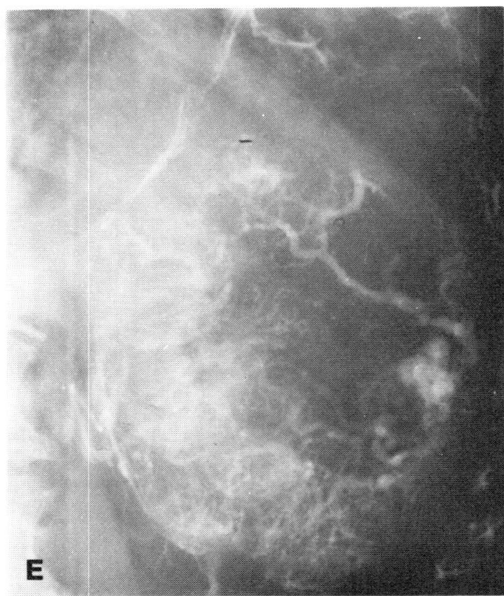

Fig. 3-10. Hypernephroma with central necrosis

A. Static renal scan. [197]Hg scan to investigate a left renal urographic suspect case demonstrates an overall decrease in tubular trapping plus a focal absence in the superolateral half of the left kidney (arrows).

B and C. Renal flow. There is perfusion of the left kidney except for a central defect (arrows). The nonperfused defect is smaller than the static defect, therefore the lesion does perfuse overall but is centrally avascular (arrows).

D. Renal arteriogram. A gross abnormality in vasculature is present with a huge lesion occupying the left superolateral aspect of the kidney and extending well beyond the renal margin.

E. Renal arteriogram with epinephrine. An area of central necrosis is identified.

Fig. 3-12. Normal renal perfusion. Rapid sequential images obtained after the bolus injection of [99mTc] Sn-DTPA. Appearance time and intensity of perfusion should be bilaterally symmetric. The central stripe of activity represents the abdominal aorta.

A. 0–15 sec. Activity is seen in both lung bases, and the abdominal aorta is just becoming visible.

B–D. 3–sec sequential scans (15–24 sec). Appearance times and intensities of renal perfusion are bilaterally symmetric.

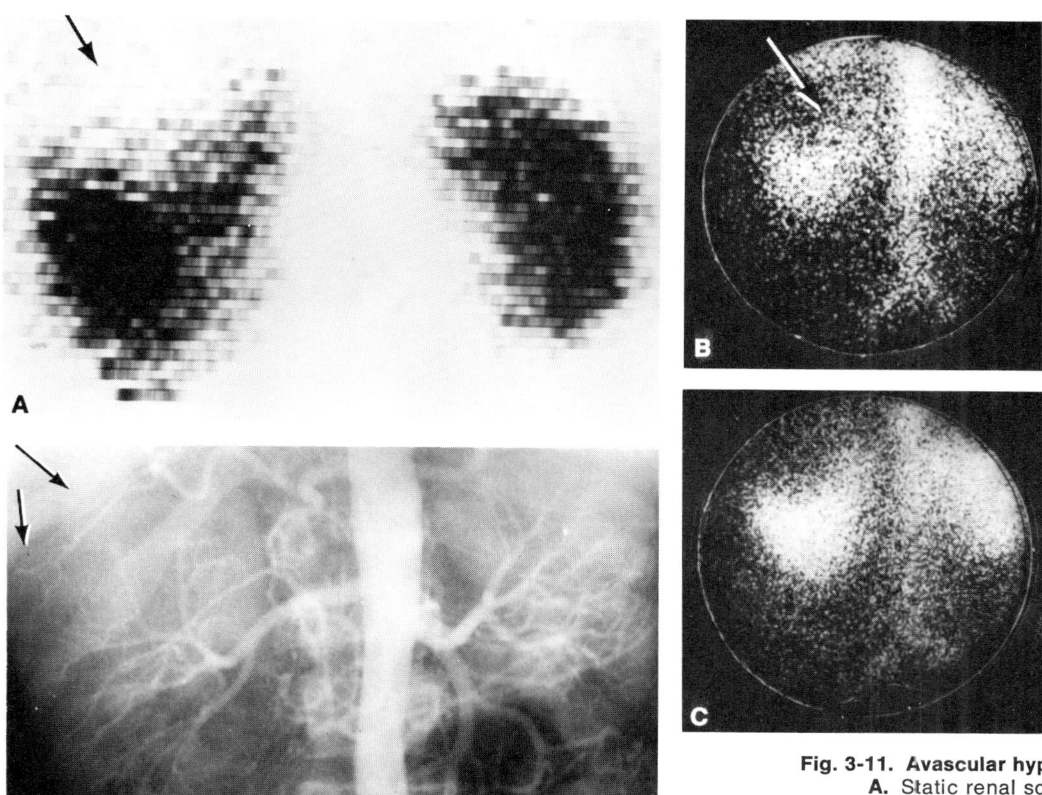

Fig. 3-11. Avascular hypernephroma.

A. Static renal scan. The large trapping defect (arrow) in the right upper pole confirms the urographically suspected lesion.

B and C. Renal flow. There is no evidence of perfusion in the right upper pole (arrow).

D. Renal arteriogram. The right upper pole is decreased in vascularity. The vessels are stretched. Questionable tumor vessels are present (arrows).

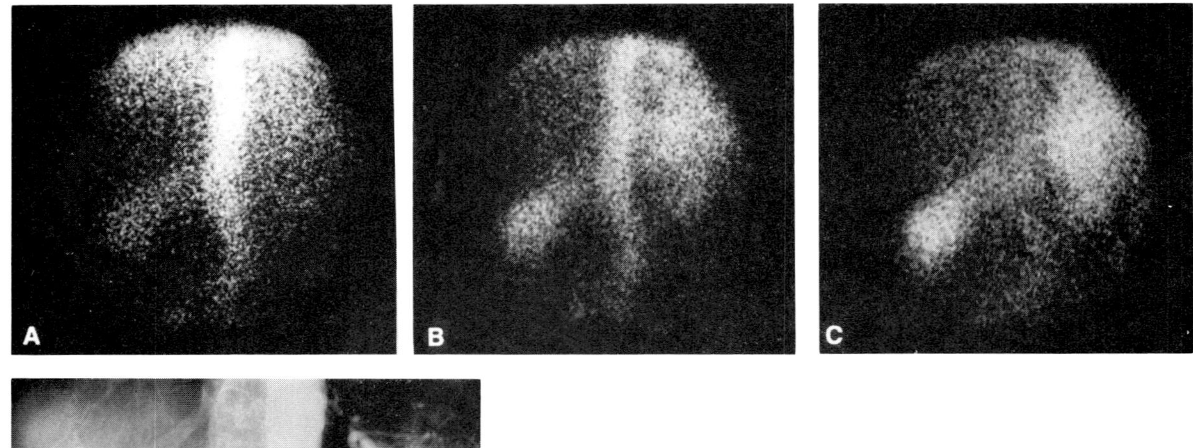

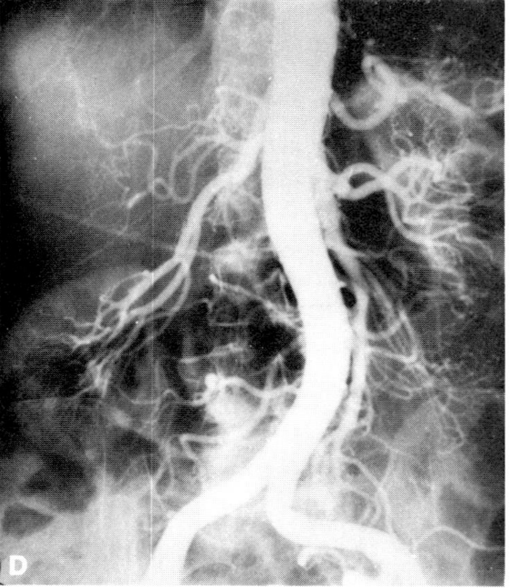

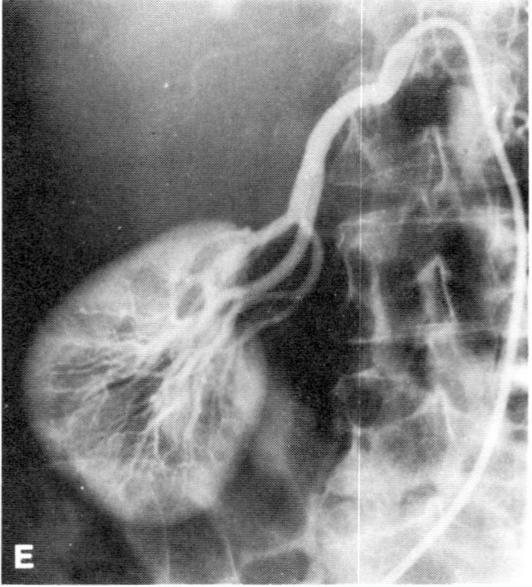

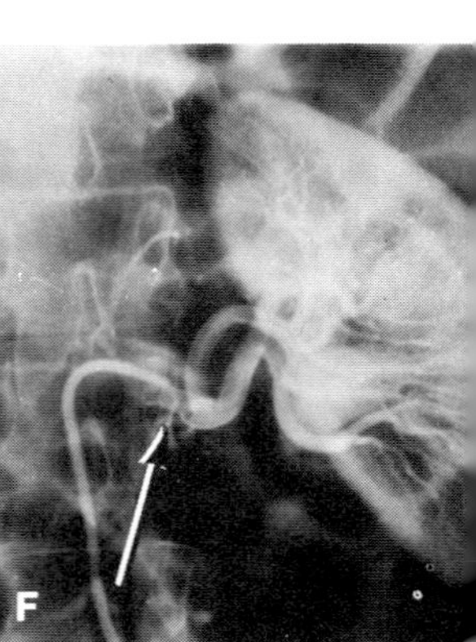

Fig. 3-13. Asymmetric renal perfusion in stenosis of left renal artery (partial)
A. Renal flow, 18–21 sec. Activity is present in the lung bases, abdominal aorta, and right kidney. No definite left kidney outline is present.
B. Renal flow, 21–24 sec. The left kidney is now seen but is less intense than the right.
C. Renal flow, 24–27 sec. The intensity (whiteness) of the right kidney is still greater than that of the left.
D. Renal arteriogram (midstream). Tortuous aorta, low-positioned right kidney
E. Renal arteriogram (right renal selective). Normal right renal artery
F. Renal arteriogram (left renal selective). Partial stenosis of left renal artery (arrow)

Fig. 3-14. Left renal artery stenosis (partial). Minute sequence pyelography. Iodinated ▶
opaque media is introduced as rapid bolus with films exposed at ½, 1, and 3 min after
injection. Normal arteries result in symmetric appearance of opaque in each kidney.
Arterial pathology should result in asymmetry.
A–C. X ray, ½, 1, and 3 min. Films are interpreted as being symmetrically equal.
D. Renal flow, 16–19 sec. Activity is in lung bases and abdominal aorta and is just entering kidneys. The activity of the right exceeds that of the left.
E. Renal flow, 17–21 sec. The right kidney is brighter (whiter) than the left suggesting more intense perfusion.
F. Renal flow, 21–24 sec. The intensity is more symmetric, but the right is still slightly greater.
G. Renal arteriogram, right selective. The right renal artery is normal.
H. Renal arteriogram, left selective. A focal narrowing is present (arrow).

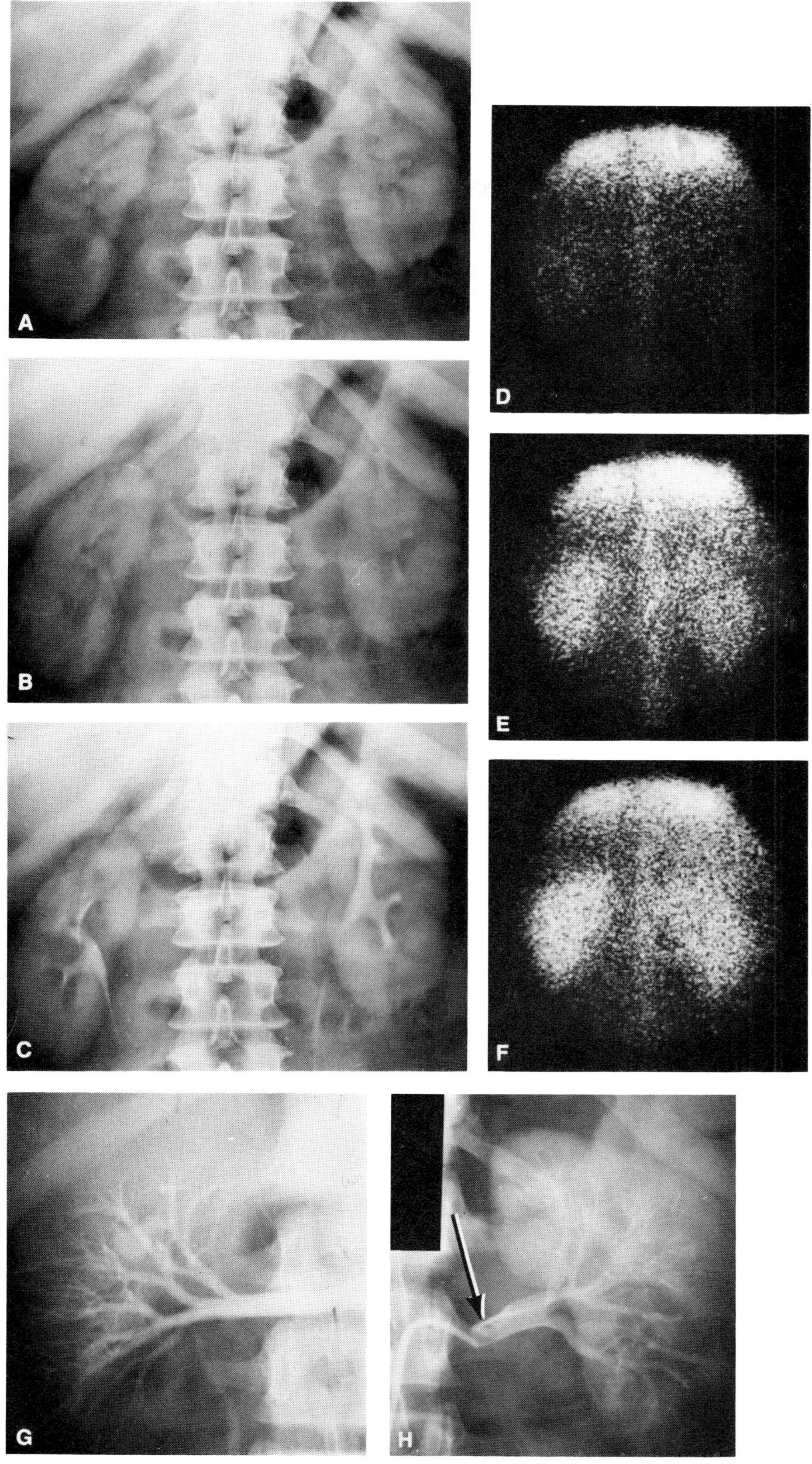

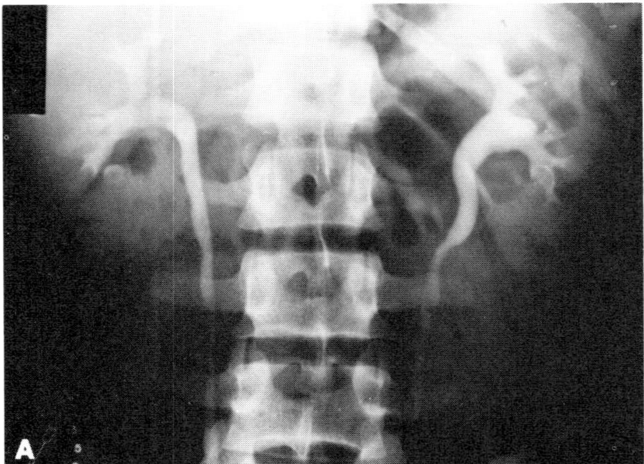
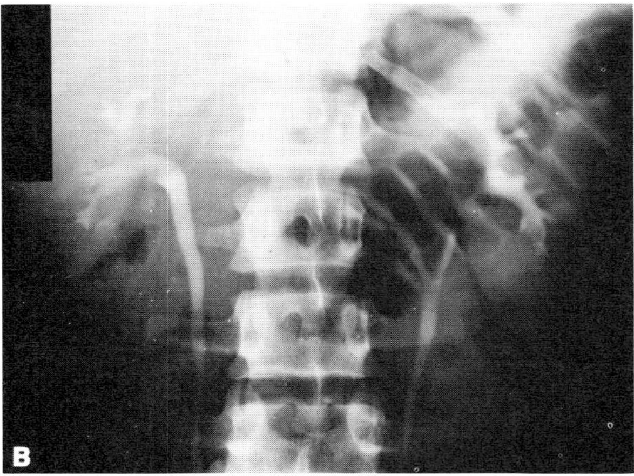
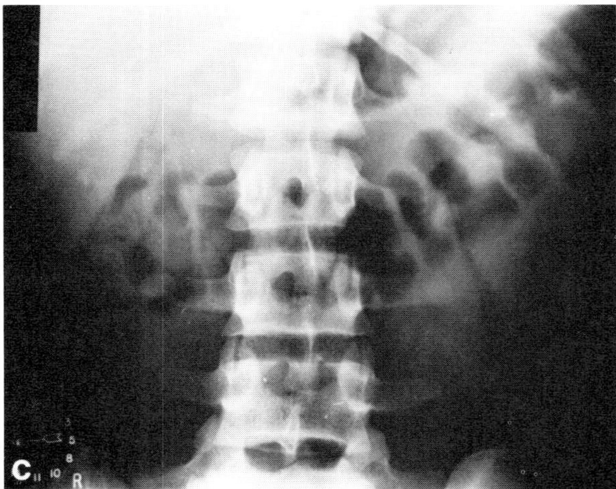

Fig. 3-15. Right renal artery stenosis (partial) and left intrarenal aneurysm. Urea wash-out. A urea infusion is initiated after the kidneys have become opacified during an IV urogram. The urea, as an osmotic diuretic, accelerates the clearance of opaque material from the collecting systems—"wash-out." If there is renal artery disease, the side of pathology will clear more slowly than the normal side.

A–C. X ray, 13, 17, and 20 min. Films identify anticipated symmetric clearance—normal wash-out.

D. Renal flow, 16–19 sec. Activity is just entering the abdominal aorta and right kidney.

E. Renal flow, 19–22 sec. The right kidney is clearly defined. The activity on the left is a combination of spleen and left kidney.

F. Renal flow, 22–25 sec. The left kidney is more easily identified below the spleen. Its intensity is still less than that of the right.

G. Renal arteriogram, right selective. The proximal right renal artery is narrow (arrows).

H. Renal arteriogram, left selective. There is an intrarenal aneurysm (arrow)

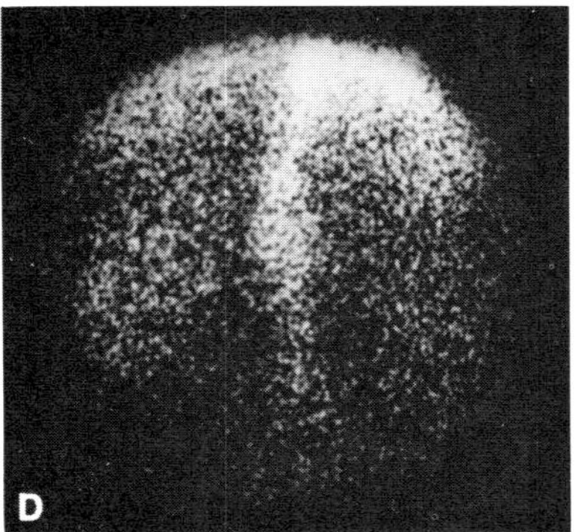
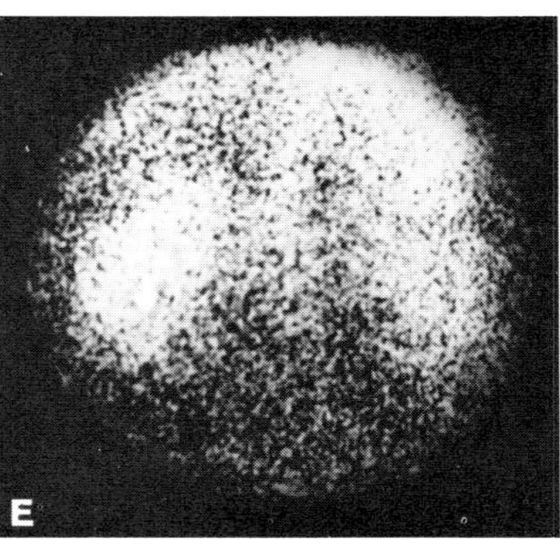
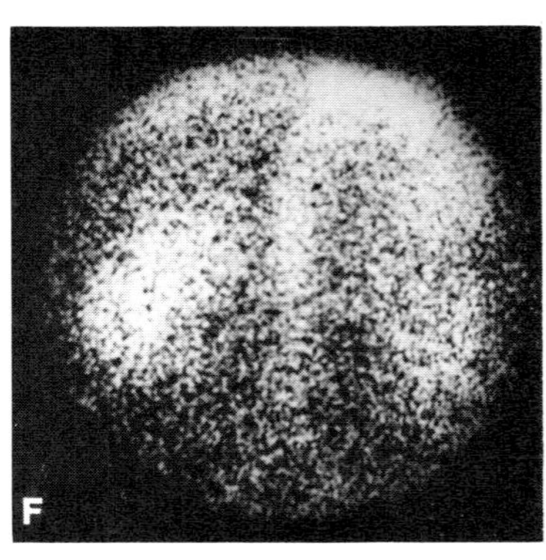

definable. These computer-assisted studies are as yet essentially investigational and unavailable for general use.

Screening techniques employing dynamic imaging of only the perfusion phase have proven sensitive and accurate. Technetium 99m injected IV as a small volume of high concentration, *i.e.,* 10–20 mCi in 0.5–2 cc, produces excellent delineation of the abdominal aorta and kidneys when imaged by the camera sequentially every 3–4 sec through 15–20 sec after the arrival of the bolus into the abdominal aorta. Judgment is based on symmetry of appearance and symmetry of intensity of activity in each kidney. The sequential images are viewed either unassisted, "eye balling," or assisted by computer analysis. When symmetry is preserved, the screening technique is considered negative for unilateral disease (Fig. 3-12). When symmetry is violated, a positive examination is described and confirmation is obtained by contrast angiography (Fig. 3-13). Although the ultimate accuracy and reliability is difficult to assess, our experience suggests that this method of approach is more sensitive than the established roentgen standbys —"minute sequence pyelography" (Fig. 3-14) and "urea wash-out" (Fig. 3-15). Additionally, the "renal isotope angiogram" can be performed in 1–2 min as compared to the 30- to 45-min roentgen procedures. Radiation dose to the patient is considerably less than with the usual 12–15 exposures necessary in the specialized x-ray studies, and the "Excedrin headaches" commonly induced by the osmotic diuretic are also obviated.

When contrasting the morbidity of an anticubital puncture against laboratory procedures that require bilateral ureteral catheterization or sampling of renal venous blood, there is no contest—it's "flow" all the way.

A routine IVP, not the hyped-up hypertensive screening type, is still a companion procedure. Although rarely helpful in identifying major renal artery abnormalities, it does serve to exclude such intrarenal diseases as chronic infection or neoplasm as the mechanism for the hypertension.

Thus, the one–two punch of conventional urography and isotope angiography is recommended. If both are negative, the search at the renal level is over. This modest routine of urography plus a minute under the gamma camera requires courageous rethinking. However, there are many who already decry the use of any screening modalities, particularly in Black males, since the yield is almost negligible and the therapy unaffected by the findings. Unable to abide this totally nihilistic approach, we offer the humble compromise of the isotope angiogram and IVP. When the results are negative, cease and desist. When they are questionable or positive, press onward with a contrast angiogram.

arterial stenosis, occlusion, and infarction

Gross vascular abnormalities such as arterial stenosis or occlusion can be suspected isotopically when combined with both the clinical picture and x-ray urographic findings. The obtained patterns are not specific of themselves. Iron ascorbate or chelating agents tagged with ^{99m}Tc are preferred since both dynamic and static phases can be obtained. In chronic arterial stenosis, similar to that described for

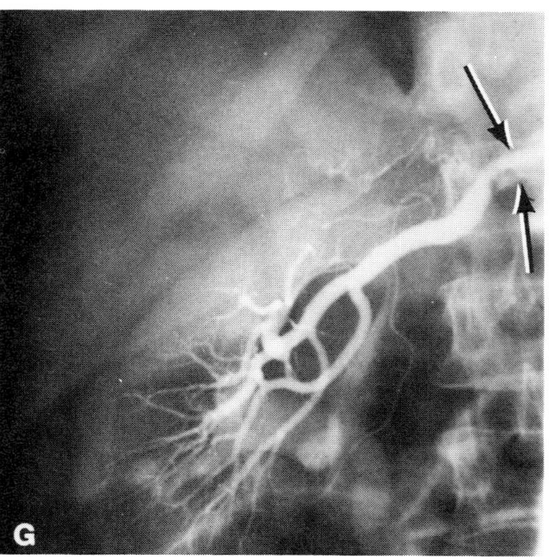

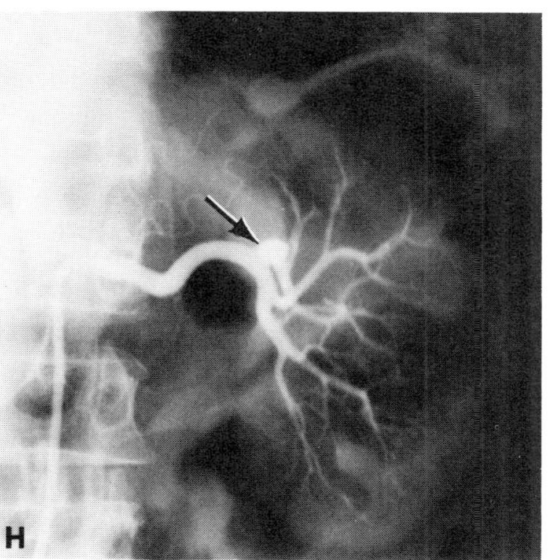

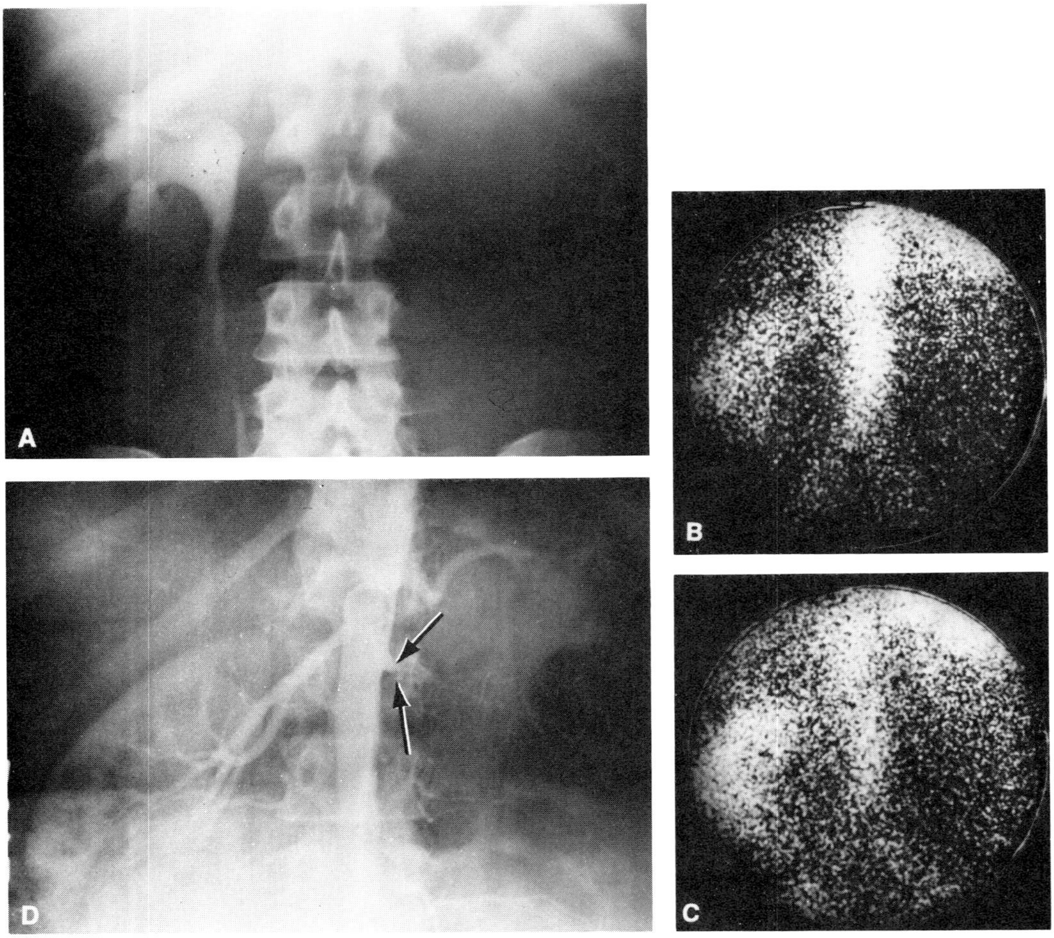

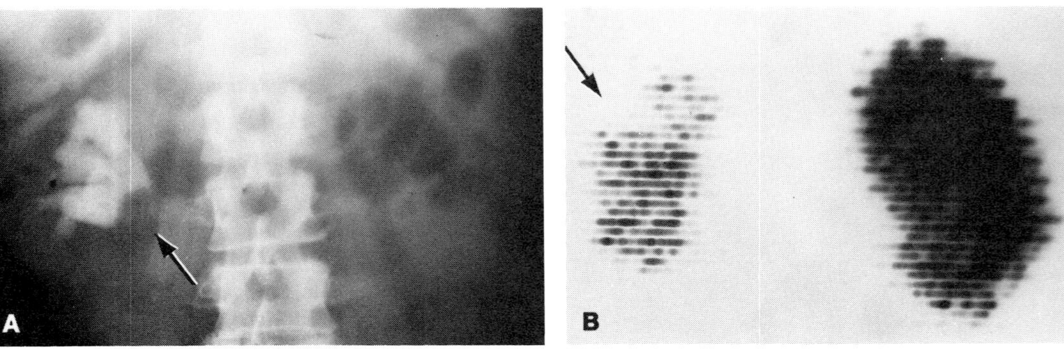

Fig. 3-16. Left renal artery occlusion (complete)
  A. IV urogram. The left kidney fails to opacify.
B and C. Renal flow. Sequential images demonstrate satisfactory perfusion of the right kidney but nonvisualization of the left.
  D. Renal arteriogram. Midstream study documents a complete occlusion of the left renal artery (arrows).

Fig. 3-17. Renal infarction. Diagnosis: Medullary carcinoma (right kidney), atrophic pyelitis (right kidney) and infarct (right kidney)
A. IV urogram. The evacuation film indicates obstruction in the right renal pelvis (arrow). The left kidney has drained.
B. Static renal scan. The left kidney exhibits normal trapping. The small right kidney exhibits poor overall trapping and a "wedge defect" at its superolateral margin (arrow). There is no appreciation of the etiology of the renal pelvis defect.

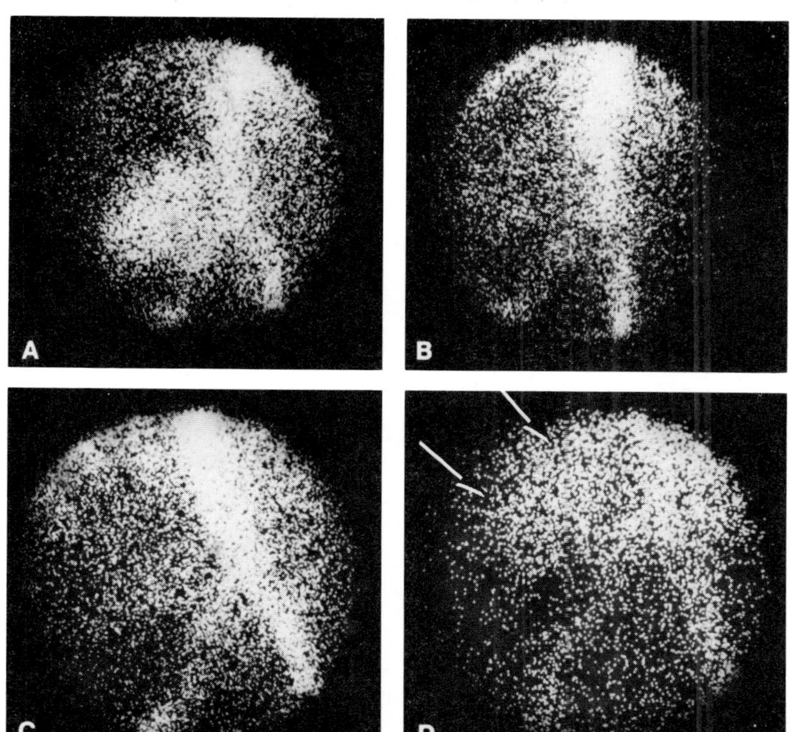

Fig. 3-18. Renal transplant– reversible rejection. Serial sequential renal flow studies with ^{99m}Tc following transplant surgery are performed to monitor renal perfusion. In this case blood flow was normal immediately after the operation, diminished by the 5th postoperative day, and almost completely absent by the 12th, but it exhibited recovery by the 30th after appropriate therapy.
A. 5/12/75. The transplanted kidney is well perfused and lies adjacent to the right iliac artery.
B. 5/17/75. The kidney is barely perceived. The patient was oliguric and febrile.
C. 5/24/75. No essential change. Perfusion is grossly decreased.
D. 6/12/75. Definite improvement in perfusion (arrows)
(Courtesy of B. Shapiro, Albert Einstein Medical Center, Philadelphia, Pa.)

unilateral artery disease, the initial flow pattern identifies diminished concentration on the diseased side. A similar pattern is obtained in disorder that affects the small intrarenal arterial tree. However, with stenosis a delayed scan in 1 hour will demonstrate improved concentration on the affected side, possibly appearing similar to the unaffected kidney's image. This is in contradistinction to the delayed images in which the underlying condition is atrophic pyelonephritis or developmental hypoplasia. In these there may also be initial asymmetry of concentration on the flow, but the concentration does not improve with time and the hour scan reveals no change. Thus, this technique offers an aid in the differential diagnosis between chronic vascular and parenchymal disease. When there is total vascular occlusion from any cause, both the flow and delayed studies will be identical, there being no visualization of the involved side (Fig. 3-16).

Infarctions can be suspected by the presence of single or multiple localized areas of diminished uptake both on flow and static imaging. These lesions can be differentiated from cysts in that the entire kidney exhibits decreased concentration in addition to the focal defect, whereas as simple cysts are characterized by a localized aberration in an otherwise "normal" organ. Infarcts are frequently peripheral in location, and their shape is usually triangular or wedgelike rather than circular or ovoid (Fig. 3-17). Differentiation of an infarct from an abscess may not be possible without clinical information.

acute tubular necrosis and renal transplant

Detection of acute tubular necrosis has recently become a common differential consideration as a consequence of renal transplantation and the need to rapidly differentiate early transplant rejection from acute necrosis. It is essential to determine when posttransplant oliguria or anuria develops, whether or not the cause is immunologic. The nonimmune mechanisms are surgical or mechanical problems such as renal arterial or venous obstruction; urinary tract obstruction; intrinsic abnormalities related to acquisition, transport, or preservation mechanisms, or to all three; and acute tubular necrosis. Multiple techniques are described both with and without computer assistance to differentiate these conditions from rejection. Probably a combination employing various nuclides is best (Figs. 3-18 and 3-19).

It has been established that when a chelating agent is used in acute tubular necrosis, the

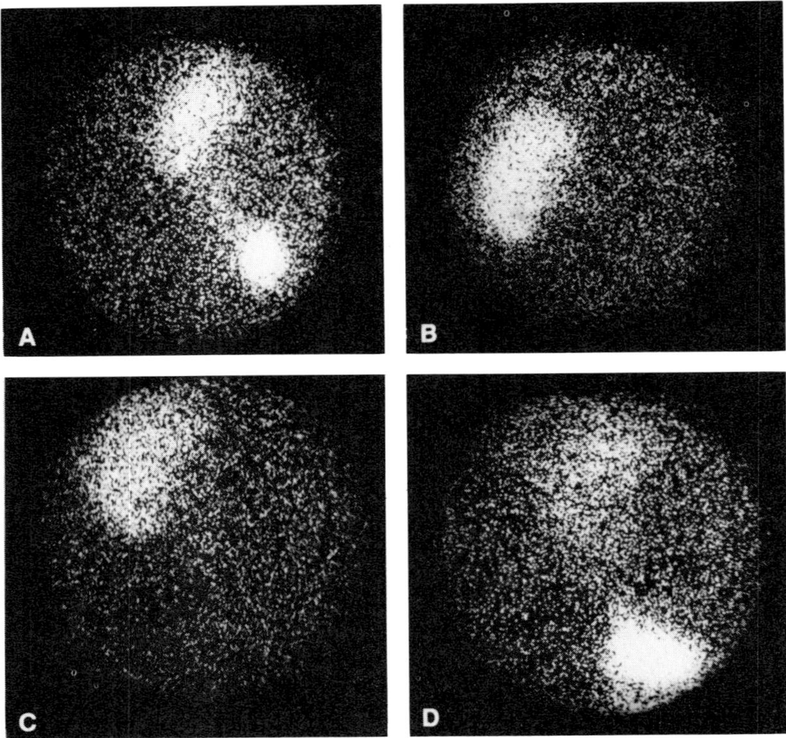

Fig. 3-19. Renal transplant–reversible rejection. Serial static images with ^{131}I sodium iodohippurate following transplant surgery are performed in conjunction with the perfusion studies to monitor the extraction and excretion of the nuclide by the kidney. The images below are from same patient as in **Fig. 3-18.**
A. 5/12/75. 12 min following ^{131}I sodium iodohippurate the tranplanted kidney is easily identified as is its ureter. Activity is present in the bladder.
B. 5/17/75. 12–min scan exhibits a decrease in extraction and no ureteric or bladder activity.
C. 5/24/75. 12–min scan is essentially unchanged. No excretion is exhibited.
D. 6/12/75. 12–min scan again demonstrates extraction and excretion.
(Courtesy of B. Shapiro, Albert Einstein Medical Center, Philadelphia, Pa.)

concentration of activity in that kidney is initially good, but on later images it is significantly impaired. When ^{131}I sodium iodohippurate is employed the exact opposite occurs; the initial concentration is poor, and the delayed scan evidences improved uptake. It has also been observed that when ^{99m}Tc is used in the pertechnetate form, there will be parenchymal retention of the nuclide for as long as 24 hours if tubular necrosis exists.

Obstruction at the arterial level may be suspected by the absolute absence of activity with any nuclide. Lower urinary tract obstruction is identified by the progressively increasing activity with time, employing ^{131}I sodium iodo-hippurate.

It has been suggested that *in vitro* scanning of the donor organ be done to detect intrinsic abnormalities not otherwise suspected. This technique employing ^{99m}Tc was successful in identifying experimentally produced defects and also in identifying lesions in otherwise "normal" donor kidneys subsequently transplanted and subsequently exhibiting failure.

Sequential examinations preoperatively and postoperatively offer the best available method of monitoring transplantation. Etiologic differentiation of postoperative complications is often possible and remedial measures can be instituted far sooner than if only laboratory values of BUN or creatinine are utilized.

inflammatory diseases

The order of merit in the isotopic detection of inflammatory diseases of the kidney is not impressive (Fig. 3-20). As discussed above, abscess, if manifested as a focal defect and associated with a definitive clinical picture, may be confirmed. Otherwise, the pattern of inflammation of any type is that of nonspecific overall decrease or absence of activity with any agent. The chelating compounds are less satisfactory than ^{131}I sodium iodohippurate in detecting the residual activity of severely damaged organs. Delayed scanning is also important if initial studies suggest nonvisualization.

However, a similar nonimpressive rating can be given to routine x-ray procedures, particularly in the identification of acute inflammatory disease. Therefore, employing both the x-ray

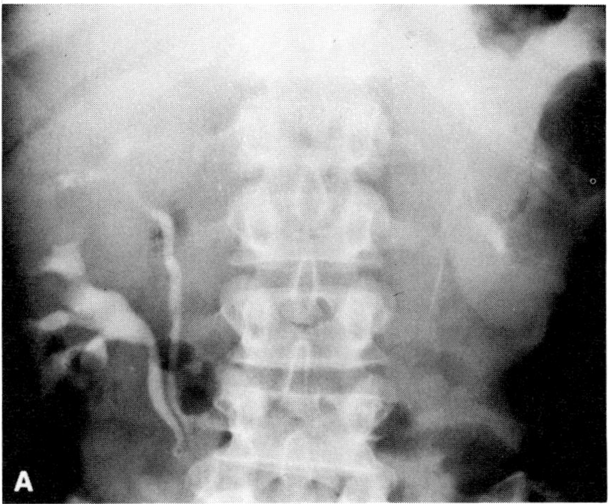

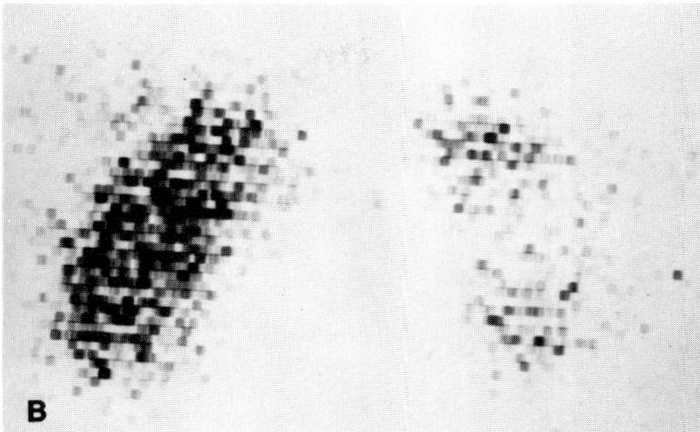

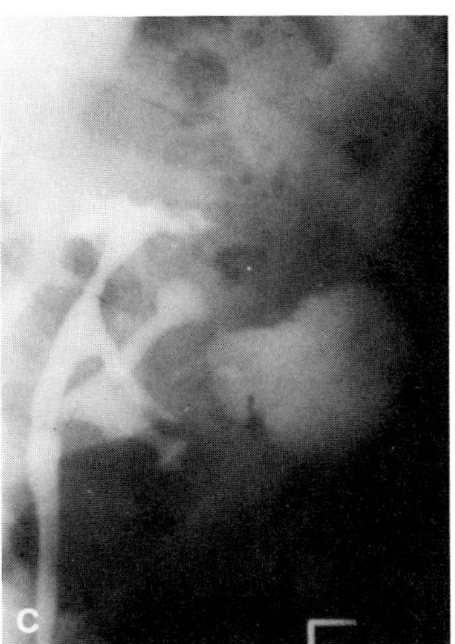

Fig. 3-20. Left renal abscess. Presenting signs were acute onset of left flank pain with associated high spiking temperatures.
A. IV urogram. Right kidney—developmental reduplication
Left kidney—probable space-occupying lesion. The lateral margin bulges, and the calyces are stretched.
B. Static renal scan. Right kidney—homogeneous trapping activity
Left kidney—diffuse loss of activity with an associated large central defect
C. Retrograde pyelogram. Left kidney—large collection of opaque in renal cortex

and isotopic approaches may improve differential potential.

obstruction

Unless urography is contraindicated or there is advanced renal functional impairment, the use of radionuclides offers little or no advantage in the diagnosis of acute mechanical obstruction. However, if either of these two factors exist, diagnosis with ^{131}I sodium iodohippurate or [99m]Tc Sn-DTPA is readily accomplished. Serial images are obtained over a sufficiently prolonged interval. Normally, the initial generalized renal activity obtained in the first 3–5 min is followed by an increased activity in the medullary structures, and the renal pelvis is easily identified.

By 15–20 min the kidney has lost most or all of its activity (Fig. 3-21). In the nonobstructive situation, the ureter is rarely imaged. In obstruction, all sequential events are delayed. If there is severe alteration in function even initial kidney detection may be prolonged and the kidney may never even be visualized urographically. Gradually, the intensity of activity increases, permitting a judgment of obstruction. If ureteric definition develops, the site of embarrassment may be further localized.

There is, however, a very significant role for nuclide investigation in advanced obstruction, not necessarily for diagnosis of the problem, but to evaluate the integrity of residual renal function. Urographic predictability of residual or reversible function in advanced hydronephrosis

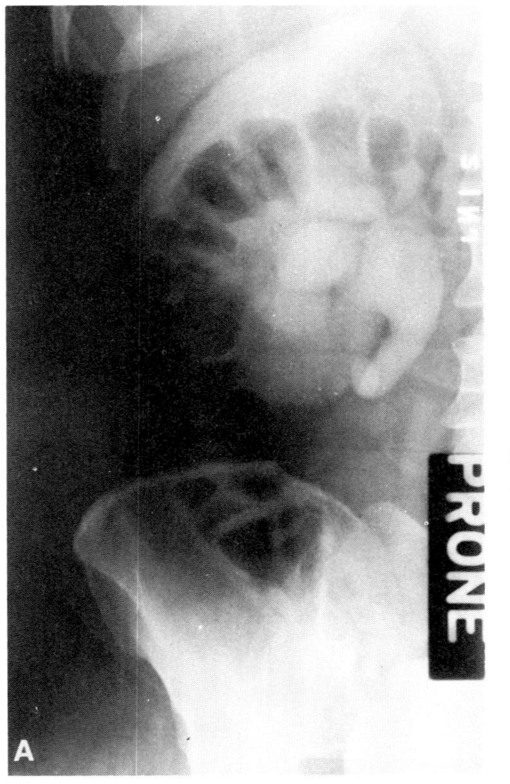

Fig. 3-21. Right proximal ureteric obstruction
A. IV urogram 2-hour prone—moderate pyelocaliectasis and ureterectasis secondary to a high ureteric obstruction
B. Sequential renal scan (^{131}I sodium iodohippurate) 5 min after injection—activity in left kidney, but no definite accumulation in right kidney.
C. 15 min later—left kidney is almost drained, and activity is now present in the right.
D. 1 hour later—left kidney is completely cleared, but there is no change on the right.
E. Renogram (^{131}I sodium iodohippurate). A dual strip chart records the entrance, accumulation, and drainage of activity in the left kidney. No drainage is recorded on the right. (Chart reads from right to left.)

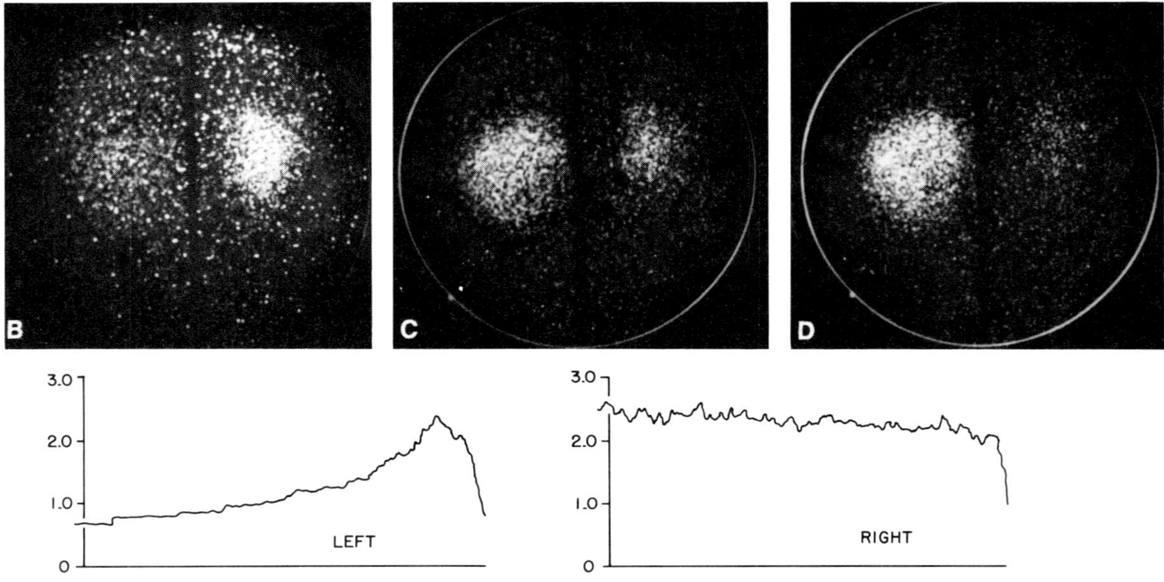

E

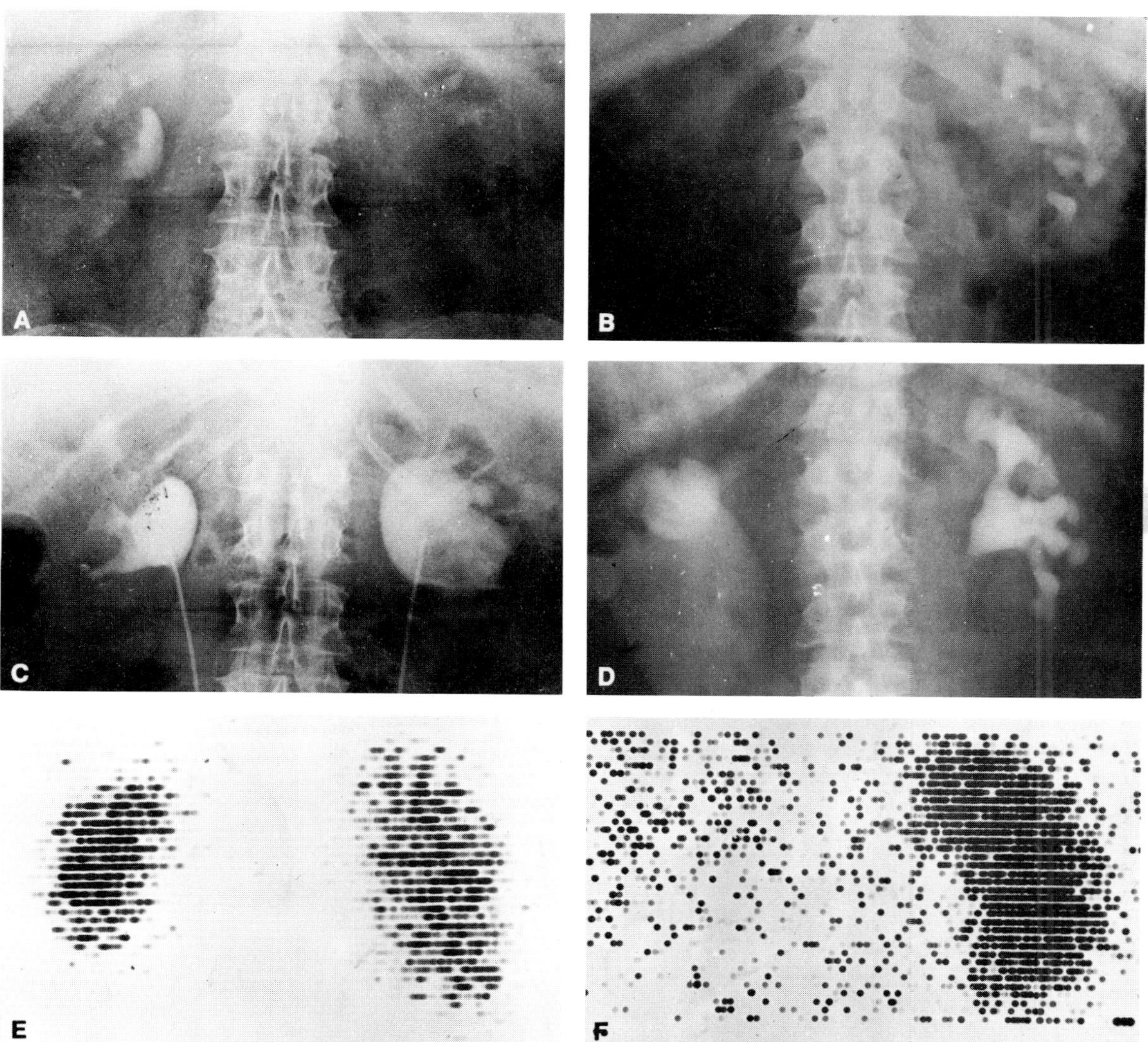

Fig. 3-22. Chronic hydronephrosis with and without residual functional integrity

A and B. IV urogram. Two patients each with chronic inflammatory and obstructive disease. At 5 min there is delayed opacification of the left kidney in **A** and of the right kidney in **B.**

C and D. Retrograde pyelogram. Hydronephrosis—similar but probably more advanced in the right kidney of **D**

E and F. Static renal scans. Marked variation in tubular trapping. The left kidney in **E** retains considerable functional integrity, but there is no observable trapping in the right kidney of **F.**

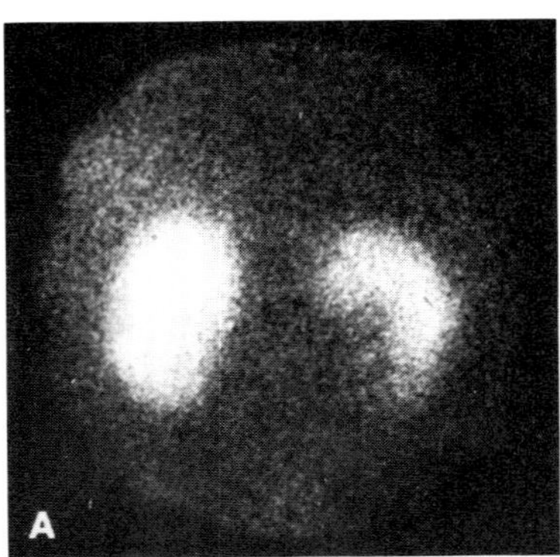
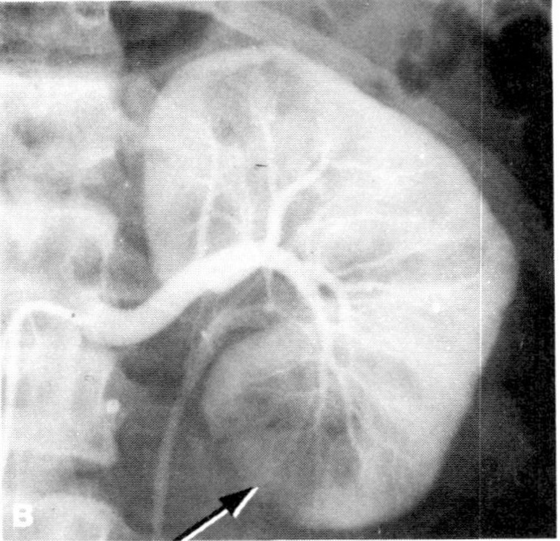

Fig. 3-23. Left renal contusion
A. Renal scan (^{99m}Tc Sn-DTPA). Defect in lower medial aspect of left kidney in patient with left flank pain and hematuria following a fall from a scaffold striking left flank region
B. Renal angiogram. Selective left renal—defect in lower pole compatible with contusion (arrow)
(Courtesy of P. Chase, John F. Kennedy Memorial Hospital, Stratford, N.J.)

Fig. 3-24. Ectopic left kidney
A. IV urogram. The right kidney is normal. There is no evidence of a left kidney in its anticipated location. Residual opaque media from an antecedent myelogram is present in the spinal canal. A questionable opacity is noted just to the left of the midline over the sacrum (arrow).
B. Static renal scan. The left kidney is easily identified in an ectopic position. Its trapping integrity is diminished.

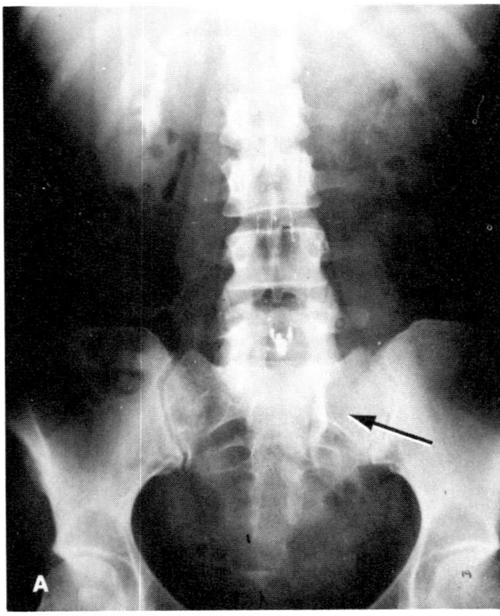
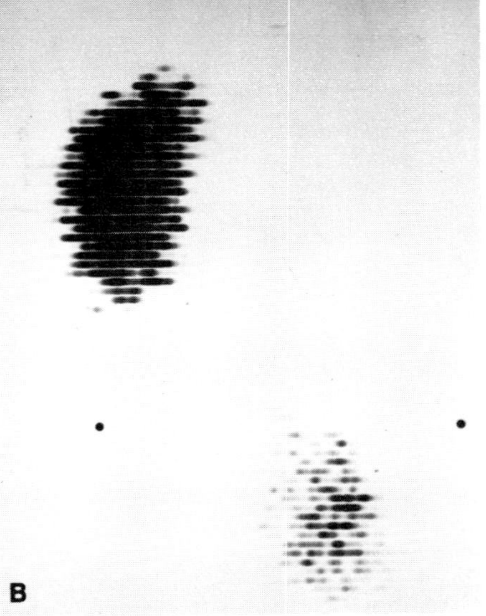

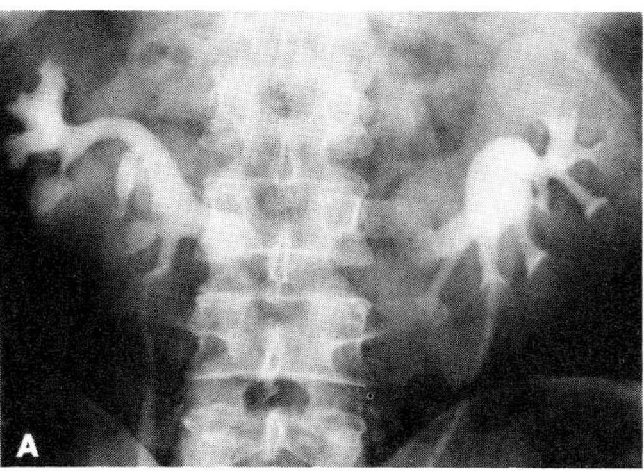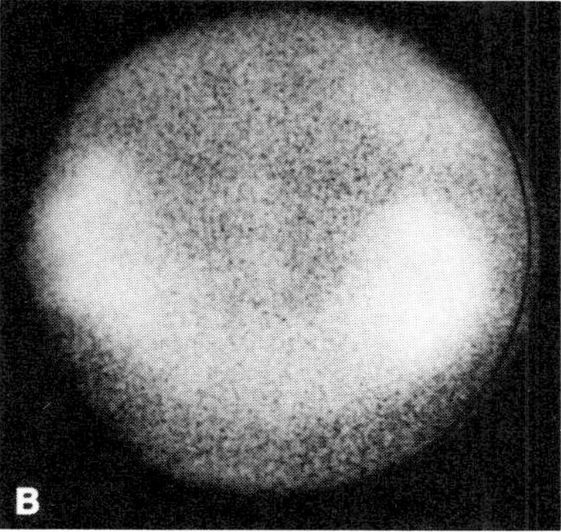

Fig. 3-25. Horseshoe kidneys
A. IV urogram. The kidneys assume an atypical axis. Probable horseshoe kidneys.
B. Sequential renal scan (^{99m}Tc Sn-DTPA). 2 min—activity throughout renal parenchyma identifying bridge at lower poles.

is not particularly accurate. Considerably better integrity than might be suspected from the urogram may be determined with either ^{197}Hg or ^{99m}Tc Sn-DTPA scanning. Occasionally, this demonstration will affect the decision concerning the mode of surgical relief.

There are examples in which the initial intent to perform a nephrectomy because of an apparent gross functional loss on the IVP was modified to a more sparing procedure after nuclide studies validated functional reserve. When a question of choice exists based on whether or not there is sufficient residual function of the organ, scanning may resolve the dilemma (Fig. 3-22).

trauma

The problem of trauma is finally beginning to receive the attention it deserves. Routine rapid screening techniques are being developed to establish the extent of involvement with a maximum of efficiency. This concern obviously extends beyond the skeletal and integumentary systems. However, the ever-present consideration of patient morbidity often deters or defers certain investigations because they are too demanding of time or patient cooperation.

Radionuclide scanning has become a most useful and effective tool in the evaluation of possible renal trauma. If the patient's condition is such that only the most minimal investigation is possible, ^{99m}Tc Sn-DTPA flow can be performed in 1–2 min. Evidence of nonfunction and grossly impaired function is immediately obtained, and appropriate measures can be initiated (Fig. 3-23).

congenital

Detection of variations in position and contour are often accomplished more easily by isotopic than by other methods. Usually the problem is unsuspected, the patient presenting for some other investigation during which the possibility of a congenital anomaly may arise: A kidney is not identified in its usual location or is not found at all; the ectopic organ is obscured by superimposed bone densities of the pelvis or is lost in the pelvic soft tissue shadows or increasing density of the opacifying bladder; a horseshoe organ is suspected (is there a functioning bridge?); an obvious ectopic kidney exists. What is the functional integrity of the anomalous organ? Most of these *whys* are answerable by static imaging. The congenital variant, if present and containing functioning tubular elements, will be both detectable and identifiable by static imaging (Figs. 3-24 and 3-25).

BIBLIOGRAPHY

GENERAL

Blaufox MD, Freeman LM: Radionuclide techniques for the evaluation of diseases of the urinary tract in children. Semin Nucl Med 3:27–53, 1973

Freeman LM: The kidney. In Freeman LM, Johnson PM (eds): Clinical Scintillation Scanning. Hagerstown, Harper & Row, 1969, pp 222–259

Haynie TP et al.: Clinical applications of renal scanning. In Quinn JL (ed): Scintillation Scanning in Clinical Medicine. Philadelphia, WB Saunders, 1964, p 231

James AE Jr, Squire LF: Kidney. In Nuclear Radiology. Philadelphia, WB Saunders, 1973, pp 108–123

MacEwan DW, Rosenthall L: Assessment of excretory urography and radioisotope renal scanning in diseases of the kidneys. Radiology 86:1010–1020, 1966

Park CH et al.: Reliability of renal imaging obtained incidentally in ^{99m}Tc polyphosphate bone scanning. J Nucl Med 14(7):534–536, 1973

Quinn JL, Maynard CD: Renal radioisotope scintiscanning. Radiol Clin North Am 3:65, 1965

Taplin GV et al.: Kidney function and disease. In Blahd WH (ed): Nuclear Medicine. New York, McGraw–Hill, 1971, pp 382–415

Wagner HN Jr et al.: The Kidney. In Wagner HN (ed): Principles of Nuclear Medicine. Philadelphia, WB Saunders, 1968, pp 628–654

PHARMACOLOGY

Brien TG, Fay JA: Letter: ^{51}Cr-EDTA biological half-life as an index of renal function. J Nucl Med 13(5):339, 1972

Farrer PA, Saha GB: ^{111}In-DTPA: A radiopharmaceutical for dynamic renal imaging and measurement of glomerular filtration rate (abstr). J Nucl Med 14(6):394, 1973

Halpern SE et al.: Clinical studies with ^{99m}Tc-penicillamine acetazolamide complex (TPAC): a new renal scanning agent (abstr). J Nucl Med 12(6):361, 1971

Halpern SE et al.: ^{99m}TPAC. A new renal scanning agent. II. Evaluation in humans. J Nucl Med 13(10):723–728, 1972

Haynie TP et al.: Localization in a mouse brain sarcoma and renal clearance in mice of DTPA compounds labeled with ^{99m}Tc, ^{113m}In, and ^{169}Yb (abstr). J Nucl Med 12(6):364–365, 1971

Haynie TP et al.: The kinetics of ^{99m}Tc-, ^{113m}In-, and ^{169}Yb-DTPA compounds in brain sarcoma and kidneys of mice. J Nucl Med 13(3):205–210, 1972

Konikowski T et al.: Renal clearance and brain tumor localization in mice of ^{99m}Tc compounds of (Sn) DTPA, (iron-ascorbic acid) DTPA, and iron-ascorbic acid. J Nucl Med 13(11):834–842, 1972

Konikowski T et al.: An intercomparison of radiopharmaceutical kidney kinetics in the mouse (abstr). J Nucl Med 14(6):417, 1973

Lebowitz E et al.: Development of ^{99m}Tc-mannitol for renal visualization (abstr). J Nucl Med 13(10):786, 1972

Lin MS et al.: Renal imaging in humans with the technetium-labeled polypeptide caseidin. J Nucl Med 13(7):517–521, 1972

Robbins PJ, Fortman DL: ^{123}I-hippuran for renal function studies—preparation from available ^{123}I (abstr). J Nucl Med 12(6):459, 1971

Winchell HS et al.: Localization of polypeptide caseidin in the renal cortex: a new radioisotope carrier for renal studies. J Nucl Med 12(10):678–682, 1971

Winston MA et al.: A critical evaluation of ^{99m}Tc-Fe-ascorbic acid complex as a renal scanning agent. J Nucl Med 12(4):171–175, 1971

SPACE-OCCUPYING LESIONS

Antoniades J et al.: Gallium 67 scanning in patients with renal cell carcinoma. J Urol 109:564–566, 1973

Black MB et al.: Double isotope scintiphotography for differentiating between renal cysts and renal tumors. J Urol 98:728–734, 1968

Braunstein P, Herinberg JG: "Hot" renal pseudotumors (abstr). J Nucl Med 12(6):421, 1971

Caplan GE et al.: The "hot" renal tumor. Radiology 91:991–992, 1968

Leitner WA et al.: Limitations of arteriography in renal mass evaluation. Arch Intern Med 130:868–873, 1972

Meringoff BN: Partial renal infarct simulating a collecting system tumor. J Nucl Med 13:125–126, 1972

Morales J: Space-occupying lesions of the kidney. Semin Nucl Med 4(2):133–149, 1974

Samuels LD: Scans in children with renal tumors. J Urol 127:132, 1972

Stewart BH et al.: Role of scintillation scanning in diagnosis of renal tumors. J Urol 87:782, 1962

Tully RJ et al.: Renal scan prior to renal biopsy—a method of renal localization. J Nucl Med 13:544–547, 1972

HYPERTENSION

Chervu LR et al.: Determination of plasma renin activity by radioimmunoassay: comparison of results from two commercial kits with bioassay. J Nucl Med 13(11):806–810, 1972

Freeman LM et al.: Rapid, sequential renal blood flow scintiphotography. Radiology 92:918–923, 1969

Halko A et al.: Computer-aided statistical analysis of the scintillation camera ^{131}I-hippuran renogram. J Nucl Med 14(5):253–264, 1973

Johnson PM et al.: Quantitative dynamic renal imaging as a screening test for potentially curable hypertension (abstr). J Nucl Med 14(6):628, 1973

Keane JM, Schlegel JV: The use of a scintillation camera system for screening of hypertensive patients. J Urol 108:12–14, 1972

Koenigsberg IN et al.: Detection of asymmetrical renal perfusion by radiopertechnetate angiography (abstr). J Nucl Med 15(6):507, 1974

Rosenthall L: Radiopertechnetate renography with the gamma ray scintillation camera. Can Med Assoc J 105:467–471, 1971

Rosenthall L: Radiotechnetium renography and serial radiohippurate imaging for screening renovascular hypertension. Semin Nucl Med 4(2):97–116, 1974

Secker–Walker RH: Practical applications of computer-assisted renography (abstr). J Nucl Med 12(6):392, 1971

Secker–Walker RH et al.: Clinical applications of computer-assisted renography. J Nucl Med 13(4):235–248, 1972

Shtasel P: Renal isotope angiography as a screening procedure for renal artery hypertension (abstr). J Nucl Med 14(6):451, 1973

Taplin GV et al.: The quantitative radiorenogram for total and differential renal blood flow measurement. J Nucl Med 4:409, 1963

Wellman HN et al: Dynamic quantitative renal imaging with ^{123}I-hippuran—A possible salvation of renogram (abstr). J Nucl Med 12(6):405, 1971

CHRONIC DISEASES AND INFECTION

Bell EG et al.: Use of ^{99m}Tc-iron ascorbate complex in the evaluation of diffuse renal parenchymal disease (abstr). J Nucl Med 12(6):339, 1971

Blatt CJ et al.: Radionuclide imaging of the kidney in tuberous sclerosis. J Nucl Med 15(8):699–702, 1974

Blaufox MD et al.: Radionuclide scintigraphy for detection of vesicoureteral reflux in children. J Pediatr 79:239–246, 1971

Braunstein P et al.: Scintiscan evaluation of prominent renal columns. Radiology 104:103–106, 1972

Conway JJ et al.: Detection of vesicoureteral reflux with radionuclide cystography. Am J Roentgenol Radium Ther Nucl Med 115:720–727, 1972

Conway JJ et al.: Direct and indirect radionuclide cystography. Semin Nucl Med 4(2):197–211, 1974

Corriere JN et al.: Urinary particle scan: a tracer technique for the study of renal infection in patients with ureterovesical reflux (abstr). J Nucl Med 11:311, 1970

Hopkins JD, Staab EV: ^{131}I-hippuran evaluation of potential renal function in acute renal failure (abstr). J Nucl Med 12(6):439, 1971

Isenstark JL et al.: Scintillation scan techniques in the evaluation of renal disease. In Quinn JL (ed): Scintillation Scanning in Clinical Medicine. Philadelphia, WB Saunders, 1964, p 245

Reba RC et al.: Radiolabeled chelates for visualization of kidney function and structure with emphasis on their use in renal insufficiency. Semin Nucl Med 4(2):151–168, 1974

Rosenthall L: Ortho-Iodohippurate-I[131] kidney scanning in renal failure. Radiology 87:298–303, 1966

Schulman N, Johnson PM: Scintillation imaging in generalized and localized radiation nephritis. Radiology 109:639–642, 1973

Staab EV et al.: The use of radionuclide studies in the prediction of function in renal failure. Radiology 106:141–146, 1973

Wagner MS et al.: ^{99m}Tc-DTPA: A comparison with ^{131}I-hippuran for gamma camera studies and ^{125}I-iothalamate clearances in chronic renal disease (abstr). J Nucl Med 12(6):470, 1971

OBSTRUCTION AND TRAUMA

Elkin M et al.: Roentgenologic evaluation of renal trauma with emphasis on renal angiography. Am J Roentgenol Radium Ther Nucl Med 98:1–26, 1966

Freeman LM: Scintigraphic studies of renal trauma and infarction. In Blaufox MD, Furk–Brentano JL (eds): Nephrology. New York, Grune & Stratton, 1972, p 281

Freeman LM et al.: The contribution of renal scanning in the evaluation of renal trauma. Radiology 86:1021–1029, 1966

Fujita K et al.: Correlation between radioisotope renographic findings and results after relief of ureteral obstruction. J Urol 107:23–25, 1972

Johnston GS, Murphy GP: The effect of acute and chronic ureteral occlusion upon renal handling of Hg[203] chlormerodrin. Am J Roentgenol Radium Ther Nucl Med 98:163–171, 1966

Kazmin MH et al.: Renal scan: the test of choice in renal trauma. J Urol 97:189–195, 1967

Kirchner PT et al.: Diagnosis of obstructive uropathy with serial Anger camera images (abstr). J Nucl Med 12(6):444, 1971

Koenigsberg IN et al.: Traumatic injuries of the renal vasculature and parenchyma. Semin Nucl Med 4(2):117–132, 1974

Raynaud C et al.: Preoperative identification of a hydronephrotic sac with sequential ^{99m}Tc-DTPA imaging: case report. J Urol 109:1033–1034, 1973

TRANSPLANT

Cantor RE et al.: Hippuran and pertechnetate evaluation of renal transplants using a scoring index (abstr). J Nucl Med 14(6):384, 1973

Conway JJ et al.: In vitro evaluation of transplant organs with radionuclide angiography during perfusion preservation (abstr). J Nucl Med 13(6):422, 1972

Davies T, Hayes M: Rapid evaluation of renal transplant function (abstr). J Nucl Med 13(11):866, 1972

Freedman G et al.: "Non-perfused" renal transplant. J Nucl Med 14(6): 395, 1973

Hayes M, Taplin GV: Comparison of ^{131}I-hippurate and ^{99m}Tc-chelates for monitoring renal homotransplant function (abstr). J Nucl Med 12(6):437, 1971

Hor G et al.: Radionuclides in renal transplantation. J Nucl Med 13(11):795–800, 1972

Rosenthall L et al.: Diagnostic applications of radiopertechnetate and radiohippurate imaging in post-renal transplant complications. Radiology 111:347–358, 1974

Weiss ER et al.: Ureteral kinking and hydronephrosis in a transplanted kidney mimicking the rejection phenomenon. J Nucl Med 12(1):43–46, 1971

Winston MA et al.: Use of ^{131}I-fibrinogen for detecting renal transplant rejection (abstr). J Nucl Med 12(6):407, 1971

MISCELLANEOUS

Blum, AS, Poppiti RJ: Detailed kidney structure with [99m]Tc Fe and pinhole anger camera (abstr). J Nucl Med 12(6):418, 1971

McKusick KA et al.: An interesting artifact in radionuclide imaging of the kidneys. J Nucl Med 14(2):113–114, 1973

Pritchard JH et al.: Radioisotope and ultrasonic imaging: a combined approach for better evaluation of renal masses (abstr). J Nucl Med 14(6):442, 1973

Torizuka K et al.: Study of intrarenal dynamic processes

with the scintillation camera (abstr). J Nucl Med 13(6):472, 1972

Tully RS et al.: Renal scan prior to renal biopsy—a method of renal localization. J Nucl Med 13(7):544–547, 1972

Wagner MS et al.: Gamma camera studies after percutaneous renal biopsy in man (abstr). J Nucl Med 12(6):470, 1971

It was a joyous day for the embattled medical masses when reliable diagnostic nuclear techniques proved capable of identifying the presence or absence of central nervous system (CNS) pathology. No other system presented a more difficult challenge to early detection of disease, and the differential diagnosis between organic and emotional etiologies was a constant anxiety. None of the usual, comfortable, atraumatic, or dependable screening modalities were available. No routine laboratory techniques existed. The spinal tap was reserved for fairly definitive evidence of disease, and even then the technical demands inherent in its performance excluded it from routine or ambulatory use. X ray, the second-line court of appeals, offered little more than the laboratory. Roentgen examination of the bony vault, the skull, had to suffice for indirect evidence of intracranial disease, and the yield, particularly in early or acute disease, was dismally low. The more-definitive procedures, *e.g.,* contrast angiography and pneumoencephalography, were reserved for the obvious problem or for the differential diagnosis of established organic disease.

Electroencephalography was a relatively unpopular procedure. Whether or not such a judgment was valid or warranted need not be debated—it failed in the role of a routine screening study.

Thus, the clinician was left to his history and his findings with the percussion hammer, straight pin, and tuning fork to evaluate what is, if not

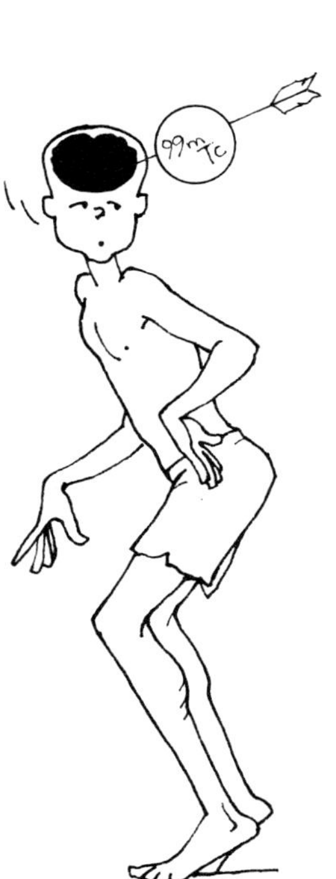

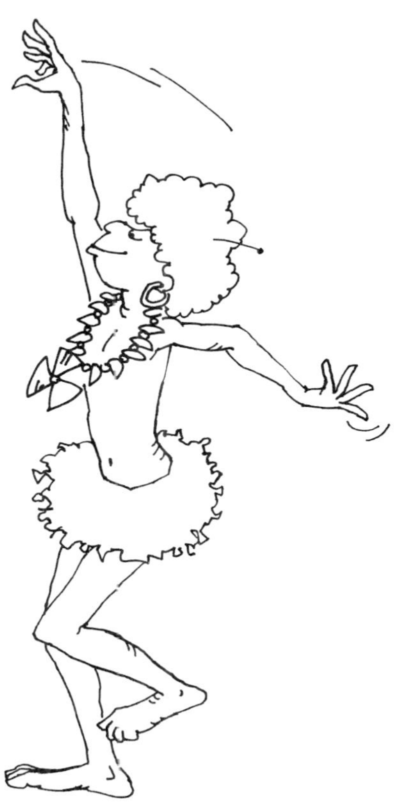

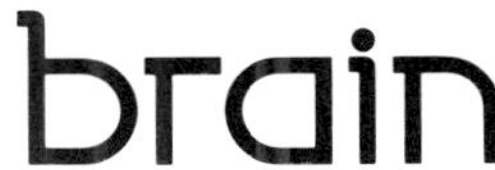

chapter 4

brain

the commonest, at least one of the commonest presenting complaints in medicine—headache. How serious was the symptom? (Tomes had been written on the evaluation of this complaint.) Were there any corroborative physical findings? (Did their absence rule against organic disease?) Should the patient be sent for x rays? (Less than 1% of all skull x rays, including those done for trauma, are positive.) Do the findings warrant consultation with the neurologist (" Why do I have to see a specialist for just a headache?''), an EEG, a spinal tap?

Into the breech marched the intrepid nuclear medicine man. Initial skirmishes were recorded as early as 1948 with the use of diiodofluorescein. The recognition of ^{131}I tagged to serum albumin as a reasonable agent in 1951 increased the activity. But it was not until approximately 1960, armed with both the proper instrument, a commercially available and reliable rectilinear scanner, and the proper nuclide, [203]Hg chlormerodrin (Neohydrin), that the battle was fully engaged. This was indeed the monumental moment. For the first time, a reasonable screening procedure was available. No invasive techniques were necessary since the agent was introduced by an IV route. No morbidity was to be anticipated. Time was not a critical factor since in most cases answers were available on the day of examination. Hospitalization was not a necessary requirement. And lastly, an order of merit of its ability to separate organic from inorganic disease exceeded 90%.

Initially, just this gross distinction of yes or no was like manna from heaven. A methodology was finally available which exhibited pathology as an area of increased activity. Often only the lesion appeared with little or no other identifiable landmarks, necessitating sketching in the outline of the head. When a perimeter of activity could be imaged, it represented distribution of radionuclide in the soft tissues of the scalp and musculature, the osseous vault, and the intracranial and extracranial blood vessels. Intracranial accumulation usually equalled pathology, with interpretation being based on the recognition of distribution patterns as being definitely positive, definitely negative, or questionable.

But man's joys and initial enthusiasms are fickle and transient. This simplistic evaluation was acceptable for only a short period. As experience increased and newer nuclides became available (particularly ^{99m}Tc in 1964) and as newer commercial imaging devices

permitted greater flexibility of picture taking (particularly the Anger Camera), interpretation became more sophisticated. It is now presumed that the detection of a definitely positive study will also suggest its likeliest cause.

The above remarks apply primarily to what has been commonly accepted as the "brain scan." Also available as a diagnostic tool is the imaging of the cerebrospinal fluid (CSF) pathways. Appropriate radiopharmaceuticals are introduced into the lumbar subarachnoid space to obtain serial images of their movement with the CSF through the basilar cisterns and ultimately over the cerebral hemispheres, where they are absorbed by the arachnoid granulations. Initially the primary indication for CSF imaging was identification of CSF fistulas and localization of sites of injury. However, considerable interest in the problems of communicating hydrocephalus have developed with the availability of a reasonably simple technique, and more and more indications for its use are being advanced. Specific imaging of the ventricles is also possible by direct instillation of nuclide into those structures.

WHAT

brain

Table 4-2 lists the choices available. Certainly ^{99m}Tc, either in the pertechnetate form or compounded as a chelate, is the most widely used agent for conventional brain scanning. Its disadvantage is that, since it is not physiologically specific to any brain process, it accumulates in both the salivary glands and choroid plexuses. Unfortunately, the criticism of nonspecificity must also be leveled at all currently employed nuclides. But be of good cheer—the pharmacologist is here—and the problem can be obviated, for the most part, by premedication with atropine to suppress salivary gland and mucosal uptake (atropine is not routinely employed since salivary accumulation is only troublesome if vertex views are obtained) and with potassium perchlorate to inhibit choroid plexus uptake. The perchlorate ion ($ClO_4{}^-$) is an analogue of both pertechnetate ($TcO_4{}^-$) and iodide (I^-) and decreases accumulation by competitive inhibition not only in the plexus but also in the thyroid. These nuisances can be further avoided by using technetium in its chelated forms, ^{99m}Tc-DTPA or ^{99m}Tc-glucoheptonate. Other radiopharmaceuticals such as ^{113m}In-DTPA or ^{169}Yb-DTPA have been considered, but none have proven superior to the technetium compounds and all are more expensive to produce.

cisternography

Iodinated I 131 serum albumin is the most commonly employed agent, but ^{99m}Tc albumin, ^{111}In-DTPA, and ^{169}Yb-DTPA also have characteristics to recommend them. Choice and decision may be based on the suspected problem. The examinations must be extended through 48 hours if the provisional diagnosis is communicating hydrocephalus, and in these cases the short-lived ^{99m}Tc agents are disadvantageous. On the other hand, when it is anticipated that the study can be completed on the same day (as, for example, when looking for CSF leaks) the short-lived agents are preferred since larger doses can be employed and these in turn improve image quality.

HOW

brain

The mechanism whereby the imaging of the brain, following the administration of a radionuclide will result in different picture patterns under different conditions is still incompletely understood. The mechanism to explain the active transport of materials from the blood to the extracellular fluid have been elaborated, but not at the brain level, where other as yet undeciphered forces maintain the extracellular fluid content in an ultrastable state. This mechanism has been fancifully described as the "brain–blood barrier." In the normal state the image pattern of the brain following the administration of a nuclide identifies that material to be confined to the intracerebral and extracerebral blood vessels, musculature, calvarium, and—probably the greatest accumulation—in the intracellular spaces of the scalp. A perimeter of increased activity thus picture frames the brain. It does not enter the brain substance. However, with disease the barrier is breeched and intracranial accumulations of nuclide occur. Just as the barrier in the normal state is not completely understood, the explanation of its violation is also unclear. Hypotheses have been advanced blaming increased vascularity,

abnormal vascular permeability, reactive edema, and altered cellular metabolism, but none have been completely accepted. Brain scanning is feasible because "simple" diffusion occurs. There is some evidence that selective uptake by tumor cells does take place, but the specificity is minimal and abnormal activity must still be considered to be accumulation primarily in extracellular fluids and small vessels. Thus, except for the relatively uncommon congenital cysts of children, the occasional acquired cysts of the adult, and the single reported case of a teratoma, all of which produce negative defects, brain disease is imaged as a positive lesion. In other words, abnormality is identified as increased activity: white on Polaroid, black on x-ray film. It is the pattern of this increased activity that is translated into a differential judgment. The pattern is analyzed as to the appearance time of activity, intensity, location, shape, size, and number. The age of the patient and all other pertinent clinical data are integrated. It is from these that decisions are made.

The radionuclides are administered IV except on those rare occasions when oral or IM routes are required. When there is available instrumentation it has now been almost universally accepted that a flow study should be an integral part of the examination. The flow or dynamic study is simply the rapid sequential imaging of the isotope transport through the head. A camera is necessary since pictures are obtained every 2–4 sec from the appearance time of activity in the carotid arteries through the cerebral venous phase for an elapsed time of perhaps 15–20 sec. Opinion is unsettled as to whether the anterior, posterior or vertex view offers the best routine yield of cerebral blood flow data. The vertex projection requires the patient to assume a somewhat more difficult position, and if pertechnetate is the scanning nuclide, premedication with atropine is desirable since in this view accumulation in the salivary glands degrades the image detail. However, most opinion is in agreement that the flow image aids in the diagnosis (Fig. 4-1).

Patient instruction should suggest that the actual performance time of the study is 30 min. The flow requires only 1–2 min, the static views approximately 5 min for each of 4 or 5 images (Fig. 4-2). However, the overall time is variable. Unless potassium perchlorate is administered IV, as has recently been advocated, there should be an average of at least 30 min delay between its administration and the initiation of static

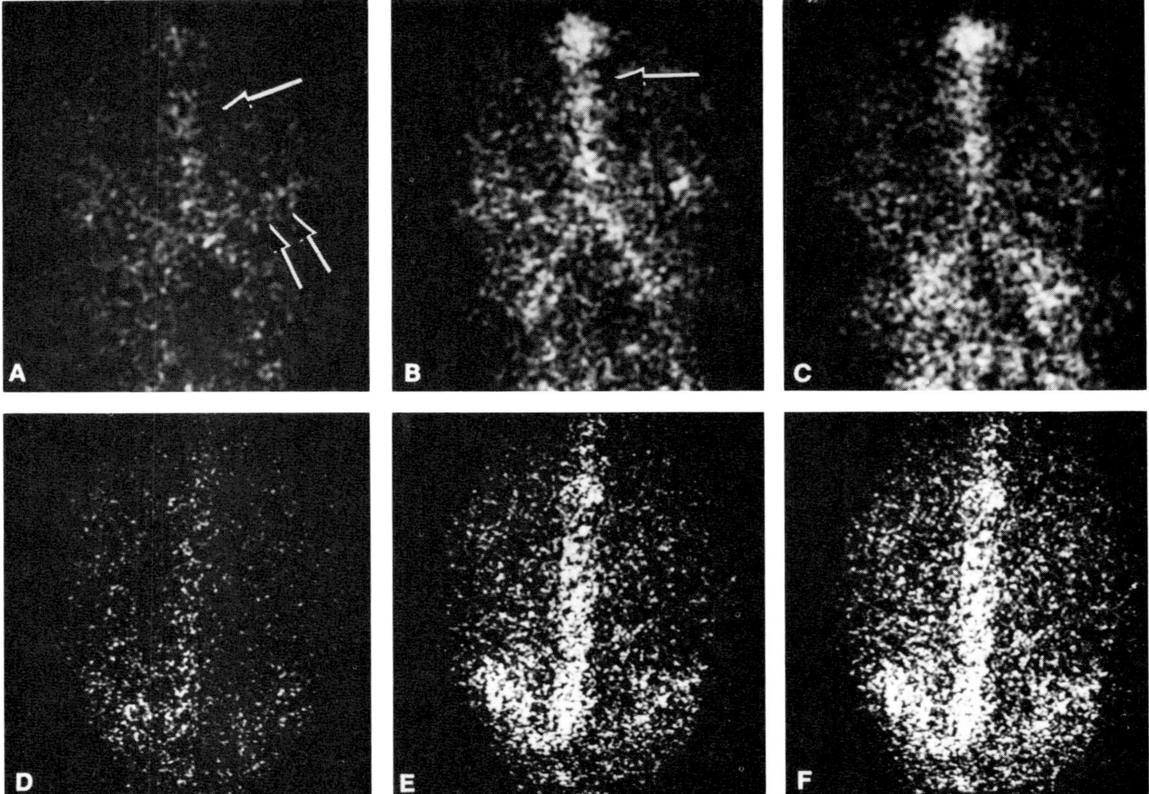

Fig. 4-1. Normal cerebral flow. Rapid sequential scans are obtained following the IV injection of a suitable nuclide. Evaluation is primarily dependent on the symmetry of perfusion. The determination extends from the early arterial through the venous phase.

   A. Anterior view, 0–18 sec. Earliest appearance and definition of the carotid arteries, the anterior cerebral (single arrow) and each middle cerebral artery (double arrow)
   B. Anterior view, 21–24 sec. Capillary-venous phase with prominence of the sagittal sinuses (arrow)
   C. Anterior view, 24–30 sec. Late venous phase with clearing of the hemispheral activity
D–F. Vertex views, sequential images 18–30 sec. Hemispheral asymmetry is more easily appreciated, but positioning is difficult (note slight rotation), and activity immediately "shines" in the salivary glands if atropine is not given.

images (Fig. 4-3). The flow portion can be done immediately. However, there is still considerable debate as to the optimal time following the flow study before static views should be obtained. Many feel that a 3- to 4-hour delay improves the detection efficiency, particularly of metastatic lesions. Others contend that, although the delayed picture images may be somewhat prettier, early scanning does not compromise diagnosis. Thus, each laboratory establishes its own schedule. The total time of the study is then the addition of the various components of actual picture taking plus delays. Two hours is probably a reasonable average. No special preparation is required. No untoward effects are to be anticipated.

cisternography

Images are obtained because the instilled nuclide moves with the CSF. Pictures identify positive activity corresponding to the localization

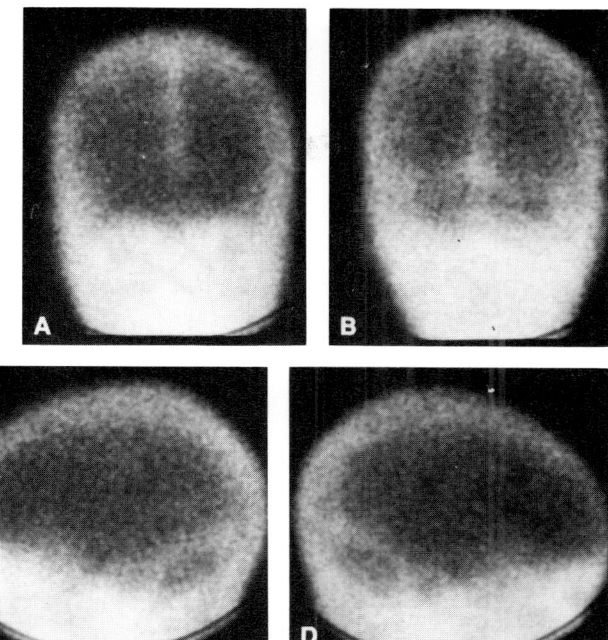

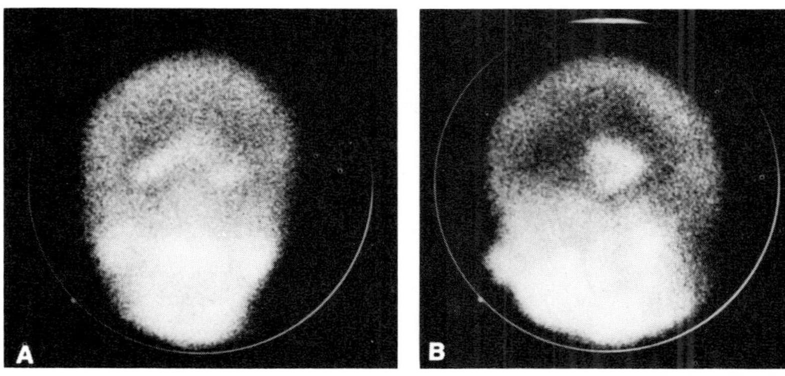

of the nuclide. Diagnosis is dependent on a
combination of flow rate and nuclide localization.
In the normal state, the ascending tracer will
reach the basilar cisterns from the lumbar
puncture site in approximately 1–2 hours. By
3–6 hours activity will be noted in the Sylvian
fissures. At 24 hours activity should be present
over the cerebral convexities and in the parasagittal area. The transit pattern is somewhat
faster in children. Unlike air, the nuclide will not
penetrate into the ventricles in a normal state.
The distribution should also be bilaterally
symmetric (Fig. 4-4).

Fig. 4-3. Normal static brain scan. Unless potassium
perchlorate is administered there will be "normal"
trapping of ^{99m}Tc pertechnetate in the choroid
plexuses.
A and B. Anterior (A) and lateral (B) views identify
   marked uptake of pertechnetate in the
   choroid plexuses of the ventricles. Note also
   the increased activity in the salivary glands.

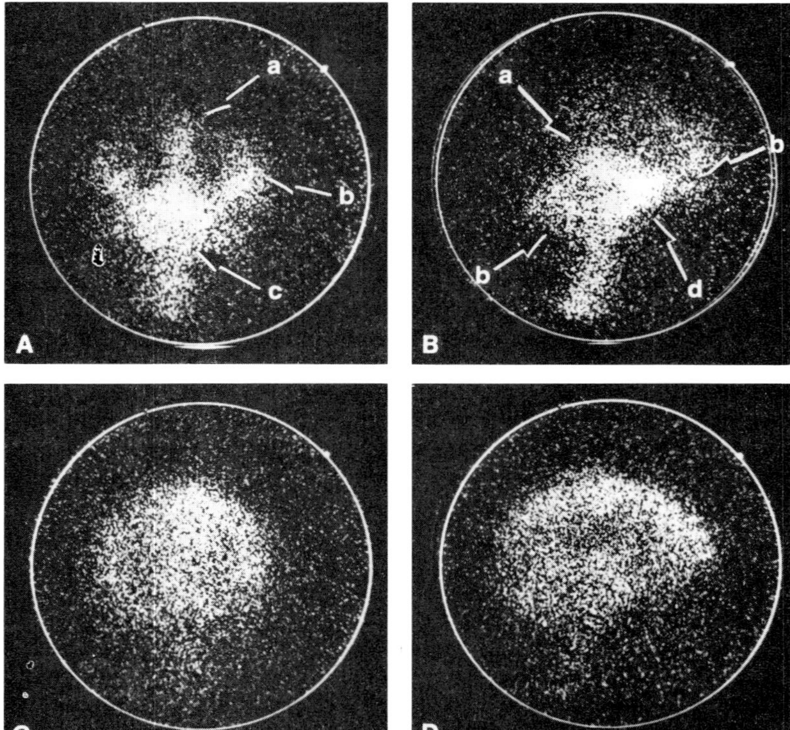

Fig. 4-4. Normal cisternogram
A and B. 4 hours. The anterior and lateral projection identify activity in the basal cisterns and sylvian fissure. The configuration is symmetric. There is no communication with the ventricles.
C and D. 24 hours. Scan views identify the progress of the nuclide to the subarachnoid spaces around the convexity of the brain.
    Key: a, quadrigemina; b, sylvii; c, magna; d, pontis

If the problem to be resolved is CSF rhinorrhea or otorrhea, imaging will begin ½–1 hour after installation and the patient will be positioned in whatever posture is known to increase the leak.

Cisternography requires hospitalization. A lumbar tap is necessary except in those very exceptional situations in which installation may be made at the cervicooccipital level directly into the cisterna magna. Thus, patient instructions and discussions should include all of the usual admonitions reserved for spinal taps, and in addition, the patient should be informed that a real possibility of technical failure exists. A warning should also be given of the possibility of aseptic meningitis. This problem has become one of the most frequently anticipated adverse reactions of any nuclear technique. Initially, the cause was thought to be a factor of albumin concentration. When this concentration exceeded 4.0 mg per injection, complications were high. However, it is now strongly suspected that the problem is a function of pyrogenic contamination. The intrathecal route of injection has been found to be 1000–4000 times more toxic than IV methods. Thus, the USP pyrogen-testing techniques may fail to identify the presence of minute amounts of bacterial endotoxins capable of producing aseptic meningitis. A specific technique for this detection, the Limulus test, is now recommended for evaluation of all materials to be introduced intrathecally, and it is hopefully anticipated that this complication will be controlled.

WHY

brain

Tumors. When the possibility of an intracranial space-taking lesion exists, x rays of the skull are almost invariably obtained. (Some reports suggest a 30% detection rate, but our rate is closer to 10%.) Identification is possible if either nonphysiologic calcification is present or manifestations of increased pressure exist. Calcifications occur in some meningiomas, oligodendrogliomas in adults, and cystic astrocytomas and craniopharyngiomas in children. Elevated pressure may cause resorption of bone as in the posterior clinoid process in the adult or sutural diathesis or altered fontanelle prominence in the infant or child. Localized hyperostosis, displacement of physiologic calcifications such as the pineal gland, and atypical patterns of vascular markings may also be suggestive. However, at best, positive evidence is only presumptive of tumor, whereas, at worst, sensitivity is poor, and false negatives are more the rule than the exception.

In the search for neoplasms, brain scanning excells because it is both sensitive to the presence of pathology and is capable of distinguishing type to a remarkable degree. The detection of the presence or absence of neoplasm is in the order of 90%. But what makes a particular collection of dots neoplasm? And what is it about those dots that permits a judgment of histology?

Neoplasms are, for the most part, spherical or ovoid. Contour is best appreciated in at least two views. The margins of the lesion are usually sharp or at least definable, particularly with a meningioma. These characteristics are violated when the lesion is invasive, as is frequently the case with the malignant gliomas (Fig. 4-5). Not only are the margins indistinct, but the tumors may extend across the midline. When this occurs the contour may assume a butterfly configuration if the process is symmetric. However, the pattern of a focal lesion crossing the midline is in itself highly diagnostic of tumor, particularly if the crossing can be localized to the region of the corpus callosum. Extension can occur through any of the intrahemispheral commissures but is most frequent at the corpus callosum since it is the largest.

Certain neoplasms have strict anatomic specificity, whereas others are unpredictable. Acoustic neuromas, pituitary adenomas, craniopharyngiomas, and papillomas of the ventricle or choroid plexuses are all predictably situated (Fig. 4-6). Meningiomas select certain characteristic sites, *e.g.,* the sphenoid wings, cribriform plate, free margins of the falx, and—

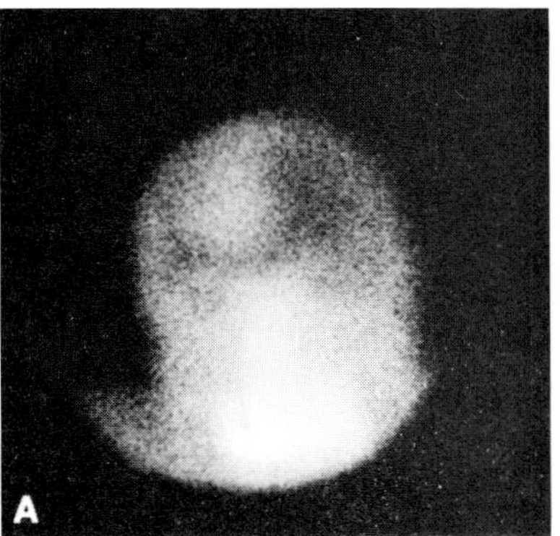
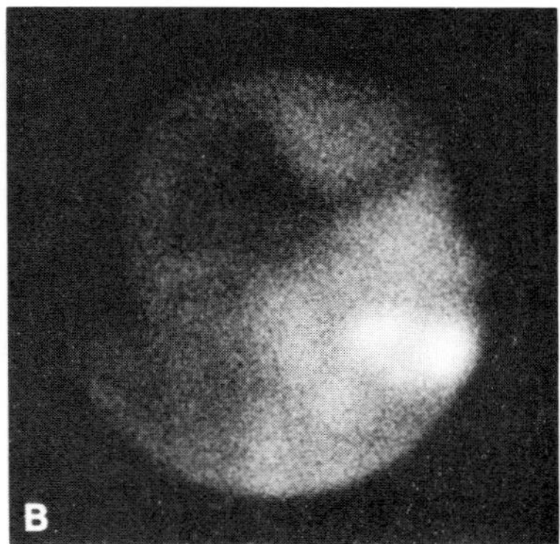
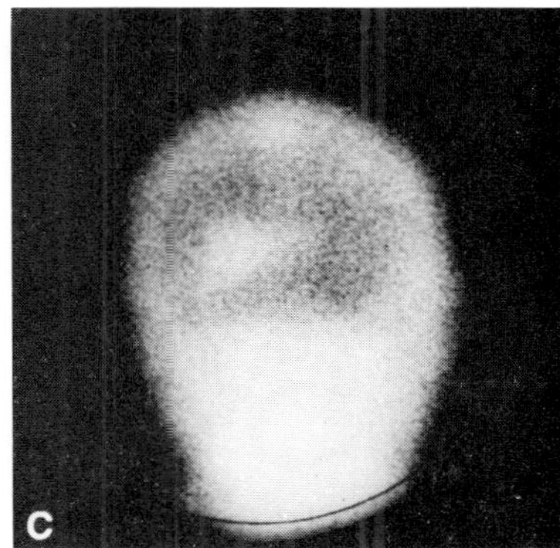
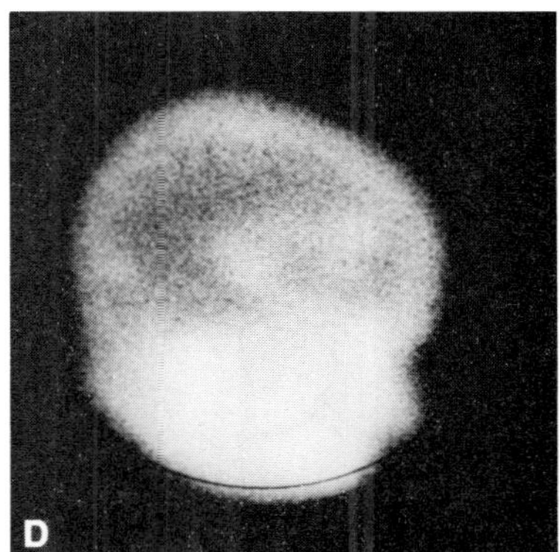

Fig. 4-5. Malignant gliomas
Diagnosis: Astrocytoma—grade III
A and B. The lesion is huge, occupying almost the entire right frontal lobe. Its margins are sharp, its contour circular.
Diagnosis: Infiltrating glioma
C and D. The lesion is triangular in frontal views and dumbbell-shaped in lateral. Its margins are unsharp.

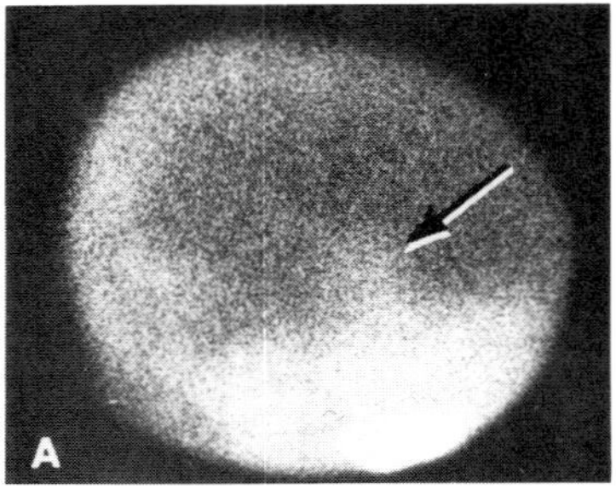

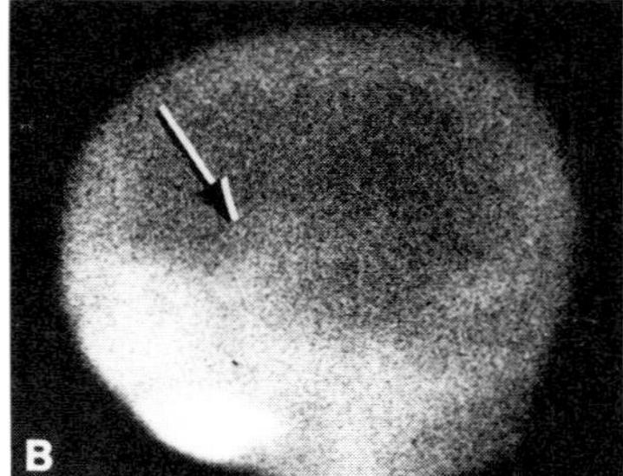

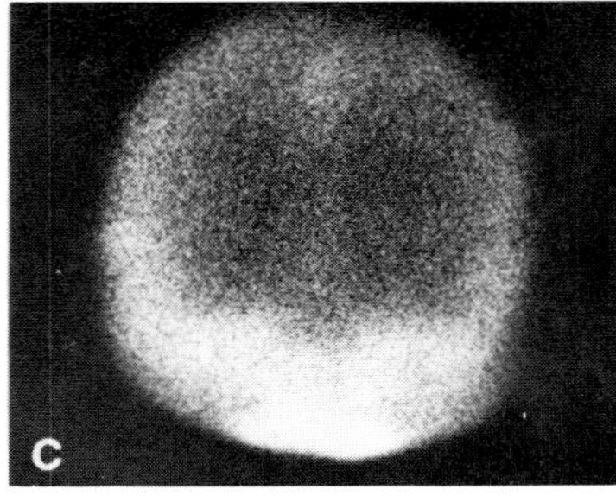

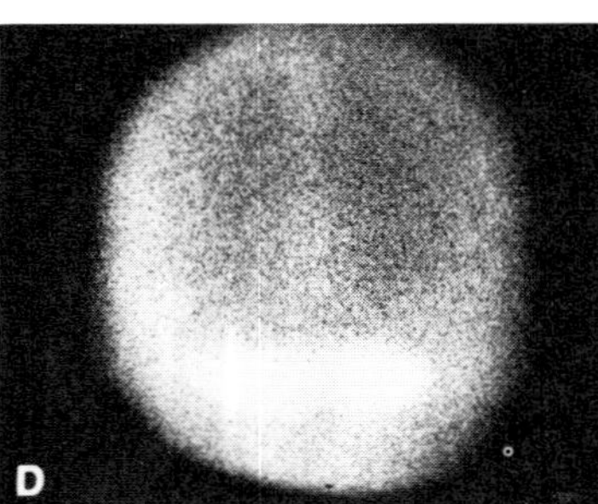

Fig. 4-6. Chromophobe adenoma of the pituitary
A and B. The lateral projection indicates an area of increased activity in the region of the sella turcica (arrow). The defect is seen almost equally well in each view, suggesting a midline position.
C and D. The anterior and posterior views do not identify the lesion. It is not unusual for an abnormality adjacent to an area of usual high activity to be obscured.

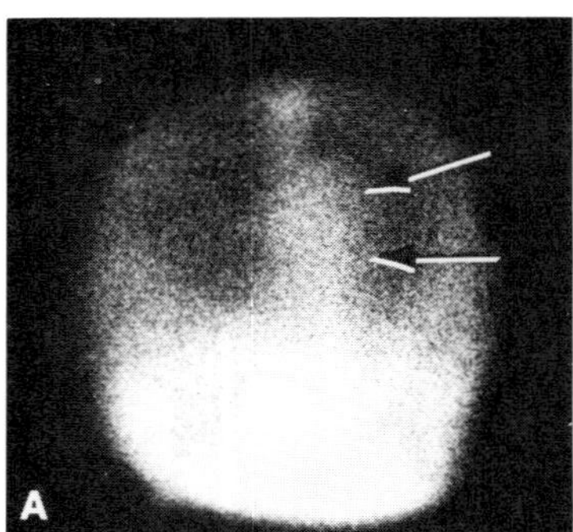

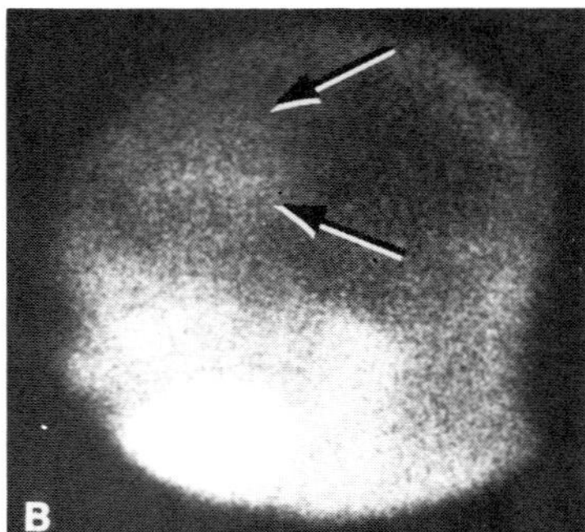

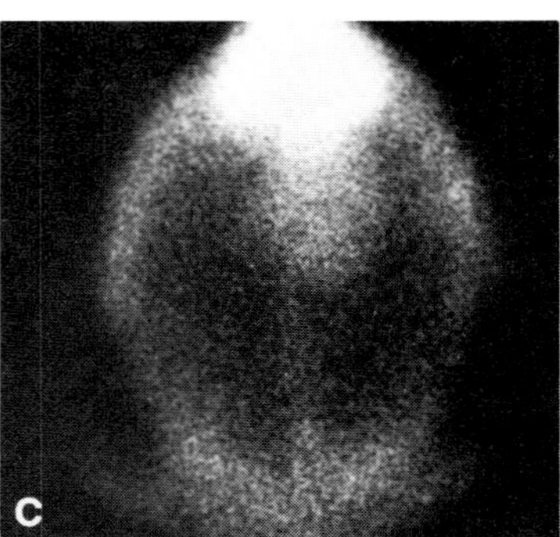

Fig. 4-7. Parasagittal meningioma
A–C. Large area of increased uptake in the left frontal lobe assuming a parasagittal location. In the vertex view **(C)** the area of marked increased uptake anterior to the lesion is activity in the mouth.

particularly—parasagittal locations (Fig. 4-7). On the other hand, glioblastomas and metastatic implants can occur anywhere. Most neoplasms in children are infratentorial. Most can be separated from the periphery in at least one view.

Location is one of the major explanations for false negative studies. Whenever there is abutment of a pathologic process against normal activity, identification is impaired. Thus lesions in the midline, along the floor of the vault, or infratentorially situated are far more difficult to identify than those that are supratentorial, peripheral, or frontal. If the history of physical deficit suggests such diseases as pituitary

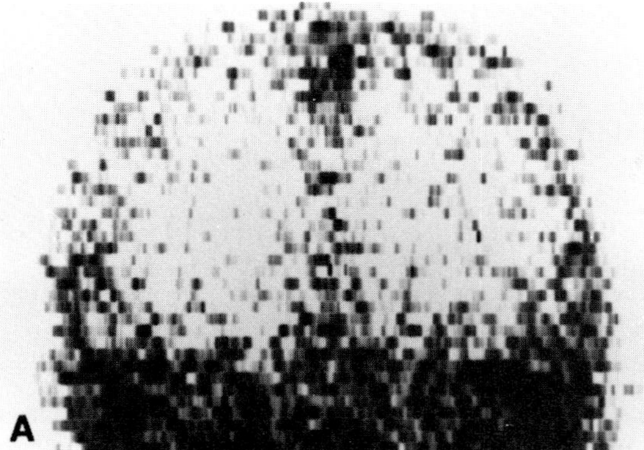
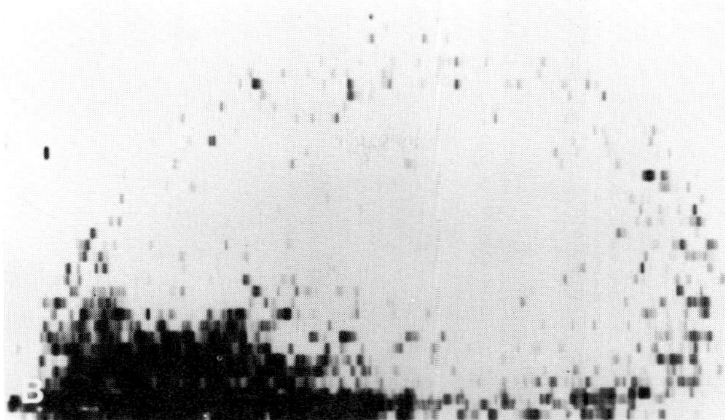
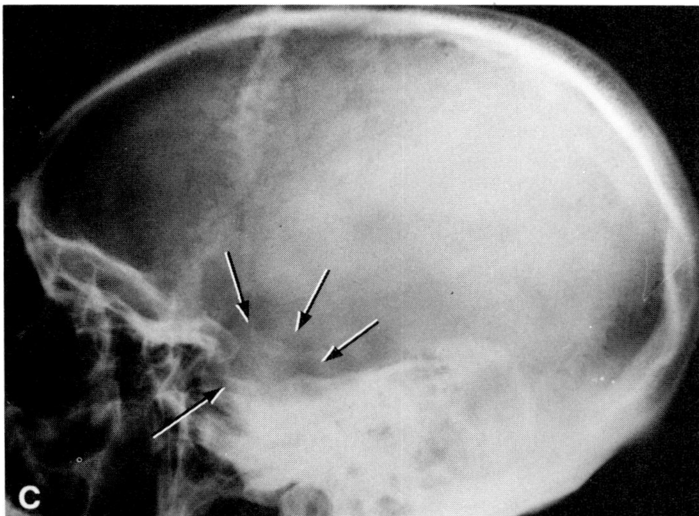

Fig. 4-8. Chromophobe adenoma of the pituitary
A and B. Scans. Posterior **(A)** and lateral **(B)** images done with a rectilinear scanner with 2:1 minification. Although the activity at the base is unsharp on the lateral view, the findings are within normal limits.
C. Lateral skull x ray. The dorsum sella, anterior and posterior clinoid processes, and floor of the sella turcica are destroyed (arrows).

adenomas, acoustic neuromas, or chordomas, a negative scan should not be accepted as final (Fig. 4-8). Contrarywise, a suspected meningioma, glioblastoma, or metastatic lesion, particularly if localized to the frontal or parietal regions, will rarely be missed and a report of a negative scan is most reliable.

Of itself, the magnitude of the defect is not of diagnostic value. If the new growth originates in a "silent" area, it may attain huge dimensions before symptoms demand investigation. Size is of importance only as it relates to the physical limitations of instrumentation. Lesions smaller than 1.5 cm will probably go undetected.

Certain neoplasms are known empirically to produce greater scan activity than others. Whether this is a function of intrinsic accumulation, increased vascularity, circumferential edema, or other factors is still incompletely understood (Fig. 4-9). A grade I astrocytoma may escape detection, whereas a grade IV is usually easily identified (Fig. 4-10). Certain metastases, such as from renal primaries, seem to accumulate greater activity than others.

If more than one lesion is detected, particularly if the general characteristics of neoplasm are suggested or a known primary exists, metastatic disease is almost invariably present (Fig. 4-11). This is not to suggest that all metastases are multiple. Lesions may be single or, perhaps what is more common, are multiple implants, all but one being too small to be visualized (Fig. 4-12).

Usually the increased activity of neoplasms presents as a homogeneous uniform pattern. Occasionally, central necrosis may occur, producing an image likened to a doughnut: a circular zone of increased activity with a lucent

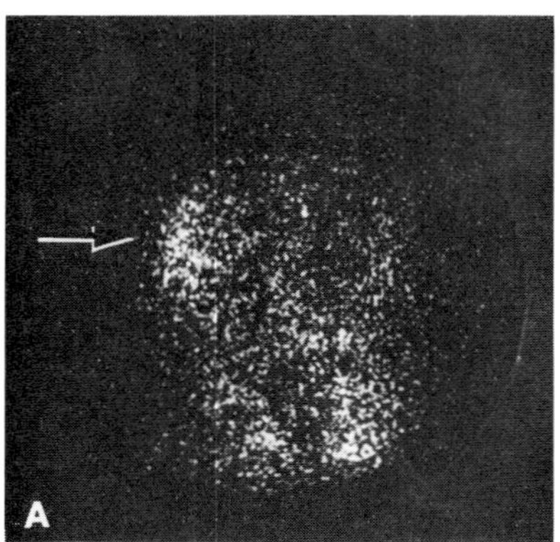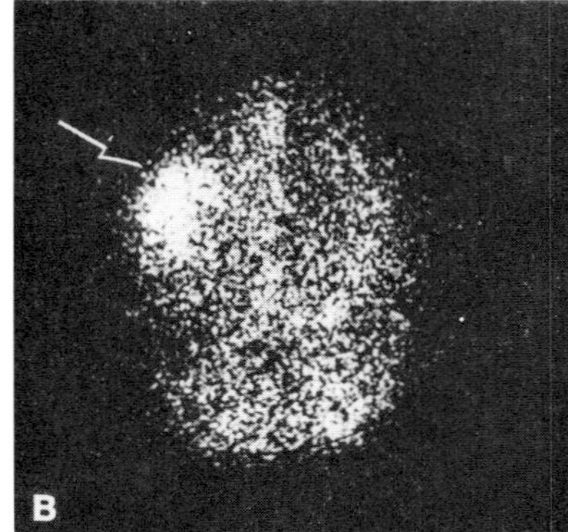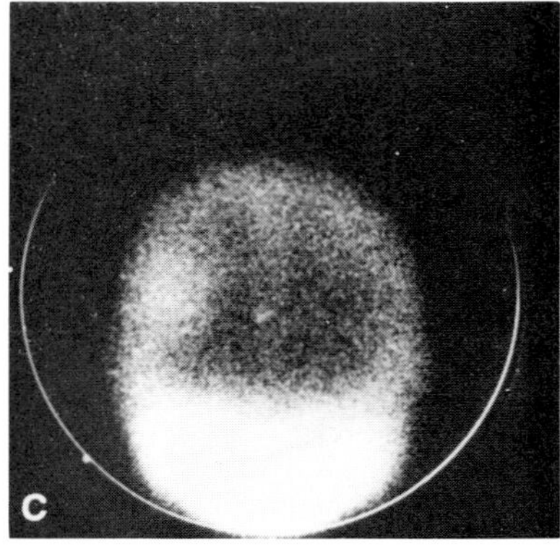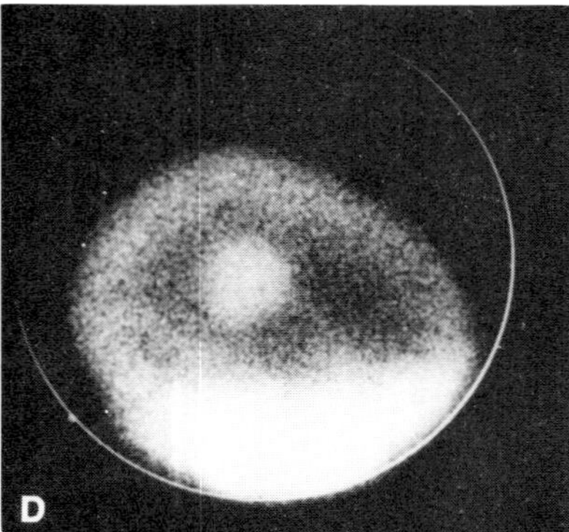

Fig. 4-9. Meningioma
A and B. Flow. Increased activity (arrow) is seen immediately in the right lateral region.
C and D. Static. Large defect of high activity is located adjacent to free margins of the falx.

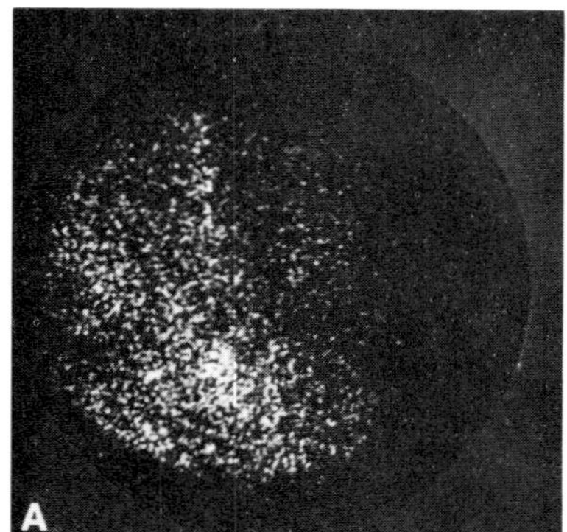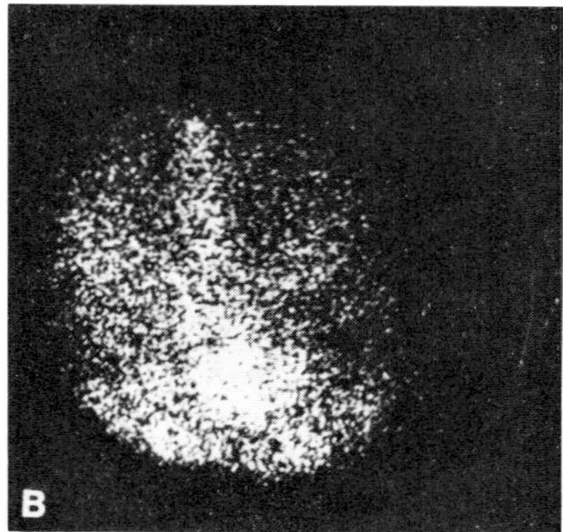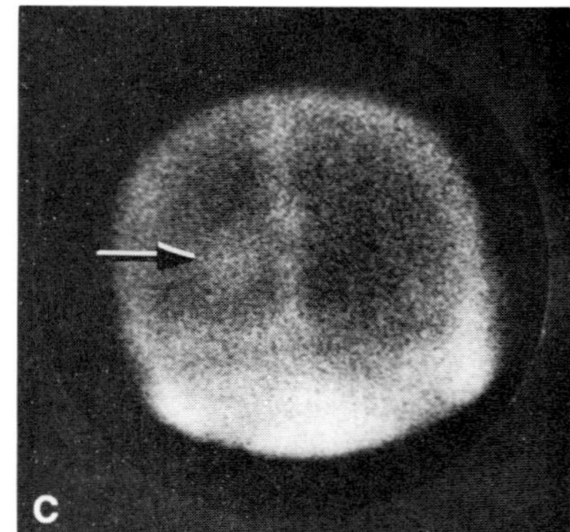

Fig. 4-10. Astrocytoma—grade III
A and B. Flow. The entire left hemisphere is underperfused as compared to the right, suggesting a vascular deficit.
C and D. Static. In the posterior view **(C)** there is an ovoid defect (arrow) with sharp margination suggesting tumor rather than infarct. In lateral view **(D)** the lesion is barely detectable as a vague zone of increased activity (arrow) above the transverse sinus.

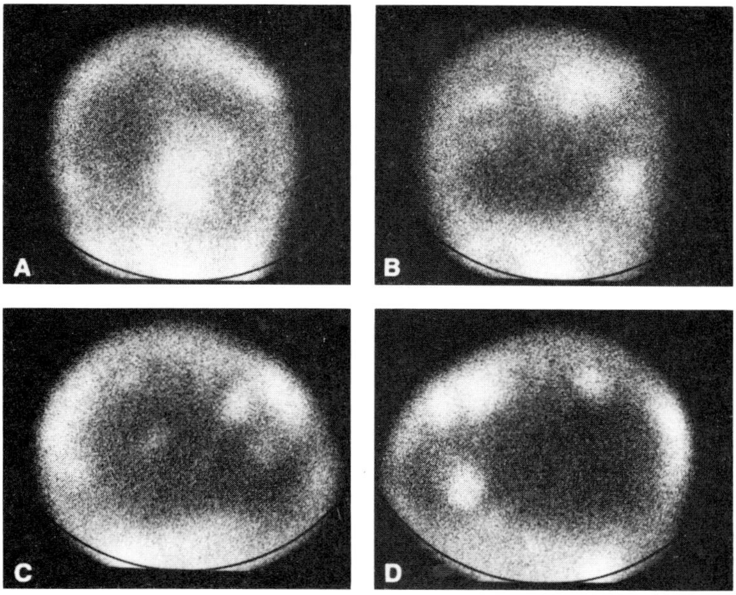

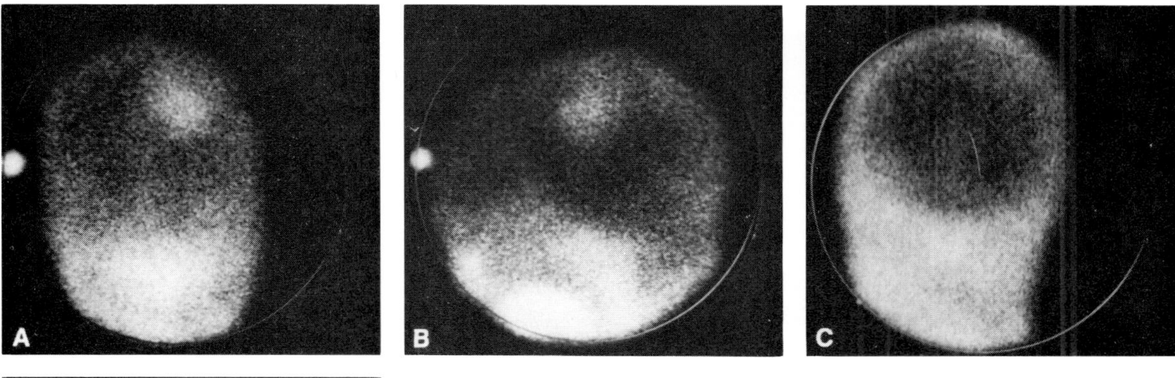

Fig. 4-11. Metastasis—breast carcinoma
A–D. Static. Numerous discrete and confluent areas of abnormally increased uptake

Fig. 4-12. Metastasis—bronchogenic carcinoma
A and B. Static. Large single defect. (Small dot at left edge is a marker.)
C and D. Static, 1 month later. Almost complete regression of the defect after 4000 rads to the lesion

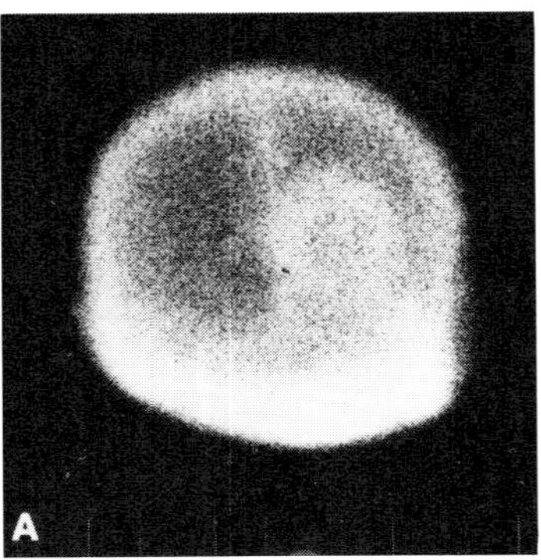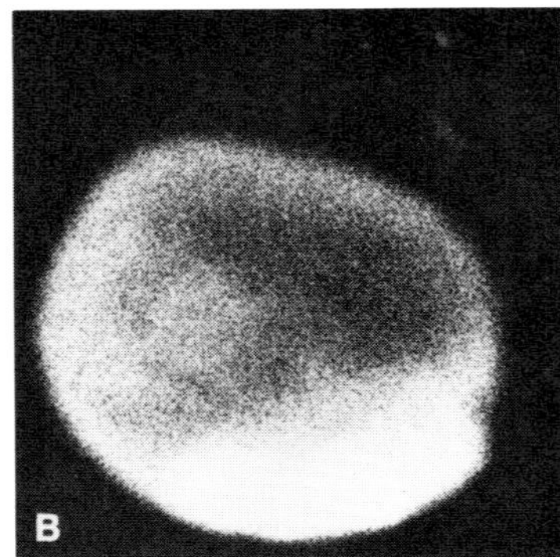

Fig. 4-13. Astrocytoma—grade III with central necrosis (same patient as in Fig. 4-10, 4 months later). Surgery refused after original study but permitted following second. In the interval the lesion had increased significantly in size and become centrally necrotic.
A. Posterior view
B. Lateral view

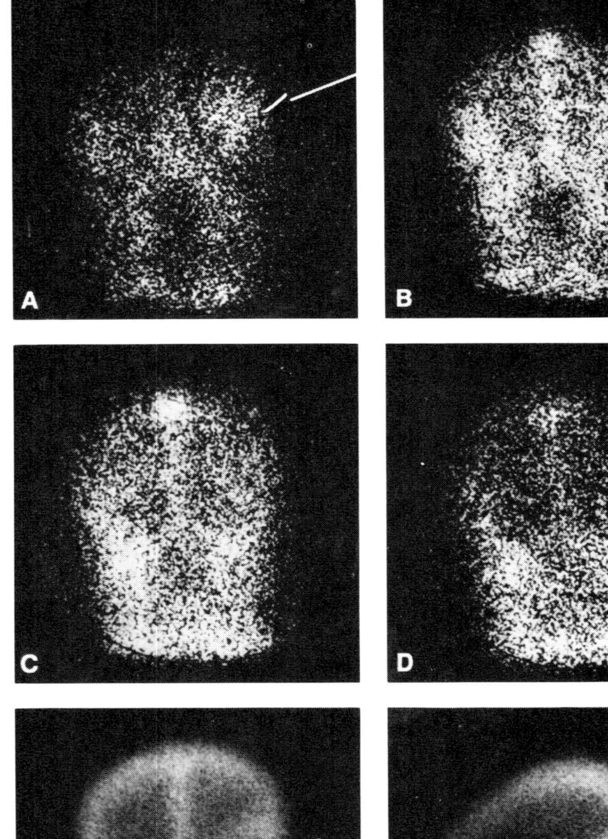

Fig. 4-14. Arteriovenous malformation
A–D. Flow. Sequential images indicate an initial increase in activity (arrow) in the left lateral hemisphere quickly fading in the late venous phase.
E and F. Static. There is a vague ill-defined area of increased activity (arrow) in the left posterior parietal region.

Fig. 4-15. Meningioma

A–D. Flow. Sequential images indicate an initial increase in activity in the midline which increases with time.

E and F. Static. There is a large, sharply defined midline frontal lesion.

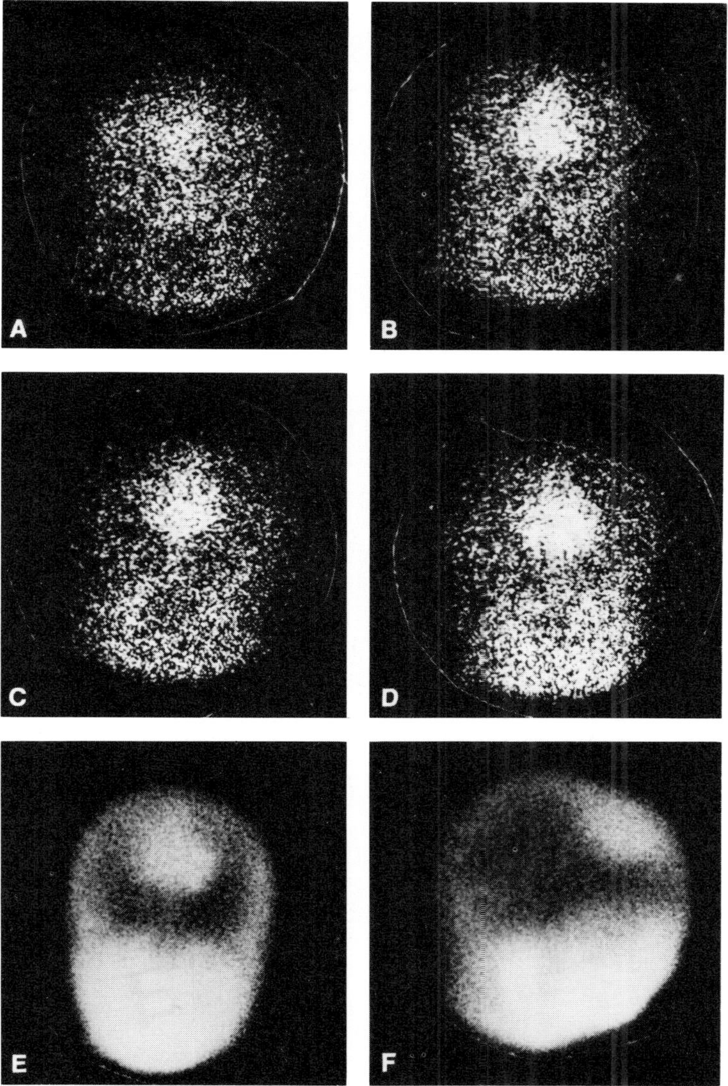

center. History should permit differentiation of this finding from the other conditions in which it is found, *i.e.,* from abscess, intracerebral hematomas, and—occasionally—even subdural hematomas (Fig. 4-13).

The routine inclusion of a flow study to complement the static images has improved differential definition. Patterns in the dynamic phase alone, but particularly in combination with the delayed images, often suggest the etiology. Increased activity on the flow scan usually separates neoplasm from defects of vascular and traumatic origins. Usually this increased activity is confused only with arterio-venous malformation (AVM). However, the AVM usually is less positive on the static images (Fig. 4-14); neoplasms, particularly meningi-omas, demonstrate increasing activity with time (Fig. 4-15).

Often when only static images are available, defects resulting from extracranial factors such as contusions or lacerations of the scalp are difficult to distinguish from neoplasm. But when the origin of the defect is extracranial, the flow study is usually "normal," whereas many neo-plasms demonstrate positive changes even during this phase (Fig. 4-16). If the differential diagnosis remains in doubt, serial examinations over a 1- to 2-week period will usually clarify the problem. The intracranial process will manifest

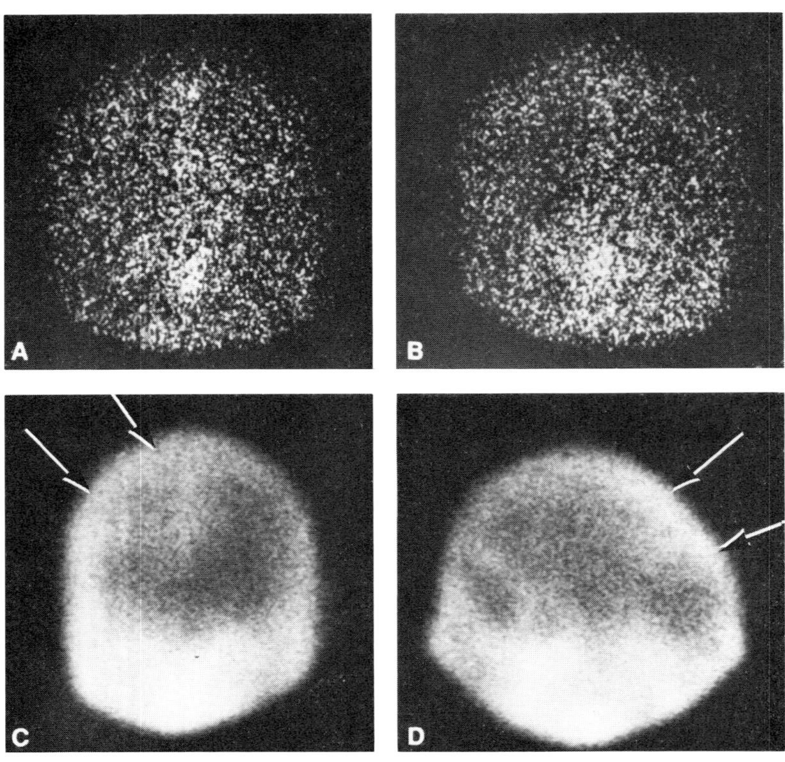

Fig. 4-16. Laceration of the scalp (right frontal)

A and B. Flow. Poor resolution of vascular structures but no evidence of asymmetric activity

C and D. Static. Vague zone of increased activity (arrows) in the right frontal region assuming the pattern neither of a mass nor of a vascular lesion

unchanged or even increased abnormality, while the extracranial lesion, if induced by trauma, will fade or disappear.

As has been previously discussed ^{99m}Tc as pertechnetate or chelated is the most commonly employed radionuclide in brain imaging. Also discussed was its lack of specificity in the differentiation of diseases. There are, however, certain radionuclides that when used in combination with ^{99m}Tc may on occasion improve identification. Where a positive ^{99m}Tc study cannot be differentiated between tumor and ischemic infarct, ^{67}Ga citrate may be helpful. This nuclide does not usually yield positive studies in vascular problems. Thus, a positive ^{99m}Tc in conjunction with a normal ^{67}Ga examination rules against neoplasm and by default suggests infarct. Unfortunately, the ^{67}Ga study requires a wait of 2–3 days after injection before the scan can be made.

Likewise, uptake from any cause in overlying bone (*e.g.,* metastasis, fracture, infection) may be distinguishable from intracranial disease. The use of one of the bone-seeking nuclides may clarify the site of abnormality. A not too uncommon clinical problem is the need to

evaluate the postoperative patient for tumor regrowth. For reasons as yet unknown, surgical calvarial defects will continue to accumulate increased quantities of ^{99m}Tc for many years. The abnormal scan thus obtained is difficult to evaluate. Is the abnormality "normal" postoperative change, residual neoplasm, neoplastic recurrence, or a combination of several? Employing both ^{99m}Tc pertechnetate and a bone-selective nuclide differentiation may be made, particularly if an immediate postoperative study has been made and is available for comparison (Fig. 4-17).

Vascular. Scanning is of value in cerebrovascular disease when the diagnosis is in doubt. Not all vascular accidents are clinically evident, and differentiation from neoplasm and trauma is often necessary.

For the most part, a vascular lesion produces a characteristic defect, being localized to the geographic distribution of the vessel involved. Exquisite mapping of defect patterns have been performed permitting excellent appreciation of both the vessel involved and the extent of the involvement (Fig. 4-18).

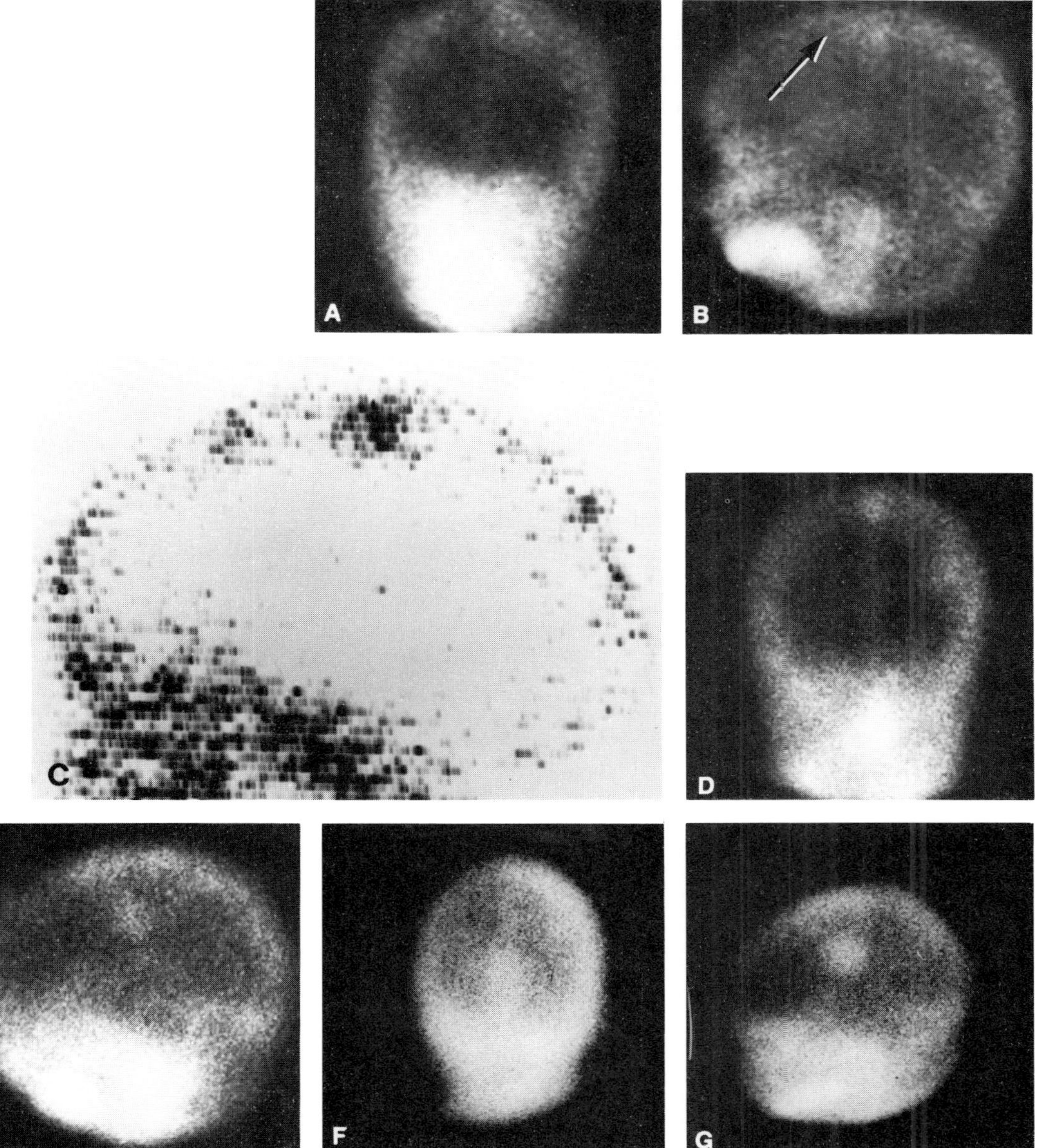

Fig. 4-17. Metastatic intracranial amelanotic melanoma and meningioma
Diagnosis: Metastatic intracranial amelanotic melanoma
A and B. Static brain scan (9/7/73). Anterior **(A)** and left lateral **(B)** views made with ^{99m}Tc suggest possible area of increased uptake (arrow) at the left frontoparietal junction.
C. Lateral bone scan (9/12/73). The lesion is better identified with ^{99m}Tc polyphosphate suggesting a calvarial defect. Biopsy revealed metastatic intracranial amelanotic melanoma.
Diagnosis: Meningioma
D and E. Static brain scan (11/21/73). Because symptoms persisted and were beccming worse after the biopsy, scanning was again performed. The defect appears more prominent than in original examination.
F and G. Static brain scan (12/18/73). Symptoms continued to exacerbate and now scan identifies an even larger lesion, perhaps slightly deeper than the original. Surgery revealed meningioma.

The presenting defect usually assumes a triangular or band-shaped contour although the pattern produced by hemorrhage is less sharply marginated than that which results from infarction. However, each is characterized by the lesion extending to the periphery.

The relationship of the time of examination to the clinical event is more significant in this type of disease than in almost all others. If the insult was hemorrhagic, perhaps 50% of scans obtained within the first week of the event will be positive. If the problem was infarction, the first week's yield will be less than 25%. Positive studies are more predictable in the second to fourth week and may never exceed 50% for the infarct or 75% for the hemorrhage. If, indeed, there is a significantly positive scan defect immediately after the clinical event, tumor as the etiologic agent should be suspected.

Additionally, the cerebrovascular accident (CVA) positive scan will begin to fade and assume a more normal appearance with time. Within 4–6 weeks of an uncomplicated course, the serial scans may revert to normal or at least reflect a changing pattern. Contrarywise, the initial lesion in neoplasm will either remain unchanged over this relatively short interval or will become worse.

Dynamic imaging improved detection. Not all flow studies of the head are diagnostic or of equal quality. Many variables, particularly the patient's age and circulatory status, account for frequent failures. Therefore, interpretation should be limited to obviously positive cases. Symmetry of activity representing hemispheral perfusion is the criterion of normality. As a rule, but not always absolute, vascular disease will be reflected by diminished or delayed activity, or by both, on the side of involvement. A "flip-flop" pattern has been described in which the side of insult is initially hypoactive (the flip) to be followed by relative hyperperfusion as the slowly filling side reaches saturation and contrasts with the already-draining normal side (the flop). Computer assistance may improve the sensitivity of detection of asymmetry. Thus, the combination of a positive flow study and negative static series is highly suggestive of a vascular accident (Fig. 4-19).

Serial examination is also of value, particularly if there is any concern whatever to the diagnosis or clinical course. A changing pattern,

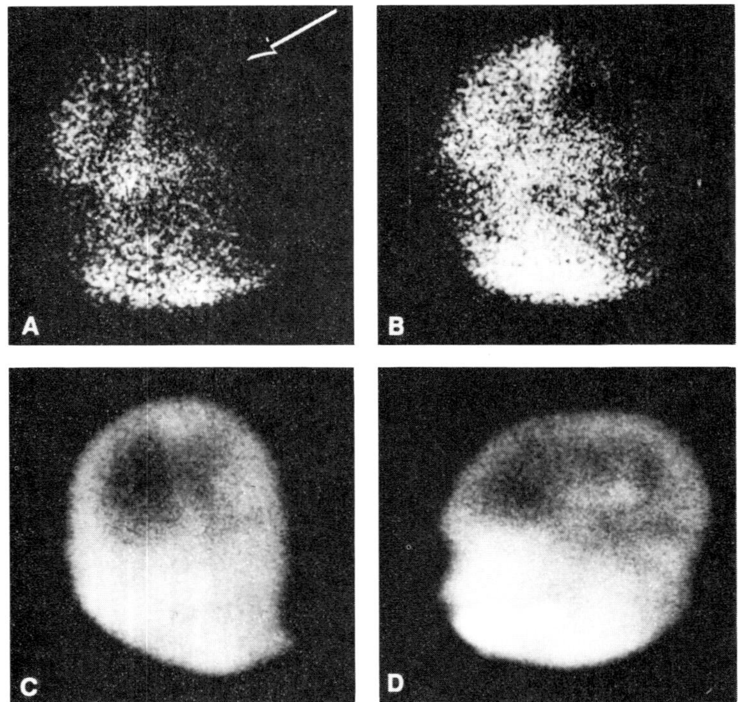

Fig. 4-18. Left middle cerebral artery hemorrhage
A and B. Flow. There is significant asymmetry in hemispheric perfusion. The activity (arrow) is considerably diminished on the left.
C and D. Static. The entire area supplied by the left middle cerebral artery demonstrates abnormal activity. The defect is grossly triangular on the lateral view and abuts both the inferior and superior peripheral zone of activity.

usually from negative to increasingly positive to diminishingly positive over a 4 to 6-week interval is almost pathognomonic for a vascular insult (Fig. 4-20). A relatively unchanging pattern, particularly if positive early, should sound the alarm that an unsuspected tumor exists. Primary vascular diseases may also be recognized with the flow study. A circumscribed zone of increased activity along a major arterial pathway may identify an aneurysm. The static images in all of these problems may be interpreted as normal (Fig. 4-21).

Trauma. Of the group of possible cerebral traumas evaluated by scanning, the subdural hematoma may be the most difficult to identify, particularly if it is of the chronic variety. More often than not there will be no accompanying skull fracture in contradistinction to epidural hemorrhage in which fracture is almost always present (Fig. 4-22). No obvious evidence of injury may exist by the time symptoms become manifest, and the patient may long since have forgotten the relatively minor traumatic event. The hemorrhage usually results from the tearing of a superior cerebral vein. The brain moving

abruptly with trauma may exert a shearing action on the veins as they enter the immobile superior sagittal sinus. The spreading clot is unlimited by any barrier and thus assumes any contour. With time, perhaps as early as 1 week to 10 days, a pseudomembrane will develop and encapsulate the fluid.

Fig. 4-19. Right posterior cerebral artery infarction
A and B. Flow, anterior view (12/19/73). Initial image **(A)** demonstrates gross asymmetry. The "avascular" right hemisphere improves in activity throughout the sequence **(B)**. The study is positive and is compatible with a cerebral vascular accident. This was also the clinical diagnosis.
C and D. Static, posterior, right lateral (12/19/73). The initial study was interpreted as normal.
E and F. Static, posterior, right lateral (1/10/74). Repeat study 3 weeks later identifies marked changes in the geographic distribution of the right posterior cerebral artery.

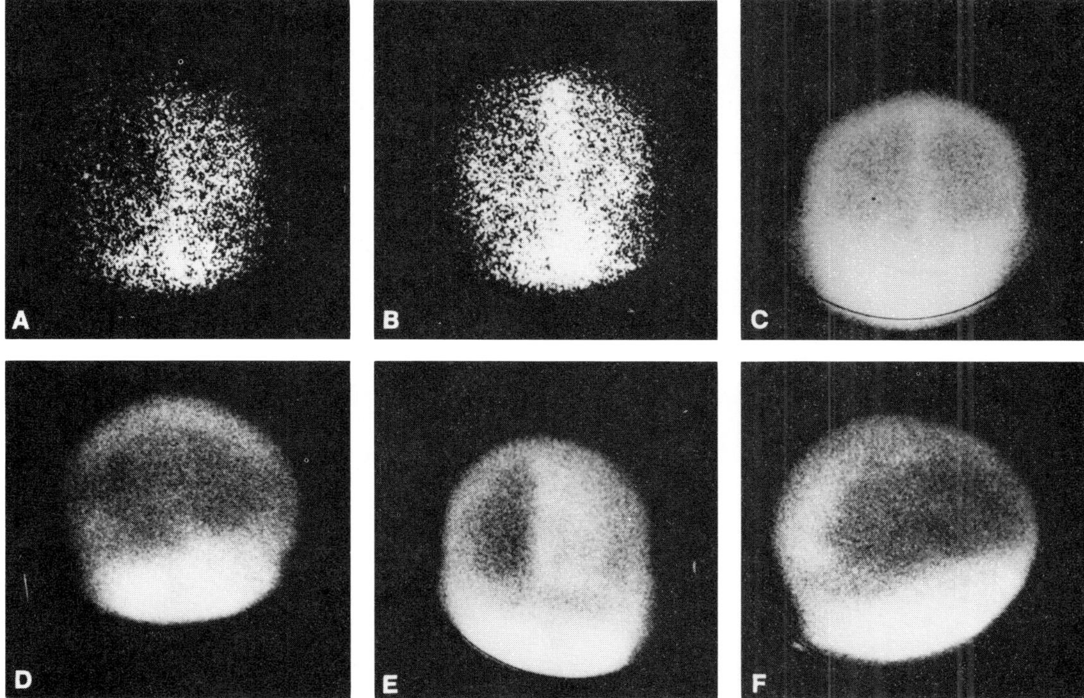

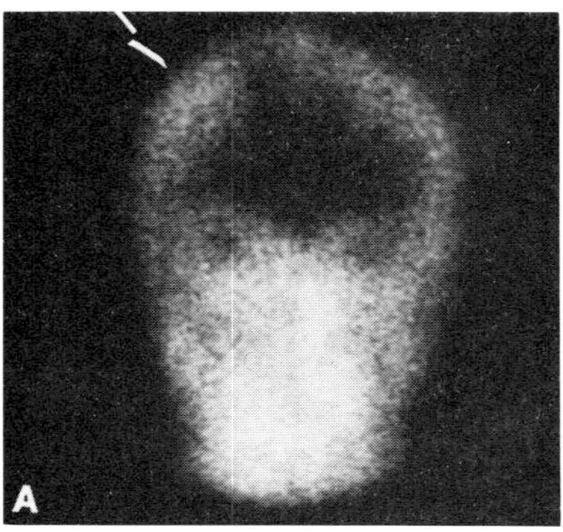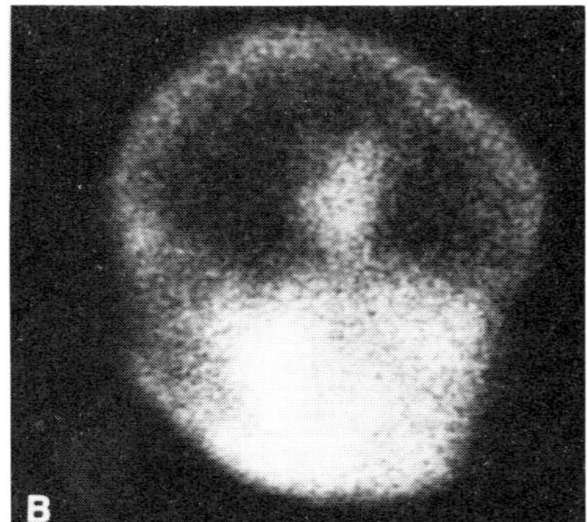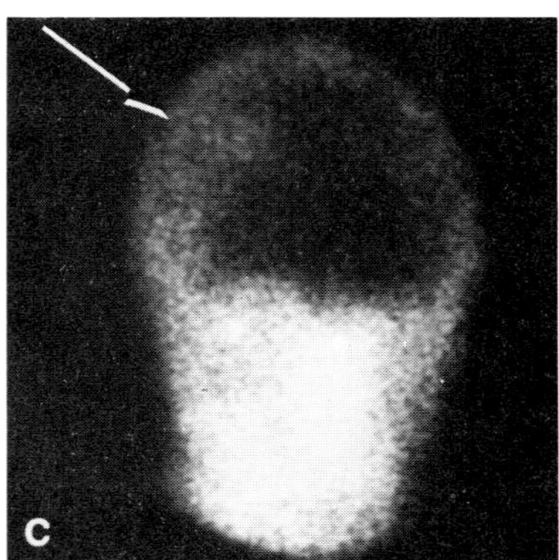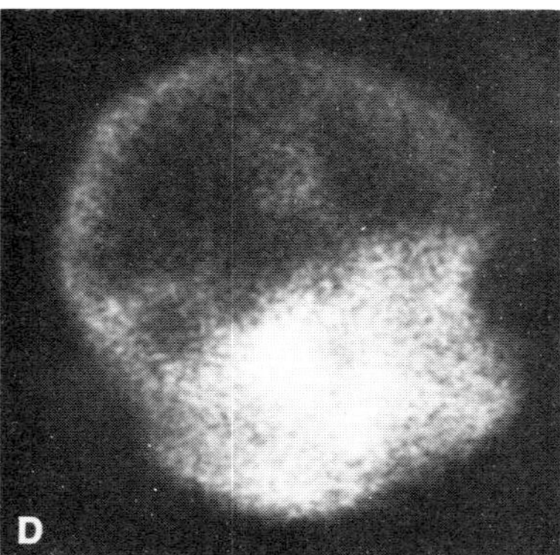

Fig. 4-20. Right middle cerebral artery hemorrhage
A and B. Static (9/10/73). The area of abnormal activity (arrow) in the **(A)** and right lateral **(B)** views has characteristics of both a mass lesion and a vascular insult. The clinical diagnosis was right middle cerebral artery hemorrhage.
C and D. Static (9/21/73). Repeat examination (11 days later) demonstrates a significant decrease in the abnormal activity (arrow), diminishing the concern of tumor.

Scanning offers an overall accuracy of over 80% in detection. Accuracy is probably better in the chronic problem, which is certainly easier to identify in the unilateral situation. Considerable unsettled discussions continue as to whether the membrane or the fluid makes the scan positive. Probably both do. Uncontested, is the agreement that the larger the lesion the greater the ease of recognition.

The classically described finding is the "crescent sign," which is evidence of the peripheral rim of activity. This is usually best seen in either the anterior or posterior view and was originally thought to be present only in those projections. However, it is not uncommon to identify changes in the lateral view as well. These vary and may simply present as increased perimeter activity or a circumscribed or diffuse zone of change. When the problem is unilateral, asymmetry of the peripheral rim will be far more obvious than when a bilateral process exists (Fig. 4-23). There is always the real danger that the bilateral involvement, diminishing the appreciation of the crescent, will go undetected (Fig. 4-24).

Again the addition of the flow study significantly complements the static views and is particularly helpful both in the detection of a bilateral problem and in a differential diagnosis of extracerebral disease (which may also create static images and a positive crescent sign). These include Paget's disease of the skull, osseous and scalp metastases, scalp contusions or hematomas or both, and even hyperostosis frontalis interna. A positive flow study will identify the inability of the vascular activity to reach the vault perimeter, and a concave defect proportional to the volume of the hematoma will result. Thus, the change is recognizable in either the unilateral or bilateral process, and the side of greater involvement may be more readily appreciated. The flow in extracerebral processes, particularly contusions or lacerations of the scalp, will be negative on at least the earlier arterial phase of the flow and the pattern of abnormality does not as a rule reflect vascular displacement (Figs. 4-25 and 4-26).

However, it must be understood that scanning rarely replaces contrast angiography. In the acute process a negative scan is not diagnostic.

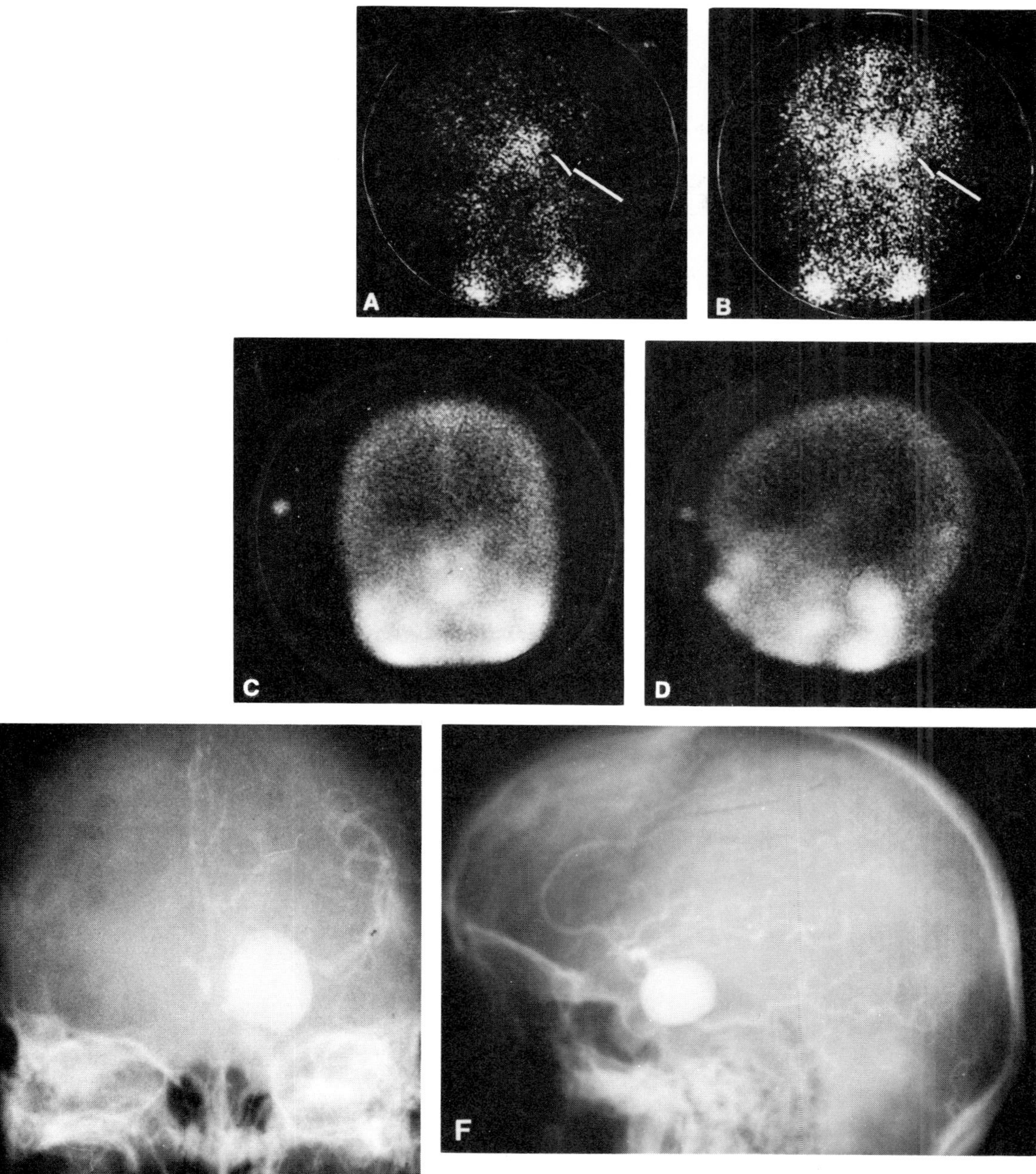

Fig. 4-21. Internal carotid artery aneurysm
A and B. Flow. Early images of the sequential series identify
a circumscribed area of increased activity (arrow).
C and D. Static. Static views were considered normal.
E and F. Arteriogram. Huge aneurysm of the internal carotid
artery

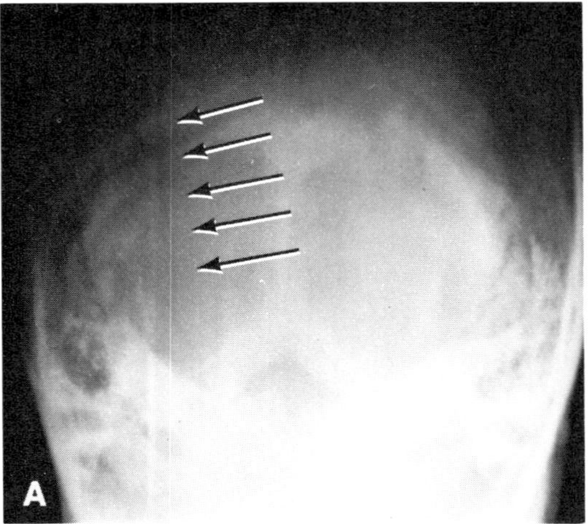
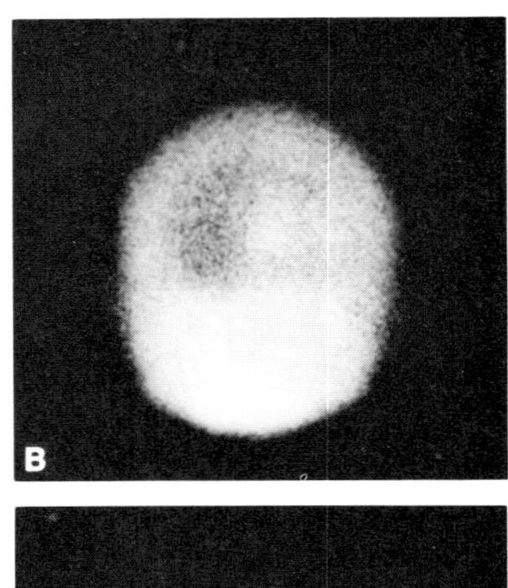
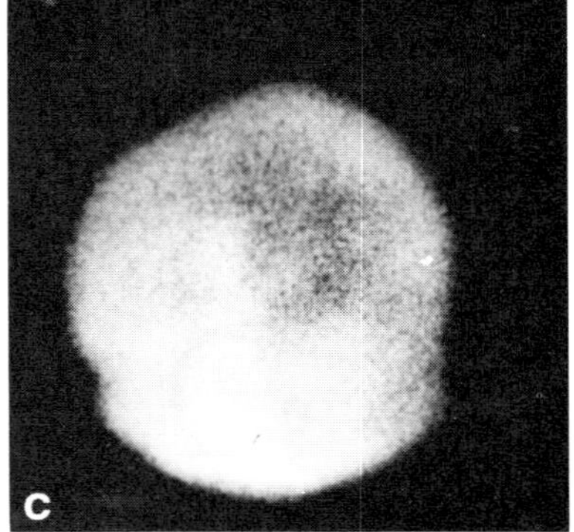

Fig. 4-22. Skull fracture and intracerebral hematoma
A. Skull x ray. The arrows identify a fracture of the right occipital bone.
B and C. Static. The entire left frontal region is obscured by a diffuse zone of increased activity that has no definitive boundaries or margins.

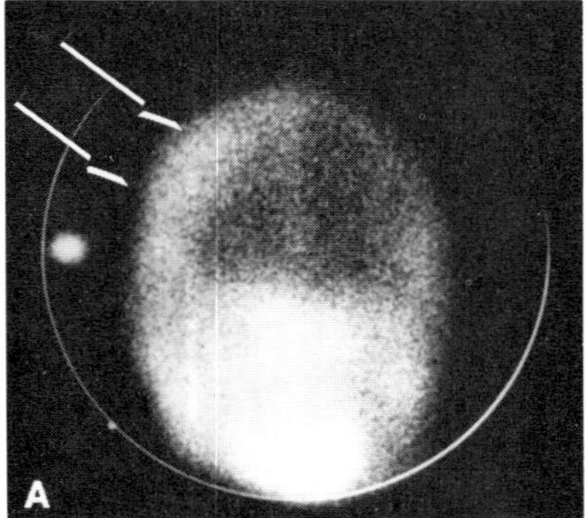
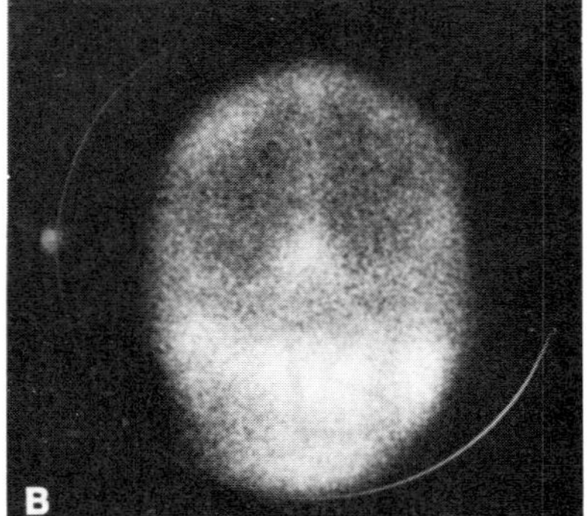
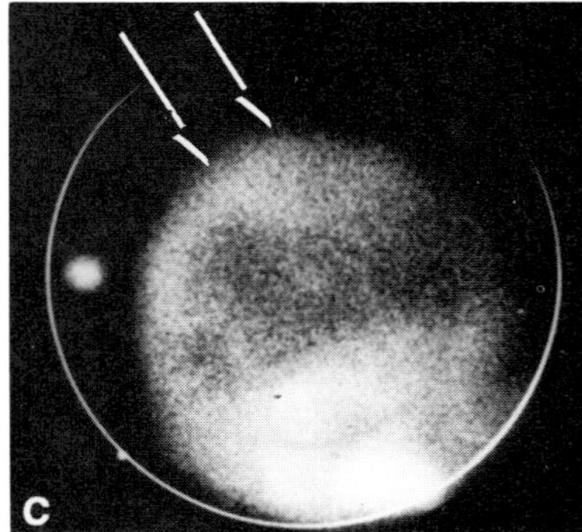
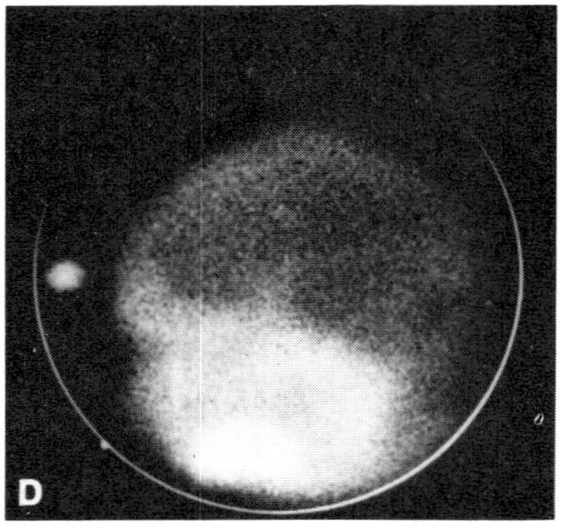

Fig. 4-23. Right subdural hematoma
A–D. Static. The perimeter activity (arrows) on the right in the anterior view **(A)** exhibits the classic "crescent sign." It is broader and more active than the contralateral region. The right lateral view **(C)** also identifies an area of increased activity (arrows) adjacent to the peripheral rim.

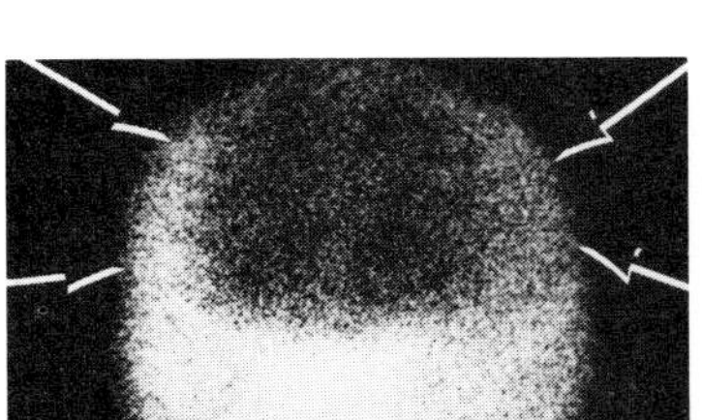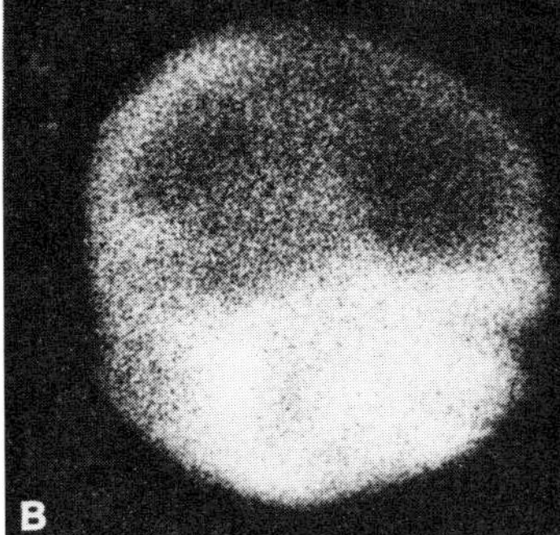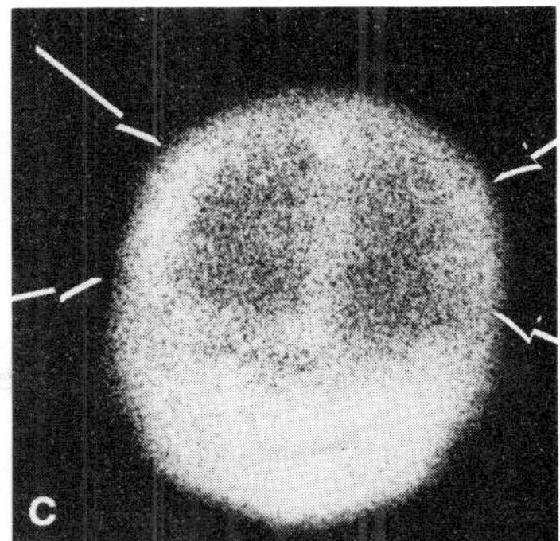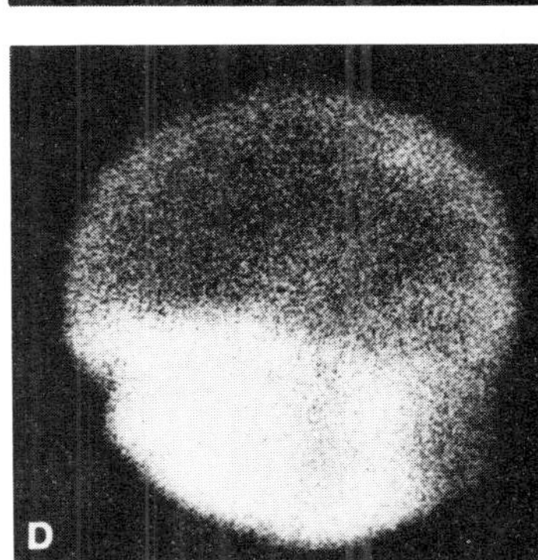

Fig. 4-24. Bilateral subdural hematoma

A. Static, anterior. The perimeter activity is more intense on the right than on the left. However, the left band is wider than the right, wider than average, and poorly marginated (arrows).

B. Static, right lateral. The entire parietotemporal region is obscured by an ill-defined zone of increased activity.

C. Static, posterior. The perimeters are asymmetric in contour and activity (arrows). Neither are normal.

D. Static, left lateral. Questionable widening of the posterior peripheral rims

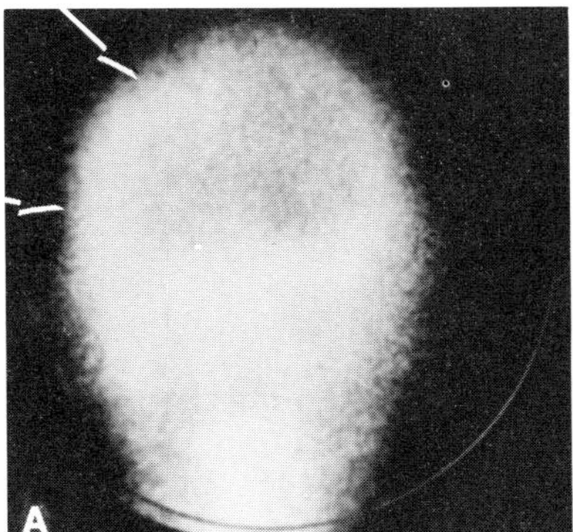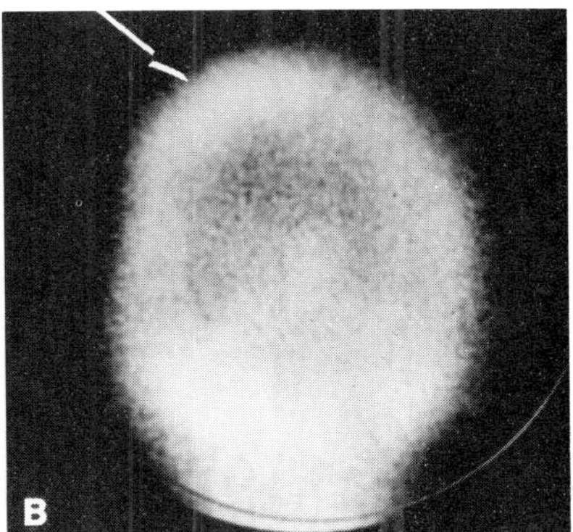

Fig. 4-25. Paget's disease of the calvarium

A and B. Static. There is gross widening and increased activity (arrows) in the right perimeter. The changes extend to the floor of the vault. The flow study was interpreted as normal.

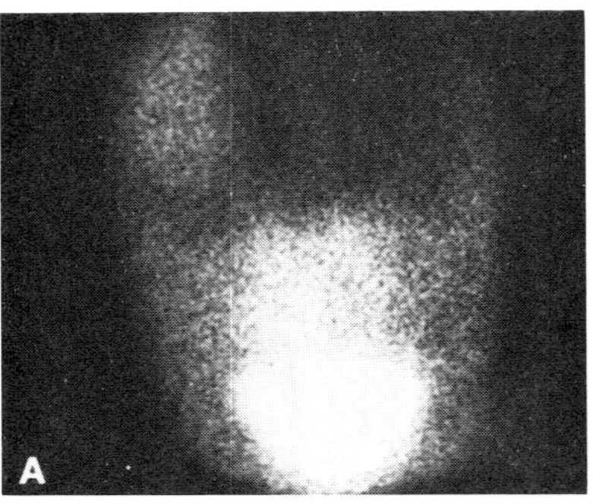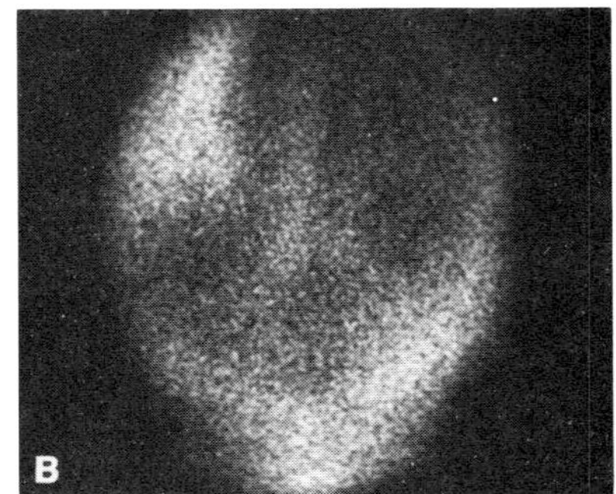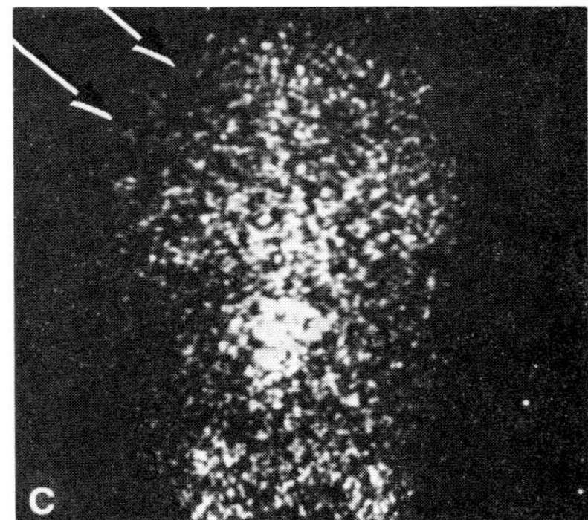

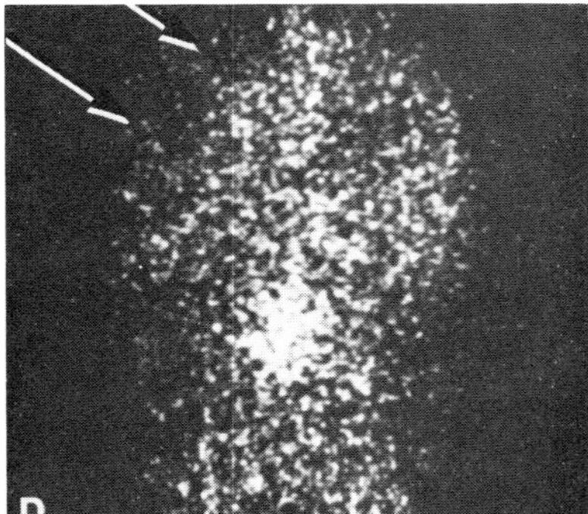

Fig. 4-26. Right subdural hematoma
A and B. Static. There is gross widening and increased activity in the right
perimeter, which does not extend to the floor.
C and D. Flow. The peripheral activity on the right (arrows) is depressed
and does not extend to the perimeter.

If the problem is clinically urgent, angiography
is indicated; if the problem is less pressing, serial
scans can be done, and if these are still negative
after 1 week to 10 days, hematoma probably
does not exist. In chronic problems, particularly
where the history may be vague, the scanning
sequence (flow plus static) is a most valuable
tool. Unless the index of clinical suspicion is
unusually high, a negative examination rarely
requires angiographic confirmation.

Echoencephalography as a screening technique is splendid only when positive. In average
hands, bilateral defects are usually missed since
there may be no obvious midline shift. Also of
particular difficulty for detection are involve-
ments of the frontal lobe.

With certain exceptions, nuclear scanning
procedures where the *why* is infection do not
rate more than a single plus or two. Add one or
two more for abscess and herpes encephalitis.
Abscess presents as a localized process and
when suspected can be recognized with an
accuracy rate of some 95%. The lesion is usually
round and extremely active. When centrally
necrotic the configuration is not unlike a

doughnut (Fig. 4-27). This "Dunkin D" sign may
also be found in degenerating neoplasms, but
the clinical picture is usually sufficiently
distinctive to permit differentiation. Also when
clinically suspected a positive scan in which
the changes are confined to the temporal lobes
may suggest herpes.

Other infectious diseases present nonspecific
findings. Patterns to recognize meningitis of
different etiologies have been described but not
universally verified. But for the heat of the
clinician's breath, associated with corroborative
chemistries and physical findings, the vagaries
on the scan might be easily passed with a shrug
of the shoulder and some garbled explanation to
the resident that some pictures are not as pretty
as others. But with the temperature of those
exhalations to warm the image a diagnosis of
"oh, yes, certainly compatible with a nonspecific
encephalitis" finds its way on to the report.

So, although the bias is not red hot, scanning
does have some value. For abscess, certainly.
It not only confirms the diagnosis but also
suggests a site of drainage if geographically
feasible. For the nonspecific infections, even

Fig. 4-27. Intracerebral abscess
A and B. Static. Large circular zone of
increased activity with a
central lucency in the left
parietal region, resembling a
doughnut

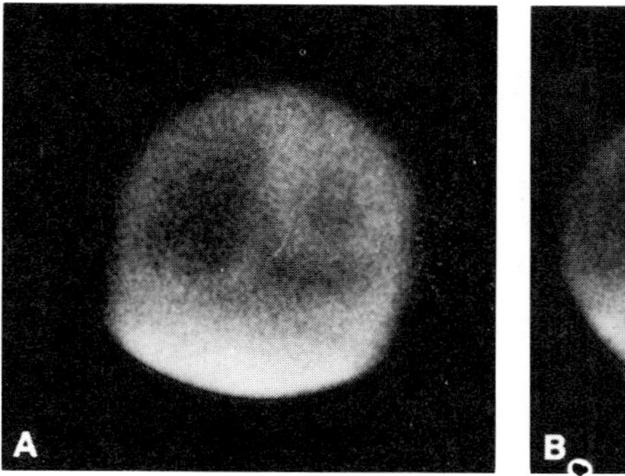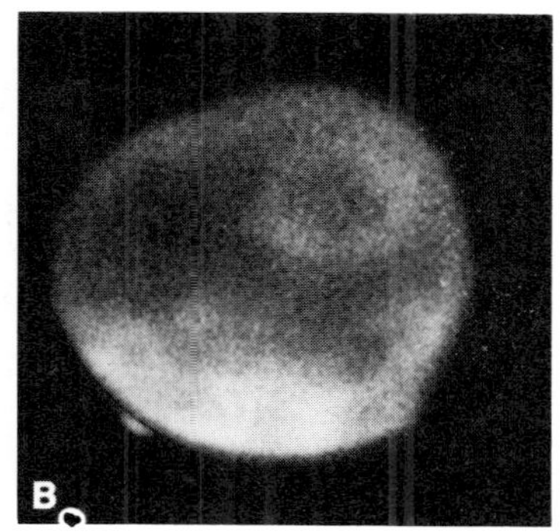

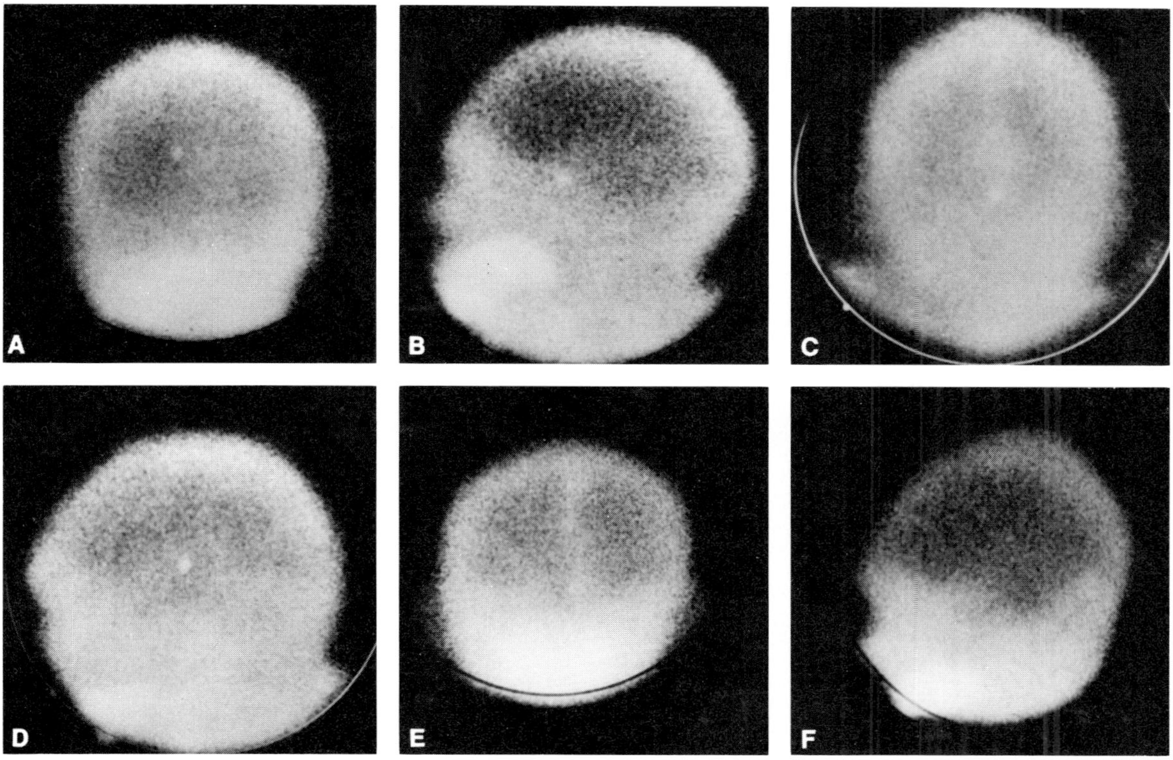

Fig. 4-28. Aseptic meningitis
A and B. Static (6/1/73). Posterior **(A)** and left lateral **(B)** images identify a
homogeneous area of increased activity throughout the left temporoparietal
region.
C and D. Static (6/15/73). 2 weeks later the findings are more abnormal. The entire
lateral hemisphere is "cloudy."
E and F. Static (8/17/73). 2 months later the scans have reverted to normal. The
clinical course and the associated laboratory findings were consistent with
meningitis.

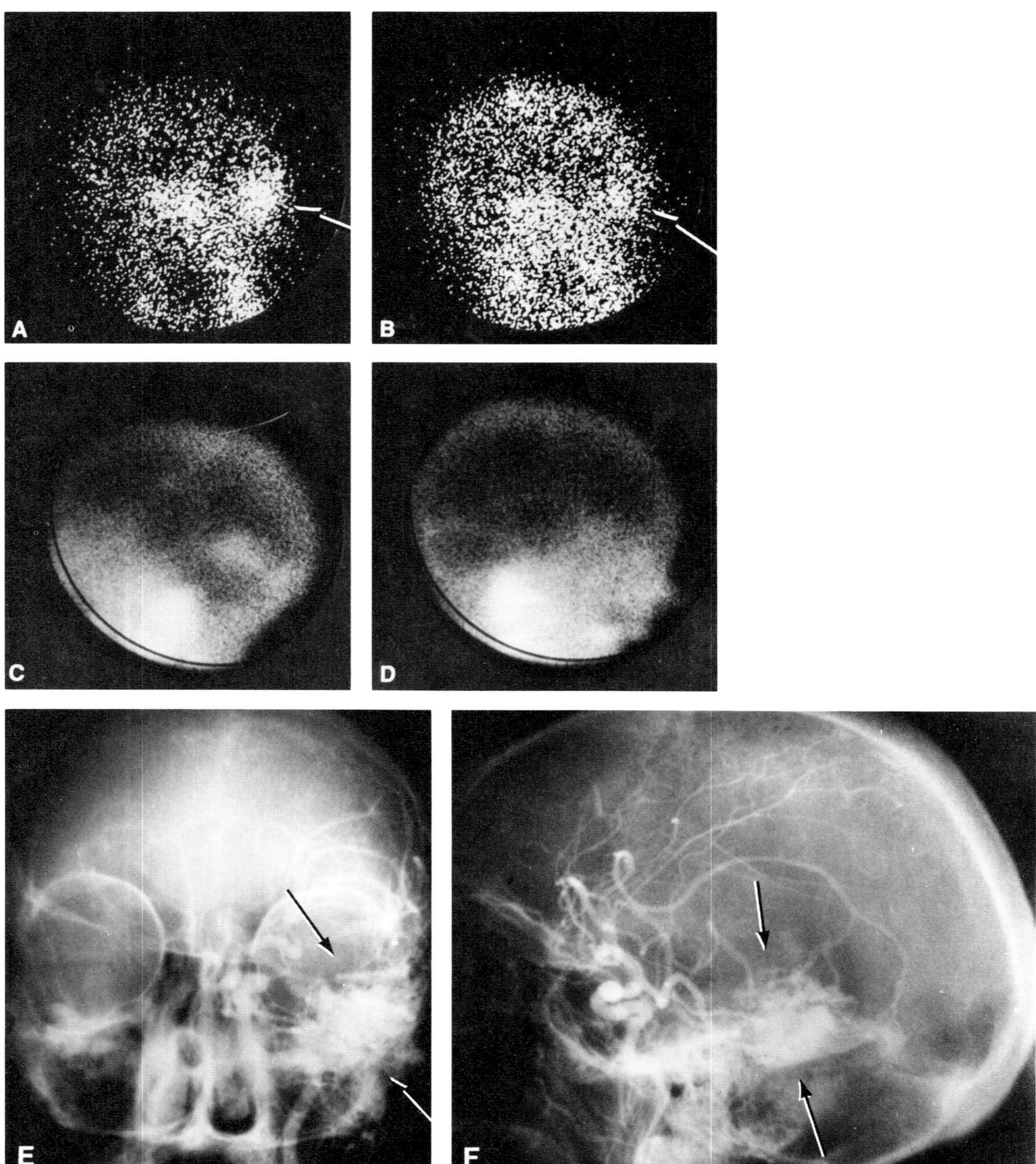

Fig. 4-29. Arteriovenous malformation

    A. Flow. In the early arterial phase there is a hot spot in the left middle cerebral artery distribution (arrow).

    B. Flow. In the venous phase the zone of increased activity (arrow) persists but is less intense.

    C. Static, left lateral. There is an abnormal collection of activity in the region of the transverse sinus.

    D. Static, right lateral. The findings are within normal limits.

E and F. Cerebral arteriogram. Bizarre arteriovenous structures

though the initial scan is vague, serial studies may prove valuable as a guide in monitoring the response to therapy (Fig. 4-28).

Congenital. Certain congenital defects can be recognized with an extremely high order of merit. Of the group, arteriovenous malformation, if studied by rapid flow techniques, yields almost 100% detection. The dynamic approach demonstrates the abnormality as a significantly increased focal zone of activity in the arterial phase. Original descriptions of arteriovenous malformation suggested that the activity fades significantly by the venous phase and the static images will be normal. The roller coaster pattern of a rapid and intense blush followed by an equally rapid detumescence is more characteristic when the malformation is small; when it is large the initial arterial flow will also "light up the burning barn," but there may be no great fading in the venous phase and later static images may be positive. When this combination is encountered it may be indistinguishable from the pattern of abnormality produced by a meningioma, which also "blushes" early and remains positive throughout. When

this differential dilemma exists, review of the conventional skull x rays is occasionally of value. Arteriovenous malformation may produce a subtle mottling and demineralization of the inner table of the calvarium which, though often initially overlooked, may be appreciated on any reinspection required by the scan findings. The arteriovenous malformation is, as a rule, less circumscribed in contour and less predictable in geographic location than is a meningioma. However, contrast angiography easily resolves and lingering differential doubts (Fig. 4-29).

Cystic lesions may be suspected if there is localized hypoactivity, particularly in the infant population. Cisternography may be more appropriate for many of these anomalies, but criteria have been offered for routine scanning for the detection of the Dandy–Walker malformations and congenital arachnoid cysts of the posterior fossa.

It should be noted that scanning is a most valuable diagnostic contribution in pediatrics. Often, the history is vague or unobtainable, and such physical events as seizures, convulsions, irritability, and the like cannot be properly evaluated. When dosage is corrected for weight, no contraindications to the procedure are

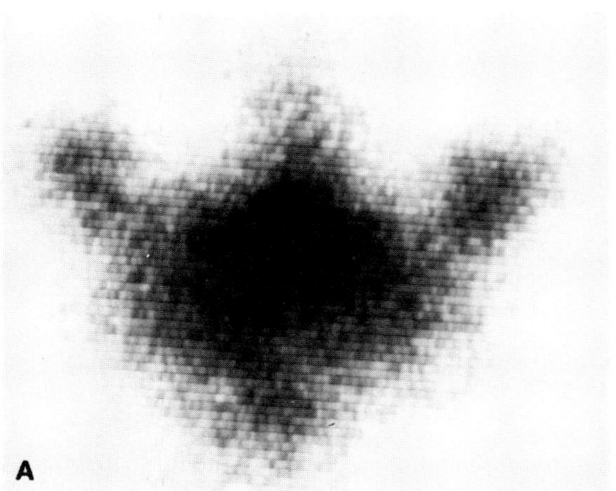
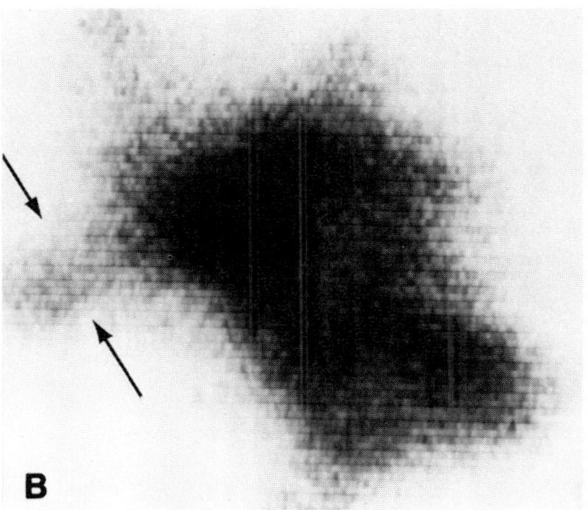

Fig. 4-30. Cerebrospinal fluid rhinorrhea
A and B. Cisternography, 6 hours. Anterior **(A)** and lateral **(B)** views employing ^{111}In DTPA clearly localize an area of atypical activity extending anteriorly to the cribriform plate and draining into the nose (arrows).
(Courtesy of J. Morales, Episcopal Hospital, Philadelphia, Pa.)

recognized. Appropriate sedation may be necessary.

cisternography

Trauma. No better way than cisternography exists for both the confirmation of the true existence and the localization of the site of fistula for suspected CSF rhinorrhea or otorrhea. The technique of examination is geared to the documentation of the process. Results are usually excellent (Fig. 4-30).

Hydrocephalus. The availability of a relatively safe and simple monitoring technique has resulted in a tremendous impetus to the study of CSF dynamics in general and of hydrocephalus in particular. Initially thought to be primarily a pediatric problem, adult forms have been recognized, and more importantly some have proven correctable with dramatic consequences. Normal pressure hydrocephalus is one such condition (Fig. 4-31). The clinical manifestations of progressive dementia, incontinence, apraxia of gait, and pyramidal tract signs are reversable

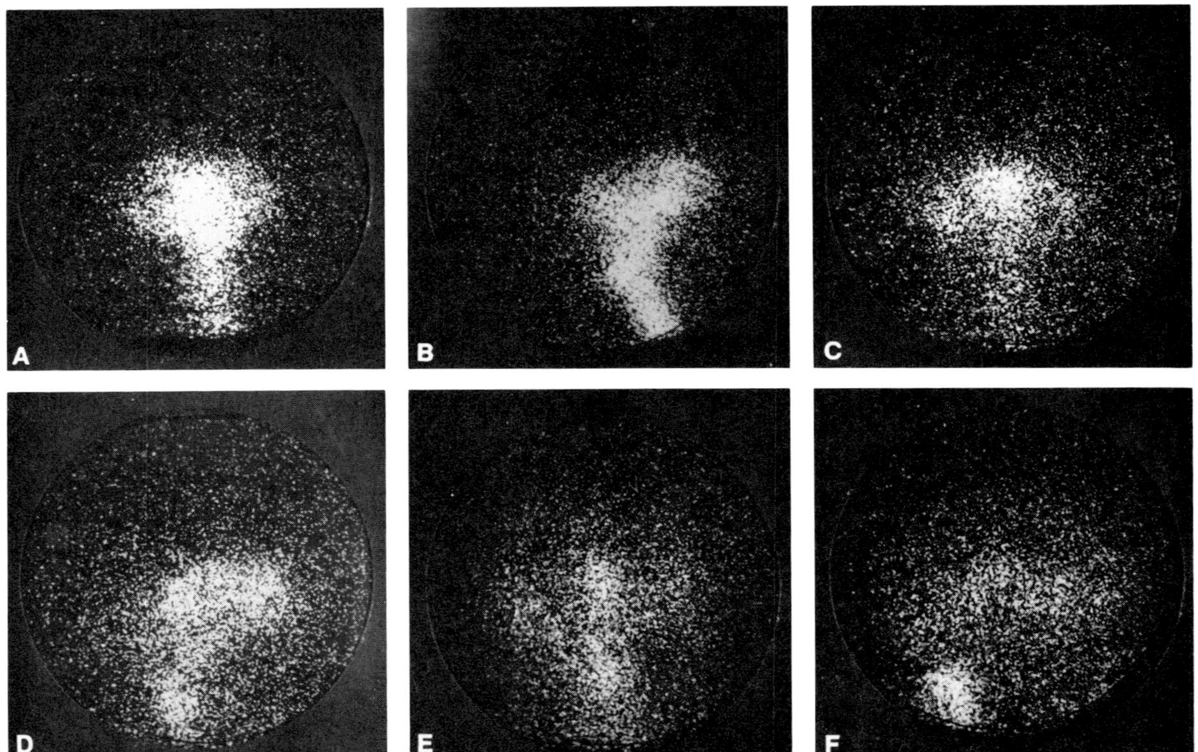

Fig. 4-31. Normal pressure or communicating hydrocephalus
A and B. Cisternography, 1 hour. Anterior **(A)** and lateral **(B)** views identify ascent of nuclide to the basal cisterns. The central activity (particularly in **A**) suggests possible activity in the ventricles.
C and D. Cisternography, 6 hours. There has been little or no cephalad transit. There is definite abnormal communication with the ventricles.
E and F. Cisternography, 48 hours. There is still no cephalad transit to the subarachnoid spaces (see Fig. 4-4).

if recognized before there has been too-extensive brain atrophy. The cisternographic criteria are sufficiently specific to differentiate this type from other nonreversible varieties. However, a normal study does not exclude the presence of correctable communicating hydrocephalus.

Tracer studies have also proven useful in the evaluation of the patency and affectiveness of ventriculoatrial and ventriculoperitoneal shunts.

Space-Occupying Lesions. Cisternography is suitable for the detection of cystic disease, either congenital or acquired. These lesions are identified as an abnormal accumulation of activity. The instilled tracer will flow into every space bathed by the CSF. Congenital arachnoid and Dandy–Walker cysts are readily visualized. Acquired posttraumatic or postinflammatory arachnoid or porencephalic collections are equally well seen.

Cerebrospinal Fluid Flow. Sites of obstruction anywhere in the CNS that are bathed by CSF can be localized. In some countries, particularly Russia, CSF flow studies are utilized routinely for lesions in the vertebral column. This technique has not as yet become popular in the United States but it has been employed on occasion when contrast agents are contraindicated. Isolated reports of detection of vertebral arteriovenous malformations and isolation of spinal cerebrospinal fistulas suggests a mounting interest in the nuclide investigation of the vertebral spaces. The possibility of intracerebral obstruction is usually the motivation for examination. It has proven of value in the detection of subdural hematomas and obstruction secondary to meningitis. It has also been used to evaluate flow following a cerebrovascular accident. Alterations have been observed in a significant number of such patients, and various hypotheses have been offered to explain this phenomenon. Perhaps the best is attributed to decreased regional flow secondary to the cerebral edema that develops within hours of an infarct. The finding raises the question as to whether or not this altered flow in an area of cerebral ischemia has any direct effect or influence on the clinical course or outcome. It is anticipated that a considerable body of data will develop in the near future as this technique gains wider acceptance.

ADDENDUM: NOTE ADDED IN PROOF

And now, having so eloquently and exhaustively described the omniscience of radionuclide screening of the CNS, this chapter should end. However, rumblings just beginning to be heard from the East require some additional remarks.

While we on the Nuclear scene serenely scanned the sensorium in an exalted mood of diagnostic-breakthrough triumph, a technologic explosion was quietly being put together in England. All of Chapter 4 may well be rendered obsolete before it even reaches the light of print by an instrument recently assembled. This mighty colossus is known as a computerized axial tomogram (CAT).

The deficiencies of conventional radiography in the diagnosis of CNS disease were discussed earlier in this section. It was pointed out that x rays of the skull offer very little information as to the integrity of its contents because there is little or no ability to discriminate between the intracranial tissues and the bony calvarium. Radionuclide techniques were successful, to the degree discussed, in identifying changes by imaging the internal distribution pattern of the injected radioisotopes. The creators of CAT have attacked the problem by producing an instrument capable of extraordinary discrimination between tissues of similar photon-absorption coefficients. Scattered radiation, a major culprit in x-ray image degradation, is almost entirely eliminated by the use of an extremely fine x-ray beam. Additionally, the tube moves across the head in a continuing prescribed pattern so that the brain is examined from some 180 different angles. A sodium iodide crystal, rather than film, is the detecting unit, and this moves together with the beam. The resultant information is computerized and after some 28,000 simultaneous equations, an image is generated. Brain sections of approximately 13-mm thickness are thus obtained. The total study produces about eight pictures representing tomographic sections of the entire brain. Approximately 20–30 minutes are required for examination. The radiation load is reported to be no greater than that of a conventional skull x-ray series.

It is still too soon to assess the impact of this instrument. That it will affect present practices is unquestioned. However, how, when, and to what degree is still to be determined.

Table 4-1. Indications, Pharmaceuticals, Methodology and Order of Merit of Radionuclide Study of Brain

Why	What	How	Yea–Nay
Brain			
Mass lesions	^{99m}Tc pertechnetate	dynamic then static	++++
Vascular	^{99m}Tc pertechnetate	dynamic then static	+++
Trauma	^{99m}Tc pertechnetate	dynamic then static	+++
Infection	^{99m}Tc pertechnetate		
Nonspecific	^{99m}Tc pertechnetate	static	+
Abscess	^{99m}Tc pertechnetate	dynamic then static	++++
Congenital	^{99m}Tc pertechnetate	dynamic then static	++++
Cisternography			
Leaks	^{111}In diethylenetriaminepentaacetic acid (DTPA) or	static	++++
Hydrocephalus	^{131}I human serum	static	+++
Mass lesions	albumin	static	++

Table 4-2. More About What

Radiopharmaceutical	Dose (mCi)	Physical Half-life	Energy Peak (keV)
^{99m}Tc pertechnetate	10–15	6 hr	140
^{99m}Tc diethylenetri-aminepentaacetic acid	10–15	6 hr	140
^{99m}Tc glucoheptonate	10–15	6 hr	140
^{203}Hg chlormerodrin	0.7–0.9	46.9 days	279
^{113m}In diethylenetri-aminepentaacetic acid	1–2	104 min	393
^{111}In diethylenetri-aminepentaacetic acid	0.5–2.0	2.8 days	173–247
^{131}I human serum albumin	0.1	8.05 days	364
^{99m}Tc human serum albumin	1–2	6 hr	140
^{169}Yb diethylenetri-aminepentaacetic acid	1–2	31.8 days	198

Why	Prepa-ration	Admin-istra-tion	Time Between Adminis-tration and Exam (hr)	Num-ber of Exams	Time for Each Exam (min)	Time for Total Study (hr)	Patient's Position	Instru-ment
Brain								
Mass	$KClO_4$	IV	dynamic: immed	1	1–2	3–4	supine, sitting,	camera
			static: 1–2	1	20–45		or re-cumbent	camera or scanner
Vascular	$KClO_4$	IV	dynamic: immed	1	1–2	3–4	supine, sitting,	camera
			static: 1–2	1	20–45		or re-cumbent	camera or scanner
Trauma	$KClO_4$	IV	dynamic: immed	1	1–2	3–4	supine, sitting,	camera
			static: 1–2	1	20–45		or re-cumbent	camera or scanner
Infection	$KClO_4$	IV	dynamic: immed	1	1–2	3–4	supine, sitting,	camera
			static: 1–2	1	20–45		or re-cumbent	camera or scanner
Congenital	$KClO_4$	IV	dynamic: immed	1	1–2	3–4	supine, sitting,	camera
			static: 1–2	1	20–45		or re-cumbent	camera or scanner
Cisterno-graphy								
Leaks	none	intra-thecal	1–6	1 or more	1–10	1–6	head depen-dent	camera or scanner
Hydro-cephalus	Lugol's I_2	intra-thecal	1	3 or more	1–10	24–48	sitting or re-cumbent	camera or scanner
Mass	Lugol's I_2	intra-thecal	1	3 or more	1–10	24	sitting or re-cumbent	camera or scanner

BIBLIOGRAPHY

GENERAL

Boller F et al.: Brain scan reliability: correlation with neuropathological data (abstr). J Nucl Med 14(6):381, 1973

Braunstein P et al.: Cerebral death: a rapid and reliable diagnostic adjunct using radioisotopes. J Nucl Med 14(2):122–124, 1973

Cowan RJ et al.: Value of the routine use of the cerebral dynamic radioisotope study. Radiology 107:111–116, 1973

DeLand FH: Nuclear medicine in diseases of the central nervous-system. Hosp Prac, pp. 57–66, December, 1971

DeLand FH, Wagner HN Jr: Brain. In Atlas of Nuclear Medicine, Vol 1. Philadelphia, WB Saunders, 1969

Handa J et al.: Sequential brain imaging as an aid in understanding disease etiology. Semin Nucl Med 1(1):56–69, 1971

James AE, Squire LF: Brain and cerebrospinal fluid. In Nuclear Radiology. Philadelphia, WB Saunders, 1973, pp 156–215

Krishnamurthy GT et al.: Clinical value and limitations of 99mTc brain scan: an autopsy correlation. J Nucl Med 13(6):373–378, 1972

Mahin D, Wagner HN Jr: The value of brain scans in pediatrics. In James AE Jr, Wagner HN Jr, Cooke RE (eds): Pediatric Nuclear Medicine. Philadelphia, WB Saunders, 1974, pp 103–114

Moody RA et al.: Brain scans of the posterior fossa. J Neurosurg 36:148–152, 1972

O'Mara RF, Mozley JM: Current status of brain scanning. Semin Nucl Med 1(1):7–30, 1971

Rosenthall L: Intravenous and intracarotid radionuclide cerebral angiography. Semin Nucl Med 1(1):70–84, 1971

Schall GL, Quinn JK: Brain scanning, in Diagnosis of central nervous system disease. In Blahd WH (ed):

Nuclear Medicine. New York, McGraw–Hill, 1971, pp 236–277

Scheinberg LC, Taylor JM: The importance of brain scanning to the neurologist and neurosurgeon. Semin Nucl Med 1(1):4–6, 1971

Zingesser LH: The brain. In Freeman LM, Johnson PM (eds): Clinical Scintillation Scanning. Hagerstown, Harper & Row, 1969, pp 158–202

PHARMACOLOGY

Buttfield IH et al.: Intravenous perchlorate in brain scanning: effects on choroid plexus and lesion visibility. J Nucl Med 14(7):543–545, 1973

Go RT, Ptacek JJ: Localization of ^{99m}Tc in choroid plexus of the fourth ventricle. J Nucl Med 14(6):352–353, 1973

Jones AE et al.: Brain scintigraphy with ^{99m}Tc pertechnetate, polyphosphate, and ^{67}Ga-citrate (abstr). J Nucl Med 14(6):412–413, 1973

Konikowski T et al.: Kinetics of ^{67}Ga compounds in brain sarcomas and kidneys of mice. J Nucl Med 14(3):164–171, 1973

Oldendorf WH: Distribution of various classes of radio-labeled tracers in plasma, scalp, and brain. J Nucl Med 13(9):681–685, 1972

Schall GL et al.: Clinical comparison of two ^{99m}Tc tracers for brain scanning: pertechnetate versus labeled albumin. Radiology 99:361–368, 1971

SPACE-OCCUPYING LESIONS

Baum S: The site of accumulation of ^{99m}Tc-sodium pertechnetate in brain tumors. Radiology 99:153–155, 1971

Blau M, Bender MA: Radiomercury (^{203}Hg) labeled neohydrin: a new agent for brain tumor localization. J Nucl Med 3: 83, 1962

Fagan JA, Cowan RJ: The effect of potassium perchlorate on the uptake of pertechnetate of ^{99m}Tc-pertechnetate in choroid plexus papillomas: a report of two cases. J Nucl Med 12(6):312–314, 1971

Handel SF et al.: Scintiphotographic evaluation of response of brain neoplasms to systemic chemotherapy. J Nucl Med 12(6):292–296, 1971

Moore GE: Use of radioactive diiodoflurecein in the diagnosis and localization of brain tumors. Science 107:569, 1948

Moore GE et al.: Clinical and experimental studies of intracranial tumors with fluorescein dyes with an additional note concerning the possible use of K^{42} and iodine 131 tagged human albumin. Am J Roentgenol Radium Ther Nucl Med 66:1–8, 1951

Moore J et al.: Positive dynamic radionuclide flow studies in intracranial tumors: correlation with angiographic studies (abstr). J Nucl Med 14(6):430, 1973

Moreno JB, DeLand FH: Brain scanning in the diagnosis of astrocytomas of the brain. J Nucl Med 12(3):107–111, 1971

Palacios E, Lawson RC: Choroid plexus papillomas of the lateral ventricles. Am J Roentgenol Radium Ther Nucl Med 115:113–119, 1972

Schwartz ML, Tator CH: Shortcomings of ^{99m}Tc-pertechnetate as a tracer for brain tumor detection as shown by well counting of human brain tumors and a mouse ependymoblastoma. J Nucl Med 13(5):321–327, 1972

Thompson RW et al.: The diagnostic value of brain scanning in intracranial lymphomas. Radiology 102:111–116, 1972

Tow D: Differentiation of brain and bone tumors with combined radionuclide technique. Semin Nucl Med 1(1):85–89, 1971

Van Houten FX et al.: Negative defect in an intracranial teratoma. J Nucl Med 13(1):122–124, 1972

Vamakli A: The pathological significance of corpus callosum involvement in brain scans. J Nucl Med 13(7):510–516, 1972

Waxman AD et al.: Gallium brain scanning and the differential diagnosis of brain tumors (abstr). J Nucl Med 14(6):463, 1973

VASCULAR

Burke G, Halko A: Cerebral blood flow studies with sodium pertechnetate Tc^{99m} and the scintillation camera. JAMA 204:319–324, 1968

DeLand FH: Scanning in cerebral vascular disease. Semin Nucl Med 1(1):31–40, 1971

Farrer PA et al.: Radiopertechnetate cerebral angiography in the early diagnosis and detection of strokes. J Nucl Med 10:401, 1969

Fisher RJ, Miale A: Evaluation of cerebral vascular disease with radionuclide angiography. Stroke 3:1–9, 1972

Glasgow JL et al.: Brain scans at varied intervals following CVA. J Nucl Med 6:902, 1965

Hawes DR, Mishkin FS: Brain scans in watershed infarction and laminar cortical necrosis. Radiology 103:131–134, 1972

Jhingran SG, Johnson PC: Radionuclide angiography in the diagnosis of cerebrovascular disease. J Nucl Med 14(5):265–268, 1973

Kahn EM, Whitney DG: Operability of the acutely stroked patient as determined by isotope brain scan. Vasc Surg 6:148–150, 1972

Kilgore BB, Bonte FJ: Scintigraphic demonstration of cerebral infarction in a "watershed" distribution. J Nucl Med 12(11):756–757, 1971

Mishkin FS, Dyken ML: Increased early radionuclide activity in the nasopharyngeal area in patients with internal carotid artery obstruction: "hot nose." Radiology 96:77–80, 1970

Moody D et al.: An improved method for visualizing carotid blood flow in the neck. J Nucl Med 12(7):520–522, 1971

Moses DC et al.: Regional cerebral blood flow estimation in the diagnosis of cerebrovascular disease. J Nucl Med 13(2):135–141, 1972

Moses DC et al: Quantitative cerebral circulation studies with sodium pertechnetate. J Nucl Med 14(3):142–148, 1973

Samuels LD: Scan visualization of mycotic aneurysm of a branch of right middle cerebral artery. J Nucl Med 13(9):695–696, 1972

TRAUMA

Gilday DL et al.: Subdural hematoma—what is the role of brain scanning in its diagnosis? J Nucl Med 14(5):283–287, 1973

Gilson AJ, Gargana FP: Correlation of brain scans and angiography in intracranial trauma. Am J Roentgenol Radium Ther Nucl Med 94:819–827, 1965

Holloway W et al.: Doughnut sign in subdural hematomas. J Nucl Med 13(8): 630–632, 1972

Hopkins GB, Kristensen KAB: Rapid sequential scintiphotography in the radionuclide detection of subdural hematomas. J Nucl Med 14(5):288–290, 1973

Hurley PJ: Effect of craniotomy on the brain scan related to time elapsed after surgery. J Nucl Med 13(2):156–158, 1972

Hurwitz SR: Brain scanning and echoencephalography in the diagnosis of chronic subdural hematoma (abstr). J Nucl Med 14(6):410, 1973

Liebeskind AL et al.: Radionuclide demonstration of spinal dural leaks. J Nucl Med 14(6):356–358, 1973

O'Mara RE et al.: The "doughnut" sign in cerebral radioisotopic images. Radiology 92:581–586, 1969

Perkerson RB et al.: The rim sign of subdural hematoma. J Nucl Med (13(8):637–639, 1972

Yeh S–H et al.: Delayed ^{99m}Tc brain scanning in the detection of chronic subdural hematoma (abstr). J Nucl Med 14(6):467, 1973

Zingesser LH: Scanning in diseases of the subdural space. Semin Nucl Med 1(1):41–47, 1971

INFECTION AND OTHER DISEASES

Fowler GW, Williams JP: Technetium brain scans in tuberous sclerosis. J Nucl Med 14(4):215–217, 1973

Jordan CE et al.: Comparison of the cerebral angiogram and the brain radionuclide image in brain abscess. Radiology 104:327–332, 1972

Lisbona R et al.: Aspergillomatous abscesses of the brain and thyroid. J Nucl Med 14(7):541–542, 1973

Maroon JC et al.: Tuberculous meningitis diagnosed by brain scan. Radiology 104:333–335, 1972

McLaughlin AF et al.: Brain scanning in intracranial infection (abstr). J Nucl Med 13(6):451, 1972

Moses DC et al.: Brain scanning with ^{99m}TcO$_4$-in multiple sclerosis. J Nucl Med 13(11):847–848, 1972

Radcliffe WB et al.: Herpes simplex encephalitis: a radiologic–pathologic study of 4 cases. Am J Roentgenol Radium Ther Nucl Med 112:263–272, 1971

Weisbaum SD, Garnett ES: Brain scan in Schilder's disease. J Nucl Med 14(5):291–292, 1973

CONGENITAL DEFECTS

Binet EF, Loken MK: Scintiangiography of cerebral arteriovenous malformations and aneuryisms. Am J Roentgenol Radium Ther Nucl Med 109:707–713, 1970

Conway JJ et al.: Radionuclide evaluation of Dandy–Walker malformation and congenital arachnoid cyst of the posterior fossa. Am J Roentgenol Radium Ther Nucl Med 112:306–314, 1971

Kuhl DE et al.: The brain scan in Sturge–Weber syndrome. Radiology 103:621–626, 1972

Rosenthall L: Radionuclide diagnosis of arteriovenous malformations with rapid sequence brain scans. Radiology 91:1185–1188, 1968

MISCELLANEOUS

Bernstein JR et al.: Accuracy of the delayed scan in differentiating calvarial from cerebral lesions (abstr). J Nucl Med 14(6):380, 1973

Gilday DL et al.: Comparison of techniques for obtaining the vertex view in brain scanning. J Nucl Med 11:503–507, 1970

Holmes RA: Value of the vertex view in brain scanning. Semin Nucl Med 1(1):48–55, 1971

Kuhl DE et al.: Transverse section and rectilinear brain scanning with Tc^{99m} pertechnetate. Radiology 86:822–829, 1966

Kuhl DE, Sanders TP: Characterizing brain lesions with use of transverse section scanning. Radiology 98:317–328, 1971

New PFJ et al.: Computerized axial tomography with the EMI scanner. Radiology 110:109–123, 1974

Park CH, Mansfield CM: Comparison of autofluoroscope brain imaging with rectilinear scanning and neuroradiologic examination. J Nucl Med 13(8):582–584, 1972

Ramsey RG, Quinn JL: Comparison of accuracy between initial and delayed ^{99m}Tc-pertechnetate brain scans. J Nucl Med 13(2):131–134, 1972

CISTERNOGRAPHY

Alazraki NP et al.: Hyberbaric cisternography: experience in humans. J Nucl Med 14(4):226–229, 1973

Banerji MA, Spencer RP: Letter: Febrile response to cerebrospinal fluid flow studies. J Nucl Med 13(8):655, 1972

Cooper JF, Harbert JC: Bacterial endotoxin as a cause of aseptic meningitis following radionuclide cisternography (abstr). J Nucl Med 14(6):387, 1973

DeLand FH: Biological behavior of ^{169}Yb-DTPA after intrathecal administration. J Nucl Med 14(2):93–98, 1973

DiChiro G, Ashburn WL: Radioisotope cisternography, ventriculography, and myelography, in Diagnosis of central nervous system disease. In Blahd WH (ed): Nuclear Medicine. New York, McGraw–Hill, 1971, pp 277–294

DiChiro G et al.: Radioisotope angiography of the spinal cord. J Nucl Med 13(7):567–569, 1972

Gilday DL, Kellan J: Use of ^{111}In-DTPA to evaluate CSF diversionary shunts in children (abstr). J Nucl Med 14(6):399, 1973

Goluboff LG: Arachnoid cyst of the posterior fossa demonstrated by isotope cisternography. J Nucl Med 14(1):61–62, 1973

Halpern SE et al.: Changes in the radioisotope cisternogram in cerebrovascular-occlusive disease. J Nucl Med 13(7):493–497, 1972

Halpern S et al.: Hyperbaric cisternography: studies in an inanimate model and monkeys. J Nucl Med 14(4):223–225, 1973

Harbert JC: Radionuclide cisternography. Semin Nucl Med 1(1):90–106, 1971

Harbert JC, James AE Jr: Posterior fossa abnormalities demonstrated by cisternography. J Nucl Med 13(1):73–80, 1972

Harbert JC et al.: Comparison between ^{131}I-IHSA and ^{169}Yb-DTPA for cisternography (abstr). J Nucl Med 14(6):405, 1973

James AE et al.: A cisternographic classification of hydrocephalus. Am J Roentgenol Radium Ther Nucl Med 115:39–49, 1972

Jonas S, Braunstein P: Neurogenic bladder as a complication of isotope cisternography. J Nucl Med 13(10):763–764, 1972

Kieffer SA et al.: Scinticisternography in progressive dementia: correlation with clinical findings, pneumo-encephalography, and results of shunt procedures (abstr). J Nucl Med 14(6):415, 1973

Larson SM et al.: The influence of previous lumbar puncture and pneumoencephalography on the incidence of unsuccessful radioisotope cisternography. J Nucl Med 12(8):555–557, 1971

Larson SM et al.: Radionuclide ventriculography (abstr). J Nucl Med 13(6):448, 1972

What accounts for the magic of the "perfect pair"? The match that was made in heaven? The devine couple? What accounts for a Romeo and Juliet? a Tristan and Isolda? Willie Mays and a baseball? John Wayne and a horse? peanut butter and jelly? gin with anything? No, dear reader, do not hope for an answer here for they represent the stuff of which dreams are made.

But there is a marriage that until recently had all of the appearances of "made in heaven" which is capable of analysis: x ray to bone.

From the 1890s, when Wilhelm Konrad Roentgen uttered those memorable words, "Don't breathe and don't move," until the 1950s this was the ultimate union of a diagnostic modality to an organ system. If x rays were good for anything, bones were *numero uno* and the *why* was even understood! The image or x-ray picture produced by passing a stream of photons through an object is dependent on the differential absorption of those photons by the object's component parts and since bone has the highest coefficient of absorption of all tissue, its image is, as a rule, sharply defined and clearly separable from surrounding less-dense structures. Fewer photons will pass through and the resulting film image will be white or whiter than those tissues allowing greater transmission and consequently increased film blackening. Thus the love affair. When diagnosis referable to the skeletal system was indicated, it was the radiologist rather than the clinical pathologist who invariably got the first call. Not that certain laboratory studies are not of value, but unquestionably it was the x ray that got down to the bare bones of the problem.

Time and familiarity have the troublesome habit of identifying flaws weaknesses, and deficiencies even in the most perfect alliance. Despite the continual improvement of picture clarity resulting from ever more-sophisticated technology and the earlier detection of subtler diseases by the sophisticated radiologist, mumblings began to be heard in the land.

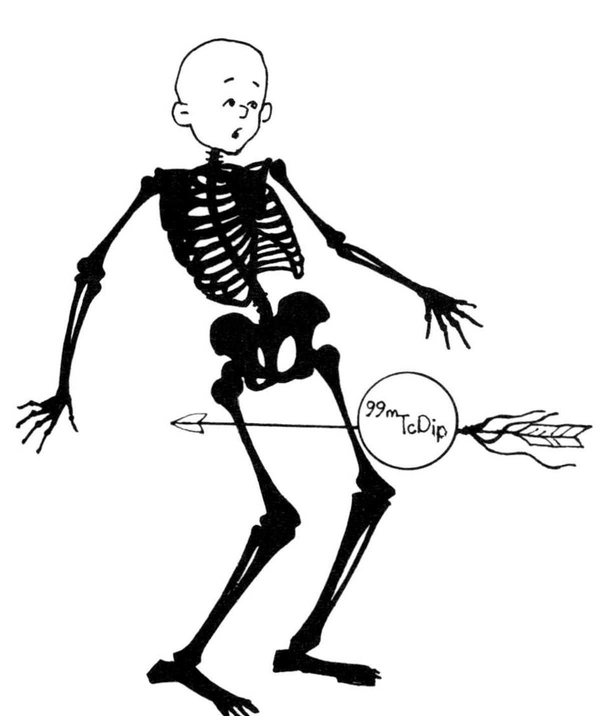

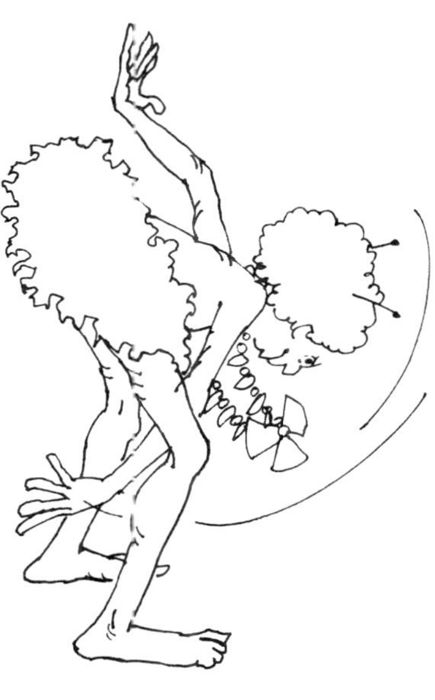

chapter 5

bone

The natives who were growing the most restless were the oncologists and oncologic surgeons, whose misgivings stemmed from almost daily occurrences of which the following is a fair representative sample. A 38-year-old female presents with a breast mass. Examination suggests a stage I process. All other studies indicate a confined problem. One of these "other studies" consists of a skeletal survey or metastatic series (the name varies from one institution to the next, but the study itself consists of a combination of views of the entire or almost entire skeleton to rule out osseous extension). Surgery is successful. Postoperative radiation therapy (if such is the practice in that particular institution) is uneventful. Yet, several months later the patient complains of skeletal pain, and now x rays are abnormal. The same chain of events can be cited changing the primary to the lungs, kidneys, thyroid, prostate, or lymphatics.

What went wrong? Was the surgery imprecise? Did the radiation fail? Was the radiologist careless? The answer slowly evolved as (d)— none of the above. The bone was already invaded by the time of original diagnosis, but the skeletal x rays were insufficiently sensitive to detect the early disease.

Wow! The situation was analogous to the ace of the pitching staff walking the end of the batting order with none out. A hurry-up call went out to the bull-pen: enter Mr. Nuclear Medicine.

With the realization that it was impossible to rely on x rays to identify early and usually unsymptomatic osseous metastasis it became imperative to identify a reliable technique. Much of the problem has been solved with radioactive nuclides and scanning, and the explanation of why this modality is successful where x ray has failed is becoming clearer. Measurements of roentgen sensitivity on the detectability of bone lesions has established that defects in spongy bone are much more difficult to identify than lesions in compact bone. Holes less than 1.5 cm in diameter experimentally drilled into vertebral bodies may go undetected, whereas small fissures produced in the cortex of the skull are easily seen. Other studies suggest that 33%– 50% of the depth of a vertebral body had to be lost before it was appreciated and that 50%– 75% of its spongy matrix were destroyed before lytic lesions were recognized. In general, it has been determined that over 50% depletion in bone calcium is necessary to obtain an x-ray

positive finding of a lytic defect, and an increase of 30%–50% over normal calcium content must exist to visualize a blastic process.

Scanning techniques treat bone not as an intersupporting structure but as an active organ system serving to regulate certain blood constituents, among these calcium, phosphorus, and hydrogen ion. In its role as a supporting framework, calcium salts are deposited in the matrix, which in turn functions as a calcium reservoir. Bone salt deposition and dissolution are normally in balance. Modeling and turnover takes place on the surface of the bone in the hydroxyapatite crystals. The comparatively small size of the crystals results in a correspondingly large surface area and establishes conditions for ion exchange of considerable reactivity. Localized increases in surface area resulting in a corresponding increase in the ion exchange at the altered site occurs as new bone is formed (radiodensities), even if bone is simultaneously being destroyed (radiolucencies).

The pathway of the exchange process has been meticulously tracked. In minutes exchangeable ions pass from the plasma through the extracellular fluid space into the special hydration shell that surrounds each bone crystal. Movement is then to the surface of the crystal, which requires hours, and finally into the crystal interior, which occurs during the next day, days, or weeks.

Thus, a mechanism becomes available to detect and measure the transfer rates, identify regions of altered exchange, and essentially detect matrix formation and resorption. Its dynamic aspect should prove to be more sensitive than x-ray to early or minimal changes.

All that was left before Go was the identification of a suitable radioactive ion that would exchange identically to the normal ionic constituents. The constituents of the hydroxyapatite crystal were calcium, phosphorus, oxygen, and hydrogen, $3Ca_3 (PO_4)_2 \cdot Ca (OH)_2$. Initial measurements with ^{32}P and ^{45}Ca proved the feasibility of scanning with this mineral. Unfortunately, each proved to be a pure beta emitter and thus essentially useless for external counting systems. In 1961, ^{85}Sr was suggested for use in photoscanning, and this proved to be a workable radioactive nuclide that satisfies the basic criteria for acceptability. It is capable of ion exchange with both stable strontium and calcium. It is a gamma emitter. It is readily available, and thus economically feasible. Bone imaging became a viable diagnostic entity. But the idyll was short-lived because ^{85}Sr was long-lived, its half-life being a horrendous 64 days! As a consequence, administered doses are in the μCi range (very, very small) to protect against inordinate whole body exposure. Its use is also restricted to patients with known malignancy. Only limited body areas can be examined at any given time because the length of the examination period is painfully long as a consequence of the low administered dose. Imaging of only the lumbar spine and pelvis as an example, averages 1–2 hours. Thus, only symptomatic areas or those suspected from previous x-ray study can be looked at. Another less than ideal attribute of this agent is its high gamma energy (513 keV), making it unsuitable for imaging with camera systems and further restricting its use.

WHAT

But from little acorns grow mighty whole body scans. As has been noted before, the genius of the radiopharmacologist took over and a host of more desirable agents are now available. It is needless to catalogue their numbers (see Table 5-2). Suffice it to identify those which at this moment are in the ascendancy. The technetium phosphate compounds, *i.e.,* polyphosphate (^{99m}Tc Sn PPO$_4$), pyrophosphate (^{99m}Tc Sn-PyP), ethylene diphosphonate (^{99m}Tc Sn-EHDP), methylene diphosphonate (^{99m}Tc Sn-MHDP), seem to have eclipsed fluorine (^{18}F) in the nuclear scene. At this moment the battle rages over the relative superiority of one phosphate over the other. Which of these complexes will emerge the winner is of no particular importance here. Indeed, it would not be at all surprising or without precedent if none of the above survived as the "one and only." We call that progress.

What is of inestimable importance is that these agents have opened up the world of bone imaging. Because of their very short half-lifes (1.8 hours for ^{18}F and 6 hours for ^{99m}Tc) high doses can be administered without fear of undue whole body radiation. Thus, mCi amounts (1000 $\times$ μCi) are permissible. This in turn markedly reduces the time of examination, so that now the entire skeleton can be imaged in less time than previously took for the limited area of concern. A whole body scan with either rectilinear or camera technique can be accomplished in less than 1 hour, and most important: the images are of remarkable detail and quality.

Another positive spin-off has been the broadening of indications. With diminished concern over radiation exposure, examination can be performed for other than metastatic searches and in all individuals rather than just those known to harbor a malignancy. Any unexplained site of skeletal symptomatology is fair game for scan review, and interest is growing in the evaluation of infectious processes, the age of traumatic lesions (particularly vertebral compression fractures), the differentiation of traumatic from pathologic fractures, the identification and selection of appropriate sites for biopsy, the evaluation of pediatric skeletal lesions, portal planning in radiation therapy, and even the study of extraosseous and soft tissue abnormalities.

However, this new ability to image the entire body, not merely the symptomatic site or the x-ray positive zone, validates again the unwritten 11th commandment: Thou mayest not accept something for nothing. The payment for this expanded vista is increased diagnostic difficulty and even misdiagnosis. Constantly to be stressed is the complete nonspecificity of increased radioisotopic uptake. A positive scan does not mean malignancy! Also to be borne in mind is that increased uptake can occur in tissues other than bone. Initially this was a shocker. One's head was turned on to the skeleton because that was what the requisition asked for and that was what the study was called, consequently, anything active in the picture had to be bone. Well, that thing called "literature" began to spew forth reports that sounded like something from Porgy and Bess—"It ain't necessarily so." Metastatic osteogenic sarcomatous lesions to the lungs were detectable. Okay, that's almost like bone. The rare osteogenic primaries arising in the soft tissue, *e.g.,* muscle and even small bowel, trap positively. Still okay, because that still was like bone. But then the dam broke. Soft tissue calcifications from many sources were capable of elevated accumulation. This was particularly evident in patients on renal dialysis or in chronic renal failure with development of soft tissue calcifications, especially in the lungs. Several cases of positive trapping in cerebral infarcts were reported, thus raising the specter of a false positive diagnosis of metastatic calvarial changes. Increased uptake has been recognized in healing wounds, irradiated tissue, sites of recent bone extraction and marrow aspiration, calcific tendinitis, soft tissue melanomas, and even in breast malignancies.

So life has been made more difficult for the intrepid nuclear interpreter, but his philosophic credo has always been and must continue to be: "Tis better to have scanned and erred than never to have scanned at all!"

HOW

There has been an associated change in the *how* if the shorter-lived agents are used. It is no longer necessary to wait days between the administration of the radioactive nuclide and the examination. Study can be initiated in 1–3 hours after administration. It is no longer necessary to perform rigorous bowel cleansing since these agents are primarily excreted by the urinary tract. Since the root of the excretion is renal, some advocate forced hydration immediately after the radioisotope is given to accelerate renal clearance and reduce renal and bladder background at the time of imaging. However, most do not feel this is of particular merit and thus no patient preparation is really necessary. Administration is almost routinely by the IV route, although ^{18}F can be given orally. Positioning is usually supine or prone.

The time and ease of examination depends on the scanning instrument. If a rectilinear unit with minification potential is available, the entire skeletal system from head to toe can be scanned in approximately 1 hour. If a dual system is used, the anterior and posterior views are obtained simultaneously with the patient supine. Minification is the term applied to the electronic trickery learned from the original head-shrinkers (the curare dart-blowers rather than the Valium couch-crouchers) that permits the image to be rendered either ½ or ⅕ actual size (Figs. 5-1 and 5-2). The advantage of this reduction is time. A 1:1 whole body scan requires 4+ hours, as opposed to approximately 1 hour for the ⅕ th size.

If the study is performed with the conventional gamma camera, multiple views are necessary to record the entire skeleton. The patient must be moved repetitively, and the examination is longer. Also, and annoying to some, is that the presentation is a number of small geographic segments as opposed to a single total image.

The image now obtained by either instrument is an excellent skeletal reproduction. Anatomic detail is often exquisite, and on a clear day it is

Fig. 5-1. Normal skeletal scans (posterior)
  A. 5:1 minification employing ^{99m}Tc polyphosphate. There is considerable activity within the urinary bladder.
  B. 2:1 minification. The pelvis and lower extremities must be viewed separately.
C and D. Selected views of the dorsal and lumbar spine employing a gamma camera. 8–12 individual views are required for total skeletal imaging.

Fig. 5-2. Normal skeletal scans (anterior)
  A. 5:1 minification employing ^{99m}Tc polyphosphate
  B. 2:1 minification
C and D. gamma camera

not uncommon to see even the vertebral pedicles and individual ribs. The activity, with only a few exceptions, is uniformly distributed. Certain sites will exhibit greater activity and must not be confused with abnormal trapping, *e.g.*, the ends of long bones (particularly the distal femurs and proximal tibias), the opposing margins of the sacroiliac joint, the vertebral angles of the scapuli. Certain anatomic relationships produce apparent intensity changes as one body part is closer to the instrument than another, *e.g.*, the dorsal kyphosis and lumbar lordosis bring some vertebral segments nearer to the anterior probe and some to the posterior.

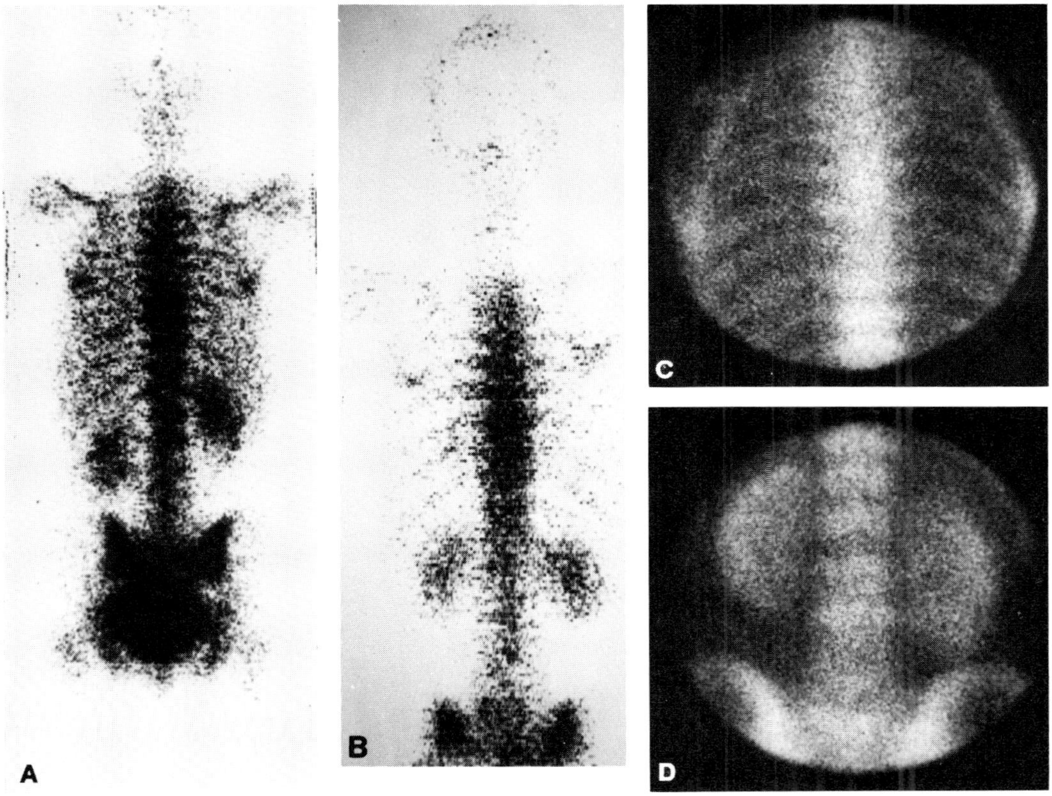

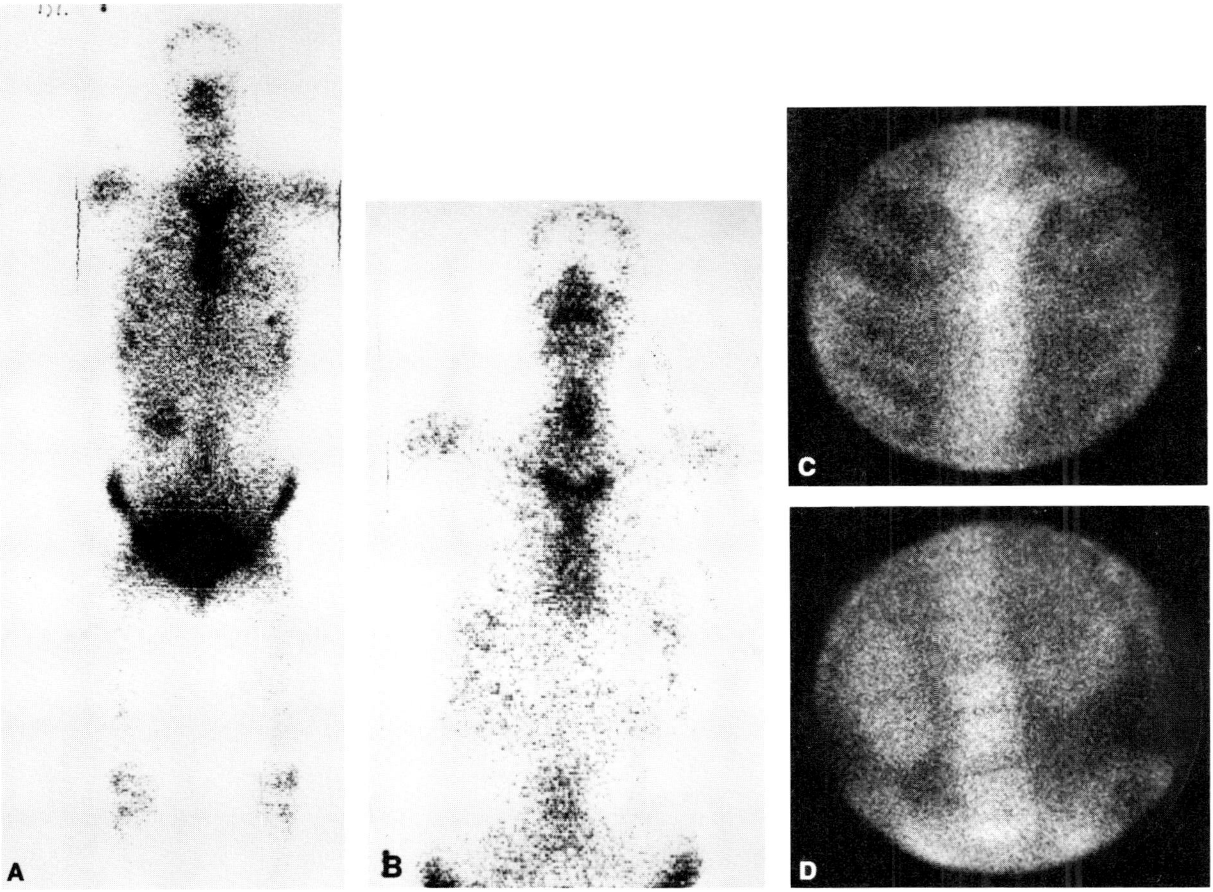

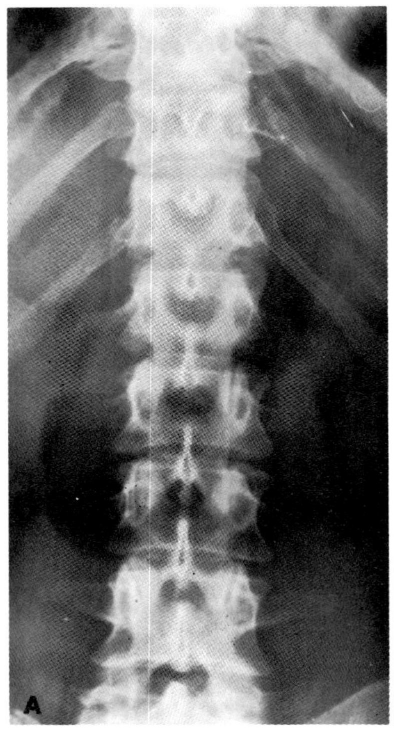
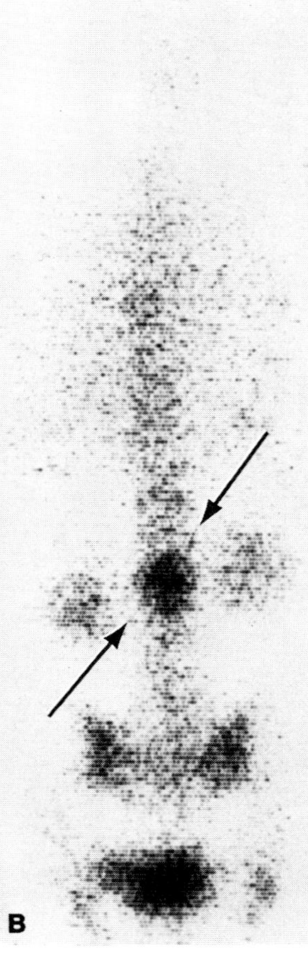

Fig. 5-3. Breast carcinoma with osseous metastasis
A. X ray, anteroposterior. The lumbar spine reveals no evidence of metastatic invasion. The study was performed as a routine metastatic series following the clinical diagnosis of breast carcinoma and in anticipation of curative surgery. The patient was symptom free.
B. Scan, posterior. Abnormal trapping activity at the first and second lumbar level (arrows)

WHY

metastatic mass

Once a primary malignancy has been established the therapeutic protocol is totally dependent on whether or not the tumor is localized. Thus, all the big guns are activated to validate this judgment. To this end, the skeletal system, a most common site of metastatic spread, is scrutinized. A most common, but by no means universal, approach is to perform a screening x-ray examination of the skeleton in an effort to rule out invasion. These search missions, which are designated in some institutions as "metastatic series," in others "skeletal surveys," fall into the category of routine work-up. It is of no consequence that the patient may have no skeletal symptoms. The order is inviolate: given a positive histology for a pulmonary or breast primary, get a skeletal survey!

Although not to suggest criticism since as with so many routinized procedures the motivating intent is noble, reexamination of the net yield of these routines often suggests that they do not best fulfill the initial intent. So, too, with the routine "metastatic series." When the patient is asymptomatic for bone pain the x ray yield in this routinely studied group approaches zero. This is not to suggest that the absence of pain is synonymous with the absence of skeletal invasion. It does suggest that there is a correlation between pain and the extent of invasion sufficient to be x ray detectable. When osseous metastasis has occurred but has produced as yet insufficient destruction to cause symptoms, it has probably produced insufficient destruction to be x ray detectable. Thus, in early metastasis the patient can be symptomatic and the x rays normal. But, and now hear this, the scans can be positive (Figs. 5-3 and 5-4). Therefore, we propose the following course (the exceptions to this routine will be identified at the end) in the work-up of the patient with a proven primary not only of the breast and lung but also of the thyroid, kidney, intestinal tract, or lymphomas.

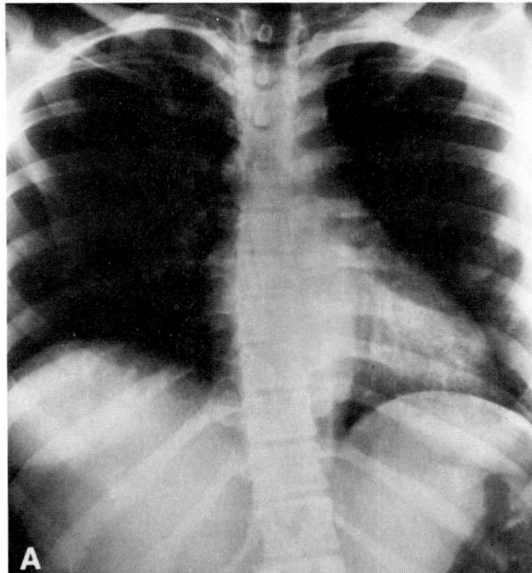

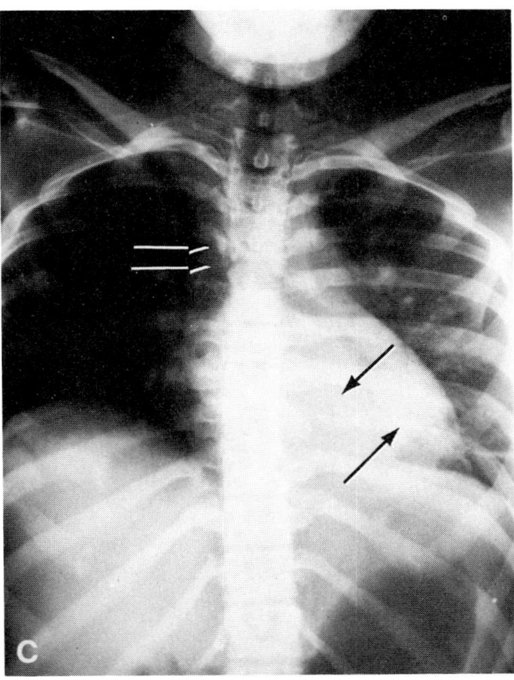

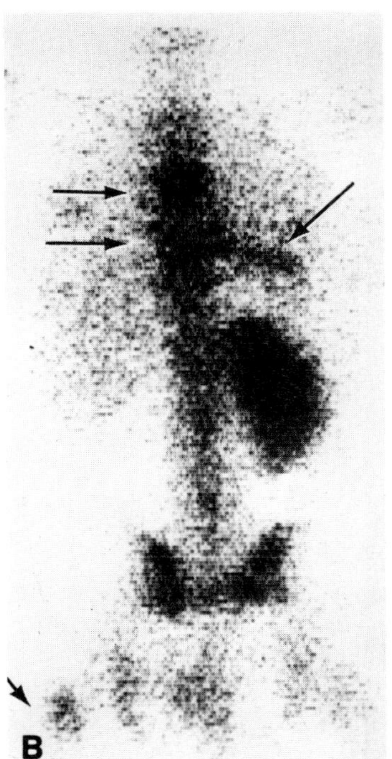

Fig. 5-4. Breast carcinoma with osseous metastasis not found in x ray

A. X ray (6/26/73). The dorsal spine and ribs are considered to be within normal limits in the screening survey for this patient with suspected breast carcinoma.

B. Scan (6/28/73). The posterior 2:1 scan identified multiple abnormal trapping sites. There are defects in the mid-dorsal group and changes in a left rib (probably 7th or 8th) and the greater trochanter region of the right femur. Additionally, the right kidney is not identified. (The scan findings initiated a review of the x rays, and the 8th left rib was then found to be questionable.)

C. X ray (8/30/73). Two months later the patient began to experience back and rib pain. The body of D4 exhibits early demineralization, D5 is sclerotic, and the posterior aspect of the 8th left rib is destroyed.

Skeletally Asymptomatic. In this group we suggest only a whole body bone scan. If that study is within normal limits, no further skeletal search is required. If the scan identifies a positive or even a suspicious area, conventional x rays of that area are mandatory. It cannot be stated too often that a positive scan is not synonymous with metastasis! Differences in scan activity merely reflect differences in ion-exchange rates. The ends of bones normally exhibit a greater exchange than the shaftal portion and therefore will normally be more active or hotter than the diaphyses. Similarly, any disease that affects cellular physiology will affect the scan's homogeneity. Thus, infection, trauma, primary bone involvement, and even extraosseous factors can all affect the local environment to produce a positive scan image. The conventional x ray works to define these mechanisms. Frequently, nonmetastatic etiologies that affect the scan are x-ray detectable. Thus, the scan hot spot may be explained by a

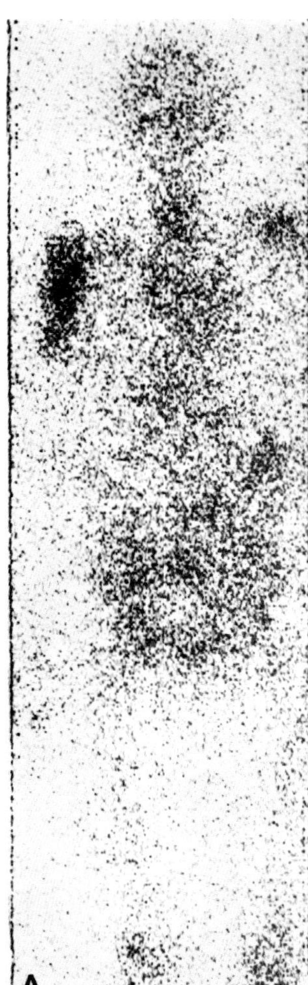

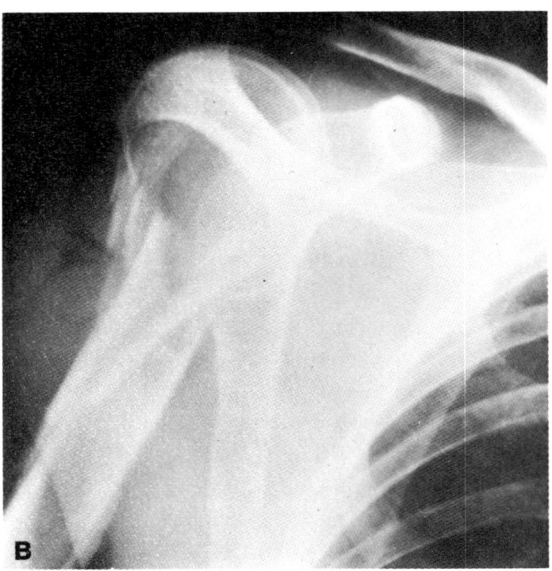

Fig. 5-5. Healing fracture
A. Scan. An alcoholic and poor historian had a history of bronchogenic carcinoma and was hospitalized because of right shoulder pain. The ⁸⁵Sr image identifies a grossly abnormal uptake in the right humerus.
B. X ray. Healing fracture of the right humerus

healing fracture forgotten by the patient since it became asymptomatic (Fig. 5-5), a localized or even diffuse Paget's disease of bone (Fig. 5-6), periosteal changes consistent with pulmonary osteoarthropathy, a site of recent tooth extraction (Fig. 5-7), and even by a subclinical arthritis (Fig. 5-8). On the other hand, an essentially negative roentgenogram of a scan positive site adds fuel to the metastatic fires and suggests a logical site of biopsy.

Skeletally Symptomatic. When this condition prevails we recommend definitive x rays of the symptomatic regions and a whole body scan. The reasons have already been defined. The site of symptomatology will be "doubly" evaluated, and if metastasis is present, other as yet nonsymptomatic areas may be discovered (Fig. 5-9).

This approach also diminishes the number of "goofs" which can occur and which are so

gleefully referred to at such seats of erudition as Tumor Boards or Department of Surgery Meetings. What is the "goof" and how is it rationalized?

In a small percentage of primary malignancies, estimated in some reports as 3%–5%, there will be clear-cut evidence of metastatic bone invasion on x ray though the scan is normal. In another small percentage of malignancies with total skeletal invasion, the scan will be interpreted as normal. In such marrow invasive disorders as multiple myeloma or eosinophilic granuloma the x rays may be horrendous though the scan is reported as normal.

Would that we could say it isn't so, but it is. At least partial explanations are available. The vast majority (and let not the word vast suggest large numbers of cases for indeed the numbers are small) of the x-ray positive–scan negative situations arise when the x-ray defect is of a

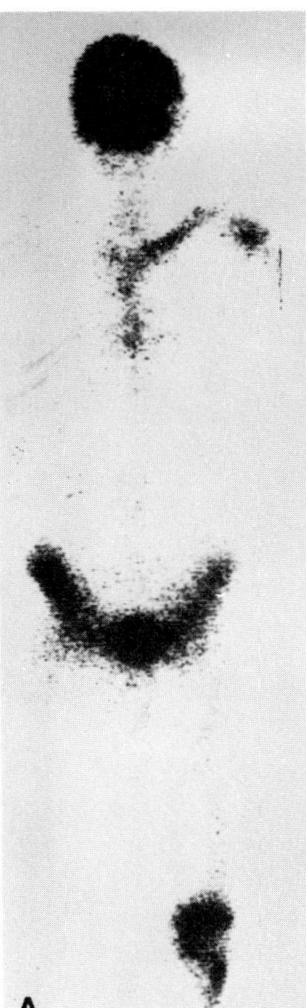
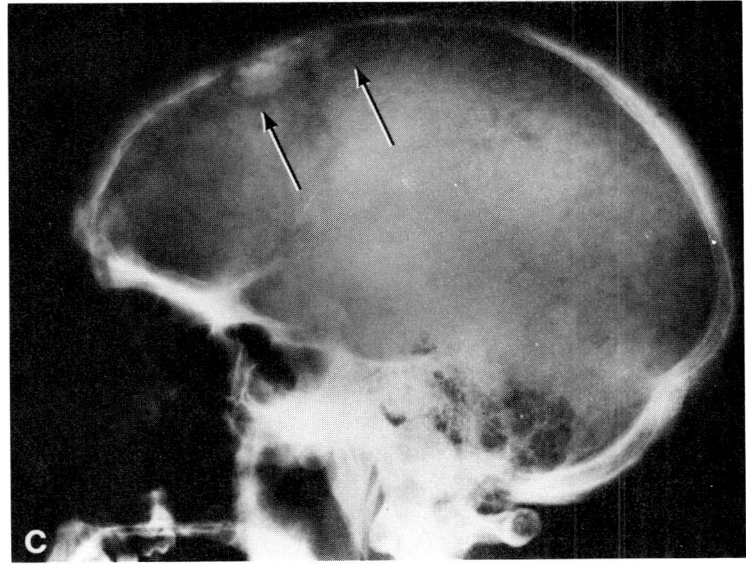
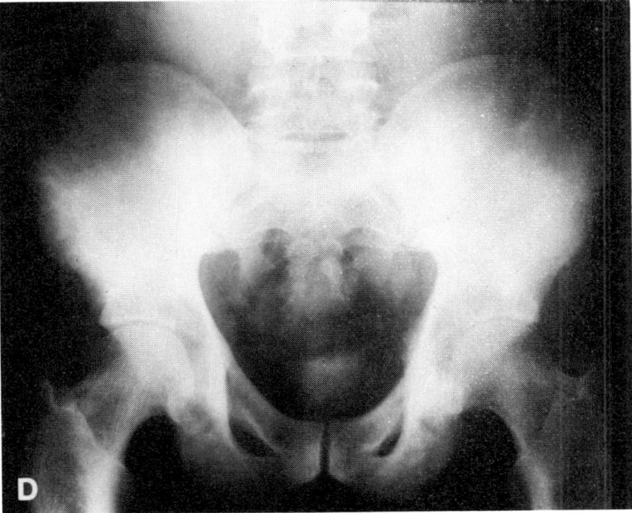
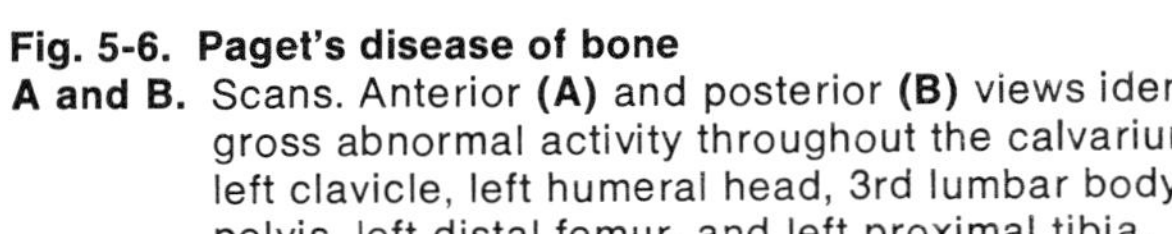

Fig. 5-6. Paget's disease of bone

A and B. Scans. Anterior **(A)** and posterior **(B)** views identify gross abnormal activity throughout the calvarium, left clavicle, left humeral head, 3rd lumbar body, pelvis, left distal femur, and left proximal tibia.

C and D. X rays. Lateral skull and transverse pelvis identify the osteolytic and blastic phases of Paget's disease of bone.

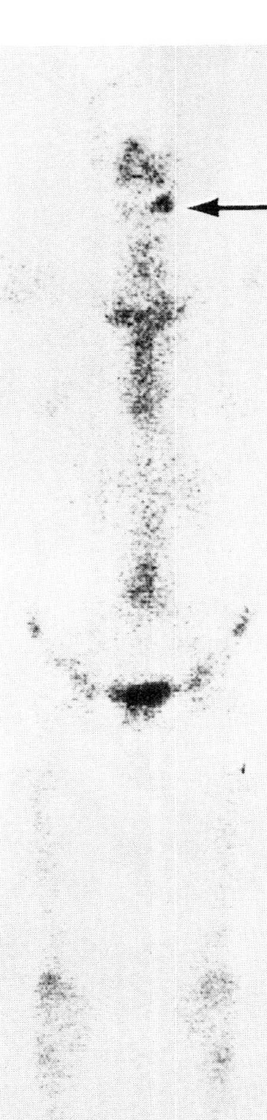

Fig. 5-7. Tooth extraction. Scan. The anterior view identifies an area of atypical uptake in the left mandible (arrow). The study was done as a routine evaluation in a breast carcinoma suspect, but the breast was found to be negative for malignancy. There had been a tooth extracted 5–6 weeks earlier.

Fig. 5-8. Arthritis compared with metastasis
Diagnosis: Degenerative arthritis
A. Scan. Posterior view identifies an asymmetric uptake pattern at the knees. The activity on the left is increased. (The pelvic activity is secondary to a distended bladder.)
B. X ray (of **A**). Anterior left knee demonstrates early sclerosis, subcortical resorption, and marginal productivity, particularly of the lateral femorotibial articulation, compatible with degenative arthritis.
Diagnosis: Metastatic carcinoma
C. Scan. Posterior view identifies a markedly abnormal uptake in the distal left femur. There is also a positive defect in the lower dorsal region and bladder distension. (The femoral shafts and knees were scanned separately due to the lateral deviation of the left femur. This explains the discontinuity of the shaftal image.)
D. X ray (of **C**). Femoral destruction from metastatic breast carcinoma

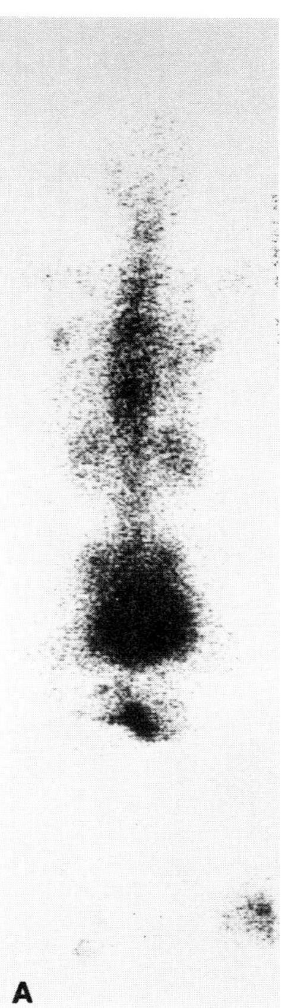

A

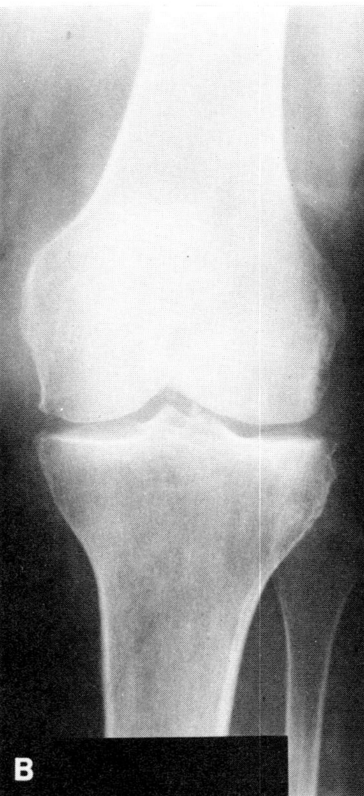

B

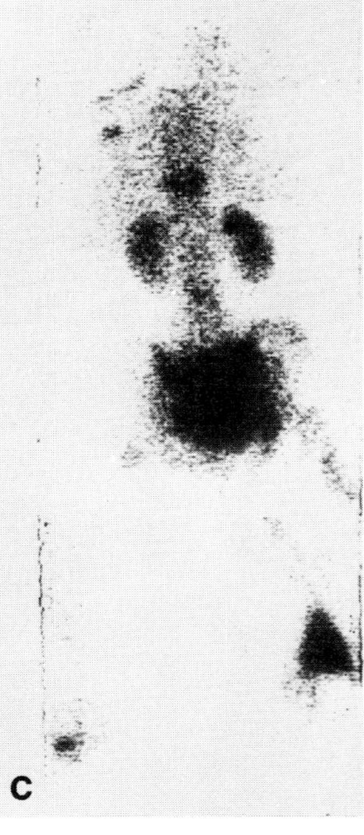

C

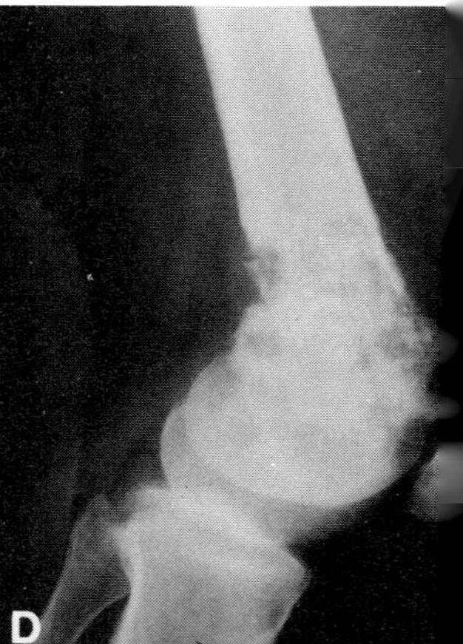

D

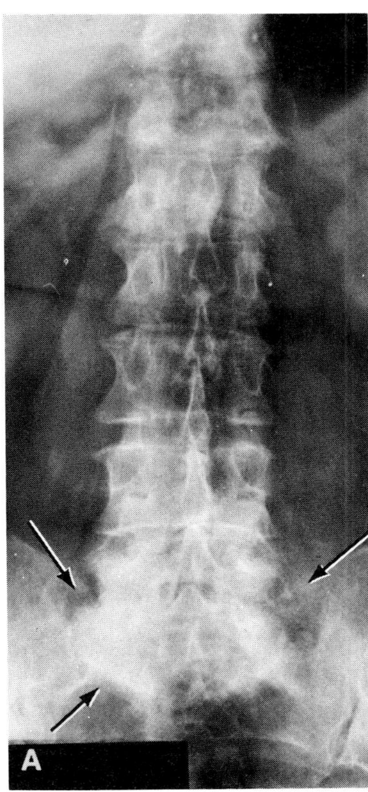

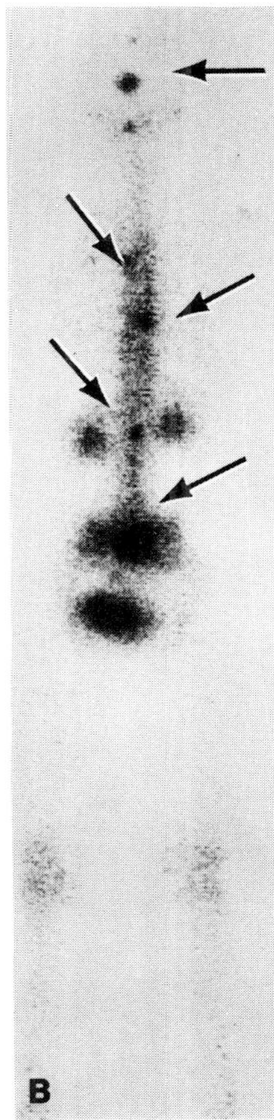

Fig. 5-9. Multiple metastatic defects—breast carcinoma
A. X ray. Both lytic and blastic changes (arrows) are identified in the lumbosacral region. This was the only site of x-ray positive findings and the only site of pain.
B. Scan. Posterior view identifies the lumbosacral changes but also suggests involvement in the calvarium, upper and mid-dorsal spine, and upper lumbar region.

lytic nature. When the scanning nuclide was ^{85m}Sr or even ^{18}F the number of misses was less than with the ^{99m}Tc compounds. Strontium and fluorine are described as true bone seekers. There is a positive ion exchange, the strontium with the calcium and the fluorine with the hydroxyl ion. Technetium tagged to a phosphate compound does not exchange but is "chemisorbed" on the crystal surface. Thus, the strontium and fluorine agents may be better able than the ^{99m}Tc compound to "find" the primary lytic defect. This is one explanation. There are others. Most lytic processes demonstrate an adjacent zone of new or reactive osteoblastic activity that many believe permits the identification of a positive scan image. When, therefore, a situation exists in which the process is so anaplastic that there has been no corresponding blastic activity (a condition not infrequently present when the primary is clear cell carcinoma of the kidney), the scan can appear normal.

Then, too, there is the "goof" of the multiple myeloma (Fig. 5-10) and the eosinophilic granuloma group that expands from the marrow out, initially sparing the cortex and thus sneaking a positive past our nuclear watchdogs (Fig. 5-11).

And lastly, the most ignoble goof of them all is the negative scan in which there is total osteoblastic skeletal replacement or total skeletal involvement from any cause. This is the one that separates out your friends—the dialogue is fairly standard and starts out with similes such as "my seeing eye dog knows that this patient is grossly metastatic but our $50,000.00 scanner says everything is fine." Explanations won't mollify him but are easily explained to you. When all of the bones are involved the scan will print out a uniform pattern of increased activity (Fig. 5-12 and 5-13). Since it is the differences between adjacent sites that signal abnormality if everything looks alike, unless the image is digitalized (which means that a count rate is obtained so that the interpreter will know that there is x times more activity than usual), the scan may be passed as an excellent normal.

Therefore, when there are skeletal symptoms the x ray–scan combination will improve the

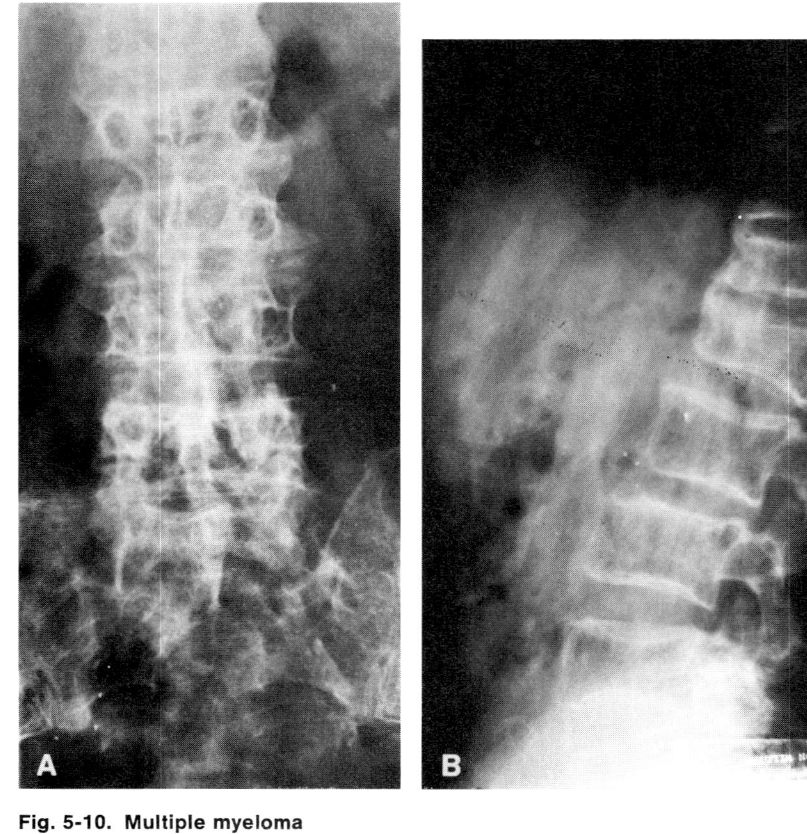

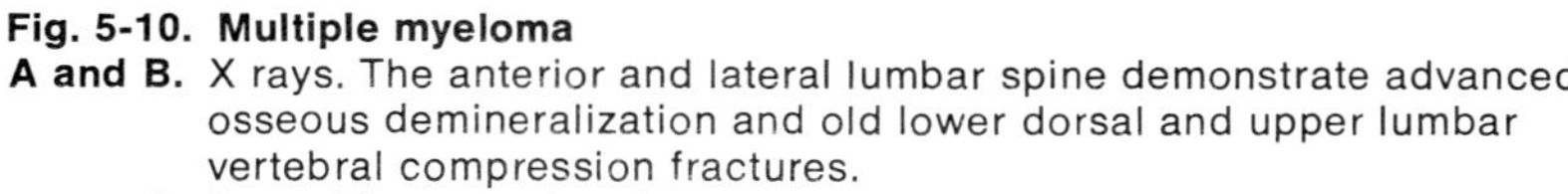

Fig. 5-10. Multiple myeloma
A and B. X rays. The anterior and lateral lumbar spine demonstrate advanced
osseous demineralization and old lower dorsal and upper lumbar
vertebral compression fractures.
C. Scan. The posterior view suggests an essentially normal study.

diagnostic yield and limit the possibility of
potentially avoidable error.

In known osseous metastasis, scanning may
still prove valuable. Often the extent of involvement is unclear and should be clarified if x-ray
therapy is contemplated. Thus, portal planning
and plotting is a distinctive indication. Along
the same lines, the efficacy of therapy to bone is
primarily subjective and rests with the patient's
report; x rays of the treated area are useless. It
is well known that the vast majority of positive
bone lesions, particularly of the blastic type,
demonstrate no change following any type of
therapy. However, the scan will reflect change.
After adequate treatment the originally scan
positive lesion will revert to normal. The same
mechanism is often useful in deciding the
activity of Paget's disease or even prostatic

extension. The dictum: "once x-ray positive,
always x-ray positive" does not hold for scans.
Rather, once scan positive, always scan positive,
but only if the pathologic process remains
metabolically active; when suppression occurs,
the scan reverts to normal.

primary mass

It is axiomatic that a patient with skeletal
symptoms should be x rayed. That is still the
first giant step on the diagnostic road to IT IS!
The x-ray findings determine the subsequent
routes. If the study is positive, the disease
recognized, its extent determined, and its
management clear, then scanning procedures
are irrelevant. If, on the other hand, the x rays
are negative or questionable, the extent of

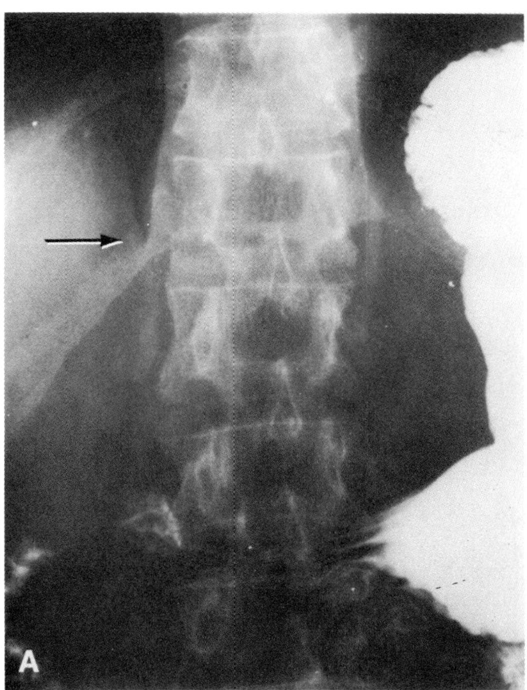
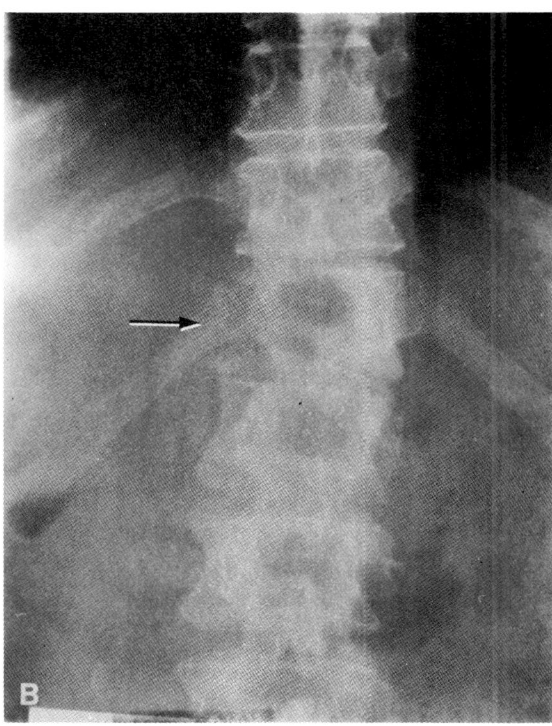
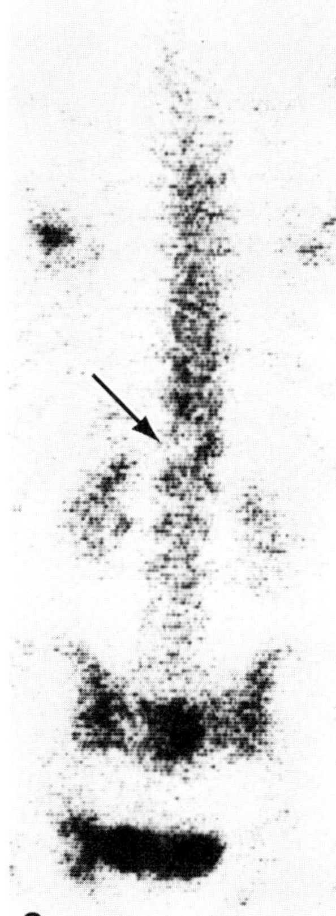

Fig. 5-11. Osteoltyic metastasis—renal carcinoma
A. X ray (1/14/74). The body of the 12th dorsal vertebra (arrow) is well preserved as noted on the GI study in January.
B. X ray (6/21/74). Five months later the right half of the body of the 12th dorsal vertebra (arrow) is partially destroyed in June. The patient had severe dorsal, right scapular, and sacral pain. X rays of the right scapula and sacrum were considered normal.
C. Scan (6/23/74). There is increased uptake in the right scapula and sacrum. There is no increased uptake in the 12th dorsal (arrow). Actually, there is a "negative" defect.

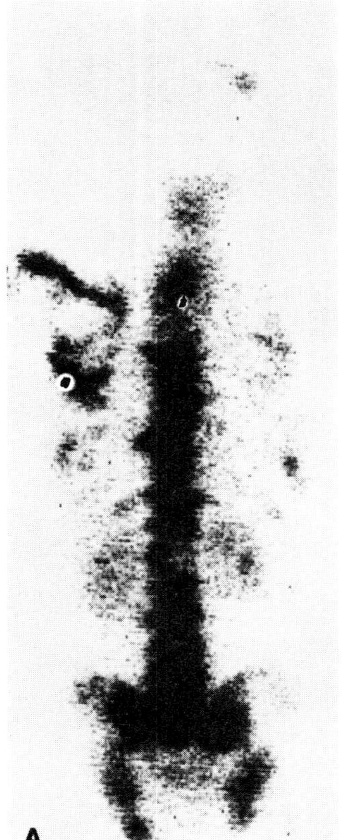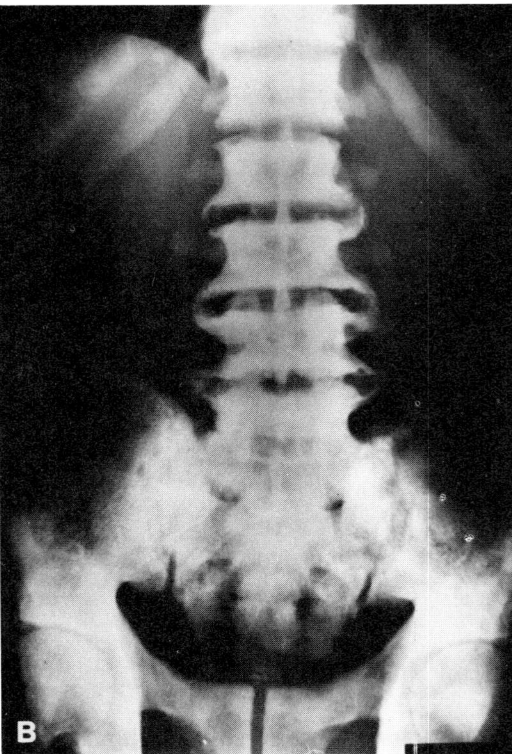

Fig. 5-12. Osteoblastic metastasis—prostatic carcinoma
A. Scan. All vertebrae are uniformly invaded. The sacral, iliac, and ischial
involvement is almost symmetric. Except for the right scapular and clavicular
changes the findings might be confused for a technically poor study.
B. X ray. Osteoblastic changes in all of the vertebrae and pelvis

involvement uncertain, and the ultimate course
unclear, then the call to the basement is
indicated.

All of the previously discussed indications
and merits obtain. Primary tumors, like their
metastatic cousins, may exist and be symptomatic
before they are x-ray detectable. Therefore, the
negative x-ray–positive symptom patient
requires imaging. If the combination becomes
x-ray negative–scan negative, the probability of
active bone disease is negligible. If the
combination becomes x-ray negative–scan
positive, then all of the big guns of differential
diagnosis are unleashed.

This approach is particularly valuable in the
pediatric group. Comparative studies of clinical
and x-ray and scan accuracy constantly indicate
far greater sensitivity of detection by scanning.
Differentiation of tumor from infection and

fracture may be difficult, but the false negative
rate is almost nonexistent.

Scanning is indicated even when the primary
is obvious on the x ray, but its extension is
unclear and management is predicated on the
presence or absence of metastases (Fig. 5-14).
It was mentioned earlier that the phosphonates
may localize in other than skeletal lesions, the
most dramatic example being pulmonary
metastasis from osteogenic sarcoma
(Fig. 5-15).
Occasionally, on a skeletal study such extraosseous localization may be appreciated. It is
mandatory that these unexplained sites of
uptake be explored. The pursuit of such coincidental "pick-ups" may lead to the diagnosis of
an unsuspected primary or metastatic focus.
This has been particularly true in the breast or
brain (Figs. 5-16 and 5-17).

Fig. 5-13. Renal osteodystrophy secondary to chronic renal failure

A and B. Scan. Anterior **(A)** and posterior **(B)** views demonstrate marked symmetric and uniform increase in uptake throughout the entire skeleton, particularly the calvarium. Note the absence of any uptake in the kidneys.

C. X ray. Lateral skull—mottled demineralization throughout

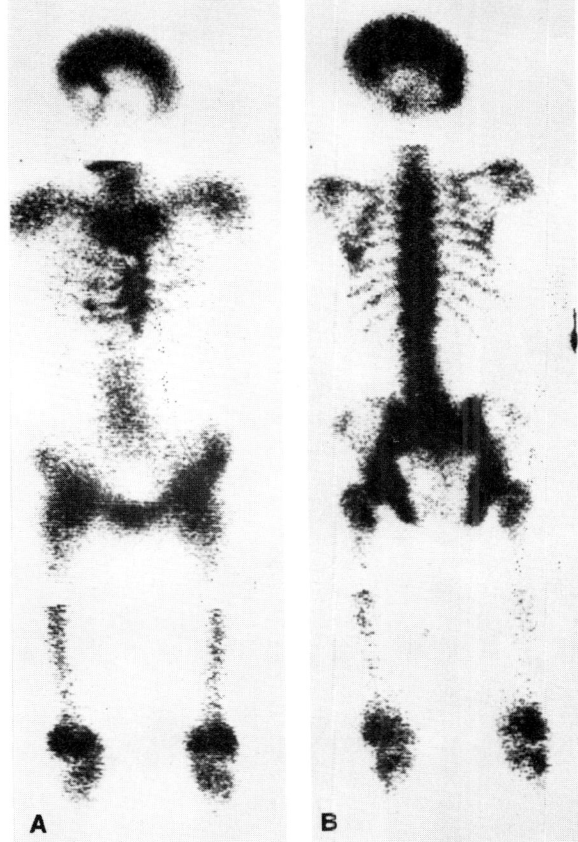

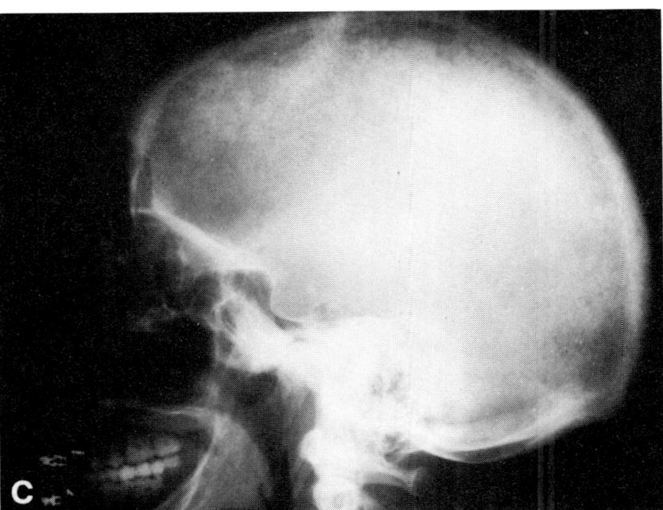

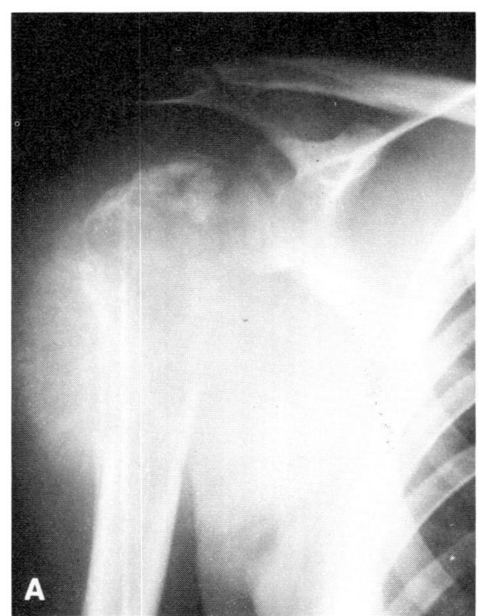

Fig. 5-14. Ewing's tumor of the right humerus with scapular and clavicular extension

A. X ray. The right shoulder film of a 17-year-old male studied because of chronic pain and a palpable soft tissue mass. The proximal humerus is almost completely destroyed by a lytic process. There is periosteal elevation and extensive soft tissue extension ("sun-burst" pattern). The adjacent scapula and clavicle appear normal.

B. Scan. A split image of the right and left shoulder region. The humeral uptake in the left is grossly abnormal. Note the abnormal uptake in the scapula and clavicle.

(Courtesy of W. Betts, Lancaster Osteopathic Hospital, Lancaster, Pa.)

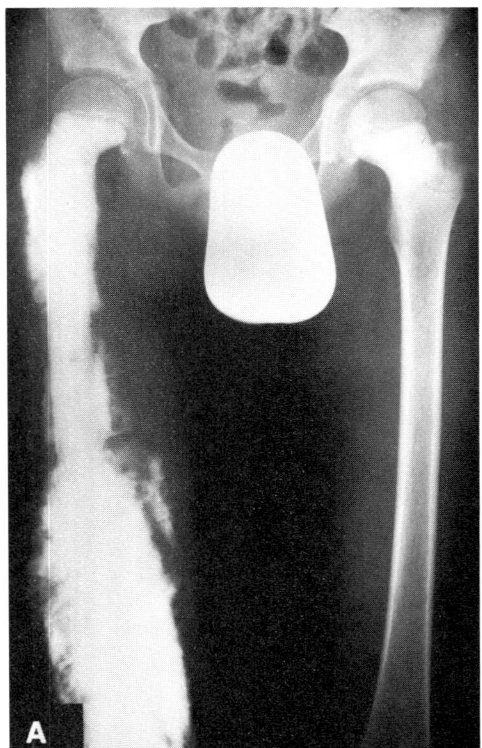

Fig. 5-15. Osteoblastic osteogenic sarcoma of the right femur with metastasis to the left humerus and lungs

A. X ray. The right femur in this 9½-year-old boy demonstrates extensive osteoblastic new bone formation extending beyond the shaft into the soft tissues.

B. X ray. Chest exhibits massive calcific metastatic deposits. Note the increased bone density of the visualized portion of the proximal left humerus.

C. Scan. Right femur trapping is grossly abnormal. There is increased uptake in the proximal shaft of the left humerus. The lesions in the chest avidly accumulate activity.

(Courtesy of D. Kuhl, Hospital of the University of Pennsylvania, Philadelphia)

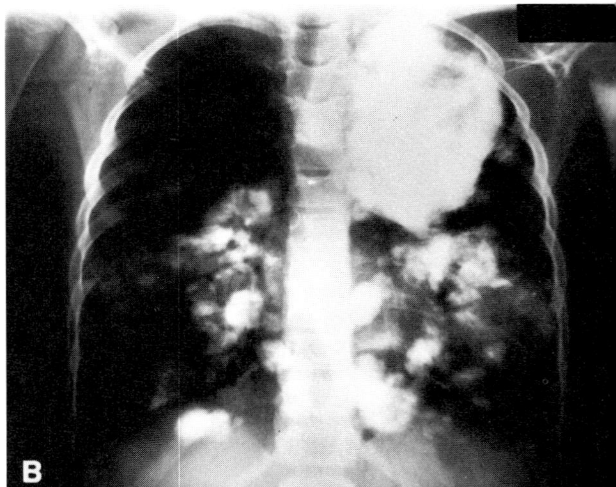

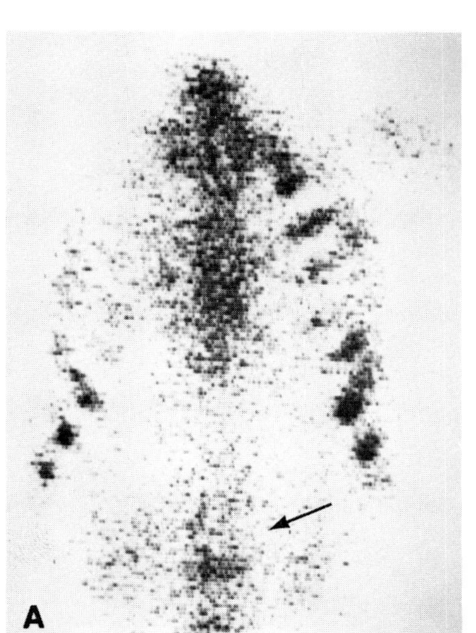

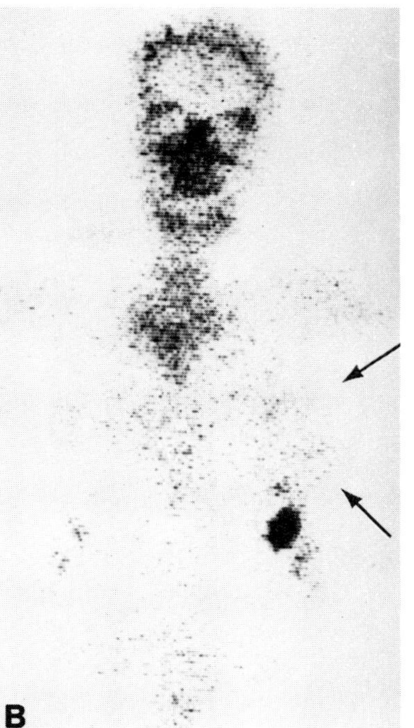

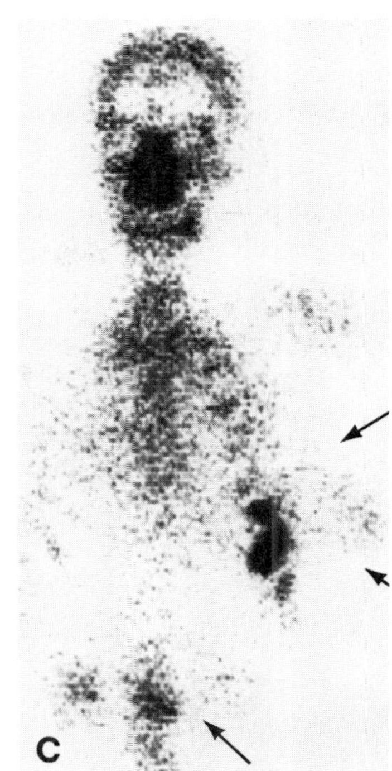

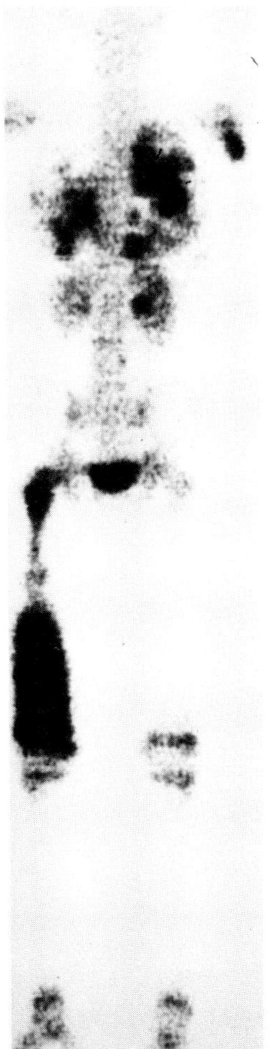

Fig. 5-16. Primary tumors—breast. Diagnosis: Breast carcinoma (second primary) and metastatic breast carcinoma to bone

A. Scan, anterior view (2:1) 9/17/73. Routine prior to simple mastectomy of right breast carcinoma. Multiple right and left rib defects are present. There is also a questionable abnormality at L2 (arrow). X-ray therapy was given to the right chest wall.

B. Scan, anterior view (5:1) 6/10/74. Recurrence of pain in left rib cage initiated recheck. Obvious abnormal uptake in a lower left rib. Also, a questionable and atypical site of activity in the left thorax (arrows)

C. Scan, anterior view (5:1) 8/26/74. Two months later the left rib defects persist. The second lumbar lesion suspected 1 year earlier is definite. The previously questionable uptake over the left thorax is now clearly abnormal and within the range of the left breast (arrows).

D. Xeroradiograph, left breast—9/1/74. An unsuspected infiltrating mass lesion

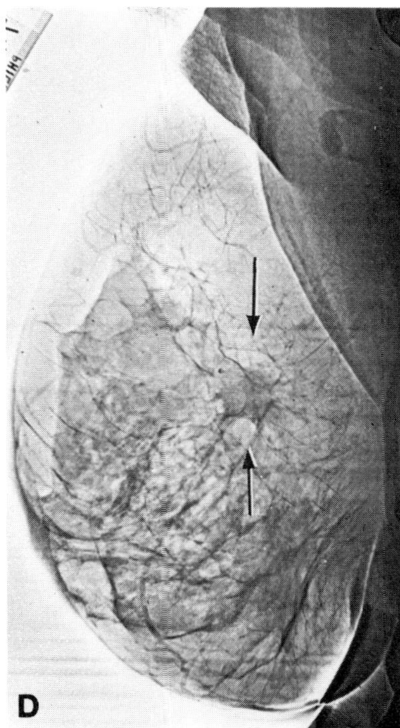

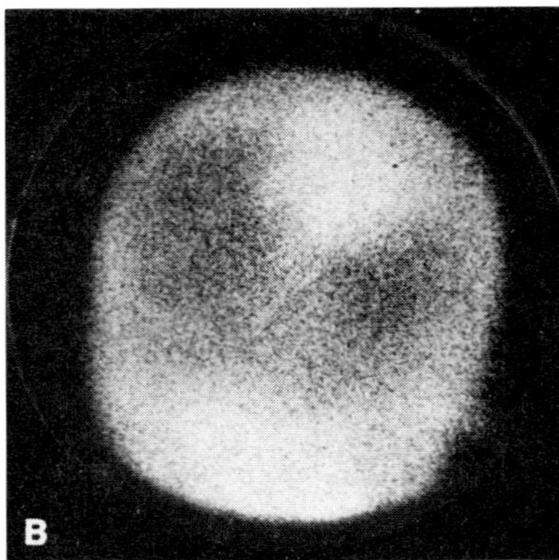

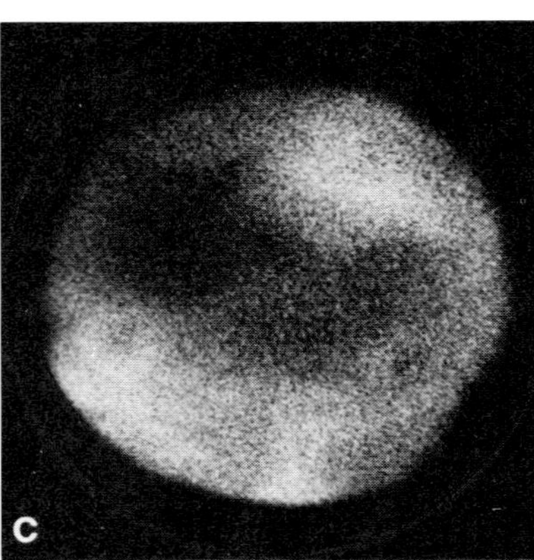

Fig. 5-17. Primary tumors—brain
Diagnosis: Meningioma
    A. Scan, posterior (5:1). Routine in evaluation of possible breast malignancy. Area of abnormal trapping noted in the calvarium (arrow)
B and C. Scan, posterior **(B)** and left lateral **(C)** brain. Gross abnormality in the left parietal region suggests a mass lesion.

infection

Osteomyelitis. Early acute osteomyelitis is often missed on x ray but almost never on scan (Fig. 5-18), particularly when the site of infection is other than in the tubular bones (Fig. 5-19). Recent reports cite the complication of spondylitis in IV drug abuse patients, whose somatic complaints (previously ignored, particularly when the correlative x rays were also negative) have now been shown with positive vertebral scans to result from hematogenously induced osteomyelitis. This is yet another example of the growing list of clinically positive patients with negative x rays being further evaluated by skeletal imaging.

At the other end of the spectrum is the chronic osteomyelitis problem. The x rays are so permanently positive that recurrence may be impossible to detect. This is not so with imaging. The scans of "burnt out" osteomyelitis will be negative; those of chronic osteomyelitis with reactivation will be positive.

Negative scans in patients suspected of harboring either acute or recurrent osteomyelitis are strong presumptive evidence that a new working diagnosis is indicated.

Arthritis. Increasing interest is developing in the use of imaging for the detection of active joint disease. The same mechanism responsible for detection of other acute bone diseases are also operable at the joint level. Detection of activity, however, may be more difficult since it must be recalled that uptake at the ends of long bones, particularly in the growing state, demonstrate higher uptake normally than the shaft portions. This is true even at the articular surfaces of flat bones as evidenced by increased activity in the region of the sacro-iliac joints. However, base lines of normal can be established so that excessive uptake is recognized. Asymmetry of joint uptake is strong presumption of pathology. Even unequal activity off the bones adjacent to individual cranial sutures may provide early evidence of premature craniostenosis.

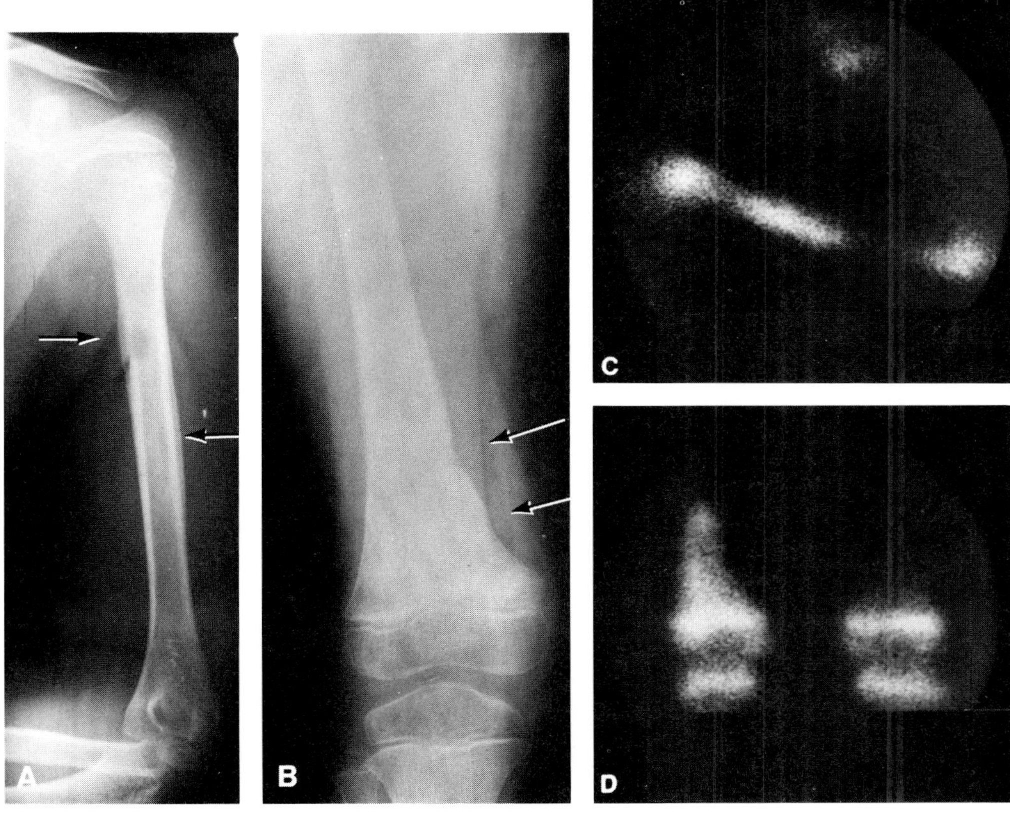

Fig. 5-18. Acute and subacute osteomyelitis of the left humerus and right femur

A and B. X rays. 7-year-old patient complained of sudden onset of pain and tenderness in the left shoulder and left knee. X rays demonstrate medullary defects, demineralization, and periosteal elevation (arrows).

C and D. Scans. Increased uptake is present in the proximal shaft of the left humerus and distal metaphysis of the right femur. Neither the shoulder nor knee joint was affected.

(Courtesy of D. Kuhl, Hospital of the University of Pennsylvania, Philadelphia)

Efforts are being expended toward establishing patterns of abnormal joint activity. Patterns purporting to distinguish the changes of osteoarthritis from those of rheumatoid disease have been reported, and criteria for the detection of ankylosing spondylitis at the sacroiliac joint level have been described. However, as of yet, although positive scan findings alone are not necessarily pathognomonic of a particular entity, in combination with x ray, they often provide a working diagnosis (Figs. 5-20 and 5-21). This group does not warrant a capital-Y yea at this time.

trauma

Is nothing sacred or immune from the ubiquitous scan? What is clearer in the diagnostic armamentarium than fracture? The quick one, two, three of trauma, pain, and x ray equals

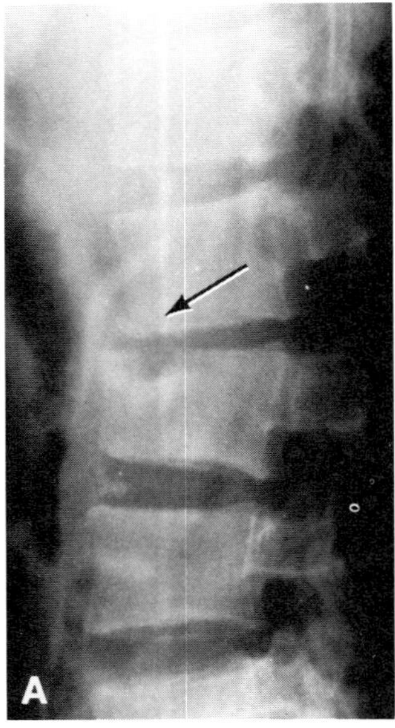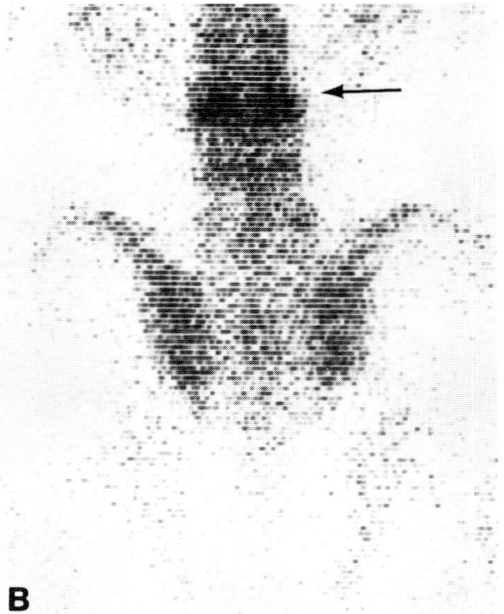

Fig. 5-19. Vertebral osteomyelitis
A. X ray. There is a lytic defect at the anterosuperior margin of the body of the 3rd lumbar segment. The intervertebral disc space between L2 and L3 is narrowed. Findings were coincidental at the time of an IV urogram.
B. Scan. 4 hours following ^{99m}Tc pyrophosphate there is abnormal uptake in the 3rd lumbar segment (arrow).
(Courtesy of R. Wallner, Hahnemann Hospital, Philadelphia, Pa.)

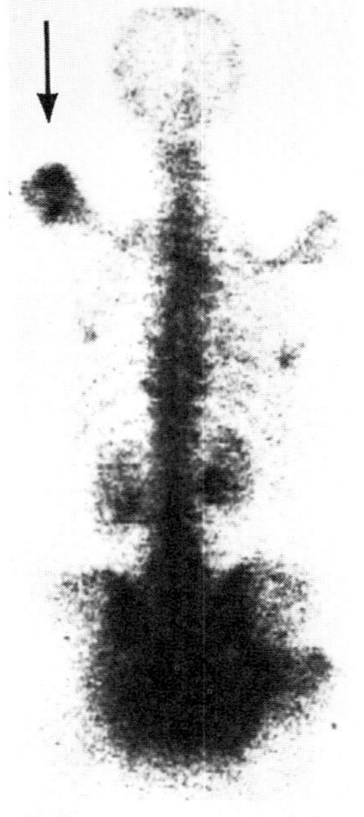

Fig. 5-20. Degenerative arthritis
A. Scan. Posterior (5:1). Pain was present at multiple sites in a patient 7 years after mastectomy for carcinoma. Abnormal activity was present in the right shoulder and right knee region (arrows).
B. X ray. Right shoulder—degenerative arthritis
C. X ray. Right knee—degenerative arthritis

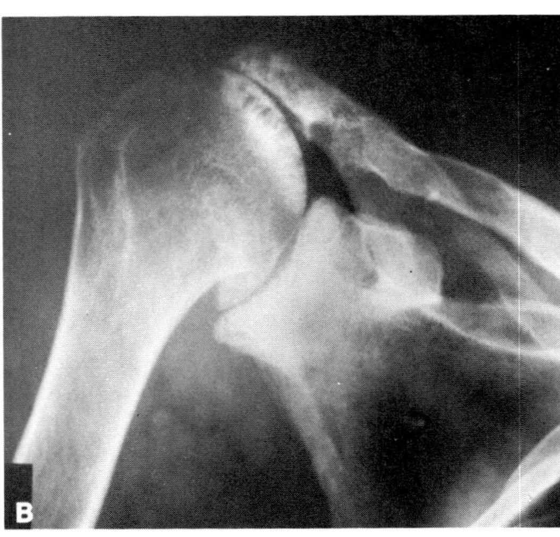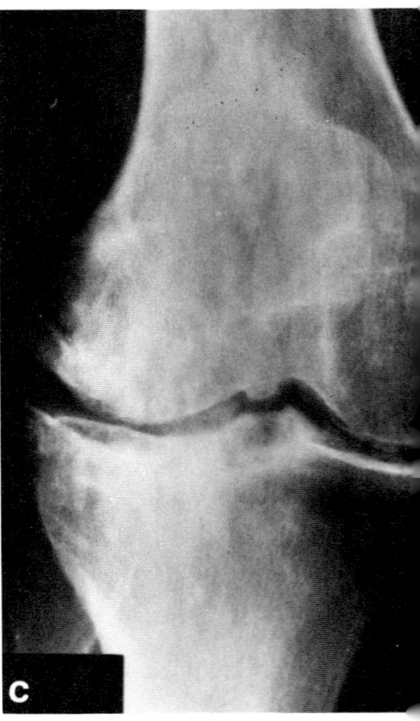

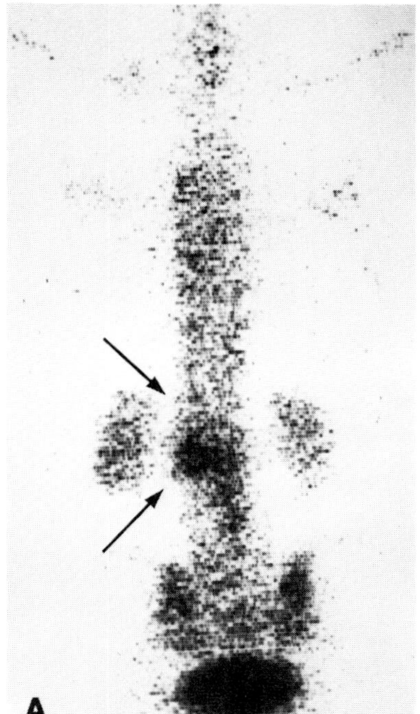

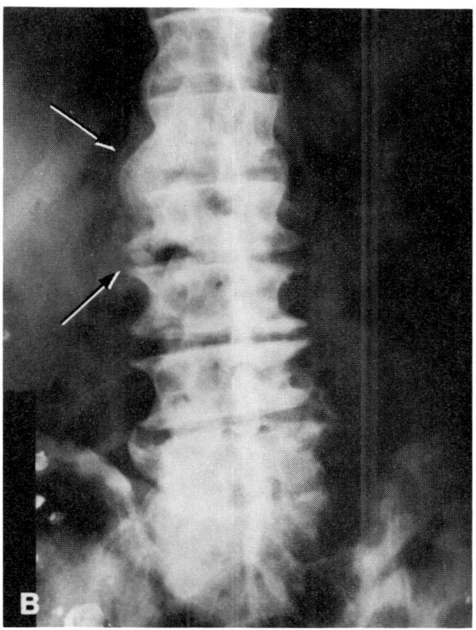

Fig. 5-21. Ankylosing spondylitis
  A. Scan, posterior (2:1). Routine work-up in bronchogenic carcinoma suspect. There
  was generalized backache. An area of abnormal activity (arrows) was present in
  the right side of the body of L1 and L2.
  B. X ray. Lumbar spine—ankylosing spondylitis and degenerative arthritis (arrows)

Fig. 5-22. Pathologic fractures
A. Scan, anterior (2:1). The patient was being treated for a right bronchogenic
  carcinoma and began to complain of right rib pain. The initial x-ray finding of the
  right ribs was interpreted as questionable due to the abnormal pulmonary
  densities. The scan identifies abnormal uptake in the lower right ribs (arrow).
B. X ray. Review after the positive scan confirms a healing fracture at the angle of
  the 7th right rib plus a new pathologic fracture in the anterior portion of the same
  rib (arrows).

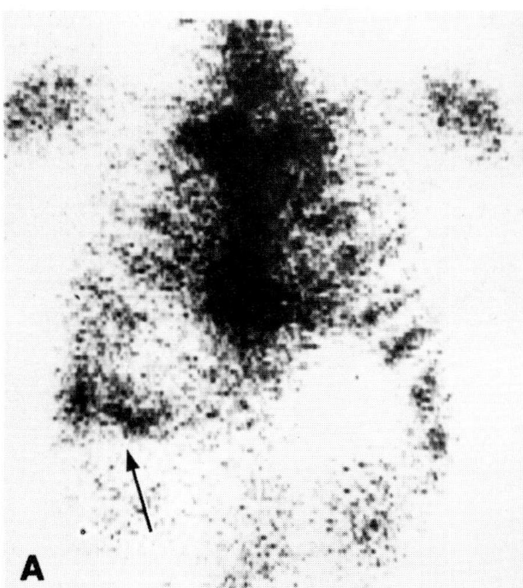

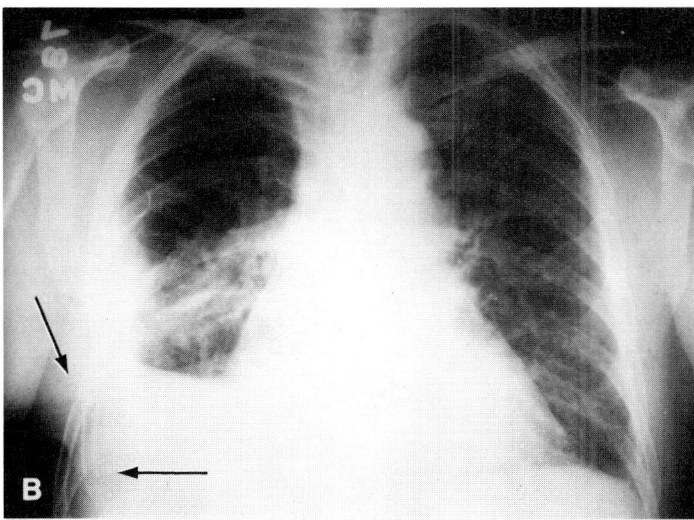

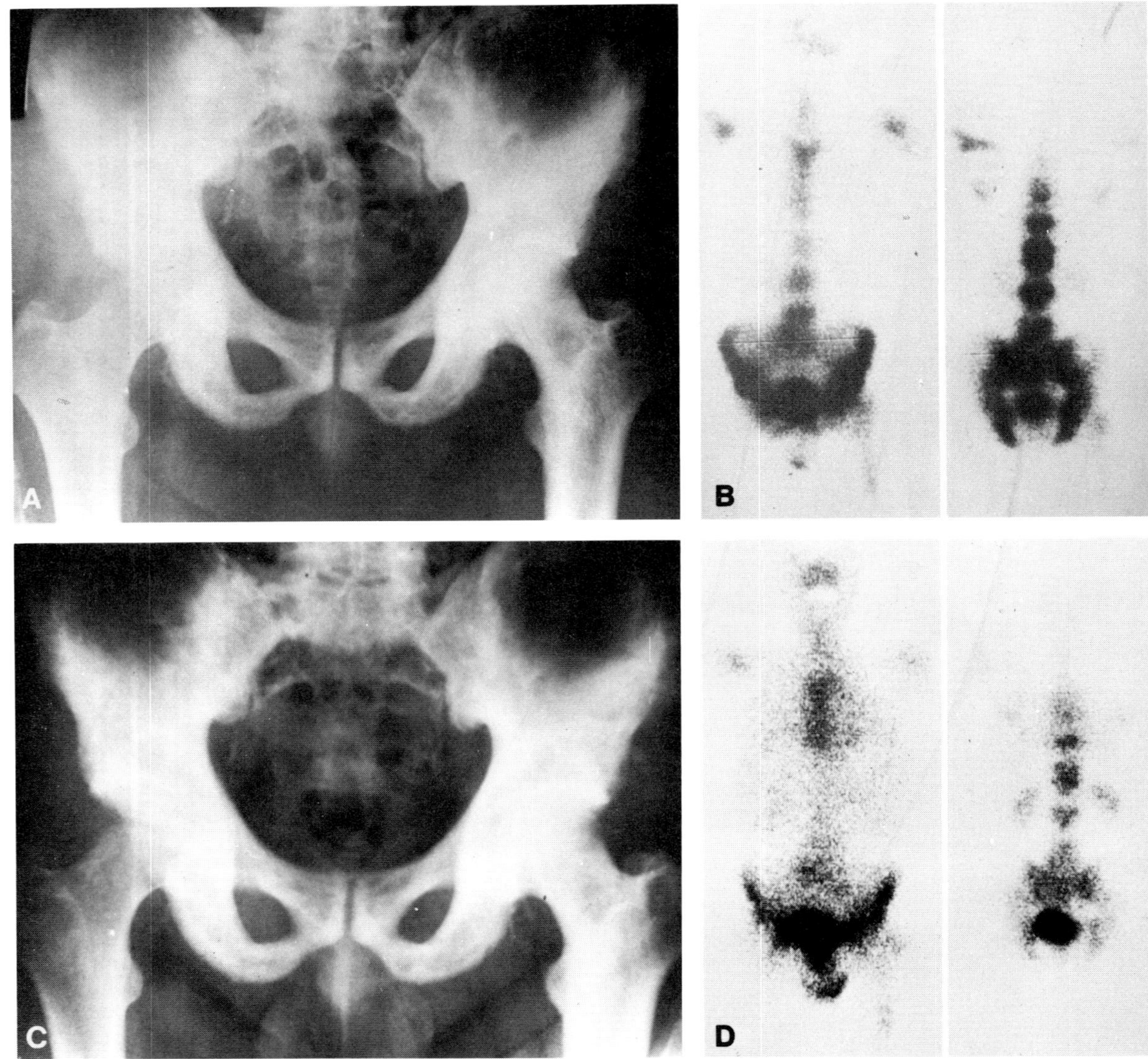

Fig. 5-23. Paget's disease with response

A. X ray. The pelvis and proximal femora demonstrate the typical increased bone density and contour changes of Paget's disease.
B. Scan. Anterior and posterior image identifies significant increased uptake in the right scapula, multiple dorsal and lumbar vertebra, pelvis, and left femur.
C. X ray, 6 months after **A.** No essential change
D. Scan, 6 months after **B.** The patient has been on therapy with definite remission of symptoms. Although still identifying abnormal sites of uptake, there is considerable improvement particularly in the scapula, pelvis, and femur.
(Courtesy of B. Shapiro, Albert Einstein Hospital Northern Division, Philadelphia, Pa.)

diagnosis. But what about when this triad equals misdiagnosis? What of the medicolegal question of how old is the injury? What of the differential dilemma of pathologic versus traumatic? (Oh for the simplicity of yesteryear!) In each of these problem areas, skeletal imaging can be helpful.

Certain fractures are difficult to identify on x ray, particularly when examined soon after the injury. It may be that the degree of trabecular or cortical damage is slight or that the involved site is particularly difficult to evaluate for minor trauma (this is not uncommon in the sternum, scapula, sacrum, and even ribs). It may be that, because of pain or other factors, the conventional techniques of roentgen examination must be limited. Regardless of cause, if immediate diagnosis is necessary, scanning may improve the detection since a positive image can probably be obtained within a day or two after trauma (Fig. 5-22).

A problem with perhaps greater applicability is determination of the age of an obvious fracture, *e.g.,* the vertebral compression fracture when previous x rays are unavailable. This question may have significant medicolegal implications. X-ray criteria may be imprecise. Scan criteria, although imprecise may improve the judgment by defining the age limits. A positive image can be obtained throughout the entire course of healing, which may frequently exist for as long as 2 years. In spite of reports of scans remaining positive for as long as 6 years after the original insult and long after all clinical symptoms have subsided, a negative scan may provide the additional data necessary to resolve a particular problem. The same mechanism of decreasing activity of uptake on the scan with healing may aid in the differentiation of traumatic and pathologic fractures. With healing, the traumatic lesion demonstrates a sequential return to normal. This is not the case when the underlying etiology is osseous invasion; these areas will remain positive on the scan.

Assessment of bone healing may become a more than didactic exercise if the use of bone grafts to replace severely traumatized skeletal tissue becomes a common practice. Allograft or Zenograft bone substitutes are being used, and scanning to monitor acceptance and healing is being attempted.

vascular

Aseptic Necrosis. Detection of bone infarction and the subsequent development of aseptic necrosis is excellent. The mechanisms responsible for positive scans and nonspecificity of the abnormal image is the same in this disease as in the others. Again it is clinical concern coupled with negative early x rays that cry out for scanning. The subsequent positive study is plugged into the jigsaw and the picture emerges.

Paget's Disease. There is some difficulty in classifying this process, and many may argue that it should be discussed under a different heading, but regardless of heading, the discussion would be unchanged. Early detection, evaluation of activity, and response to therapy are all superbly accomplished by imaging (Fig. 5-23). As has been repeated almost *ad nauseum,* the findings reflect metabolic variation and vascular environment. Thus, early detection can be accomplished and the state of the process evaluated. A positive scan with a normal x ray is the pattern of early detection. A normal scan with a positive x ray may suggest a quiescent process.

Table 5-1. Indications, Pharmaceuticals, Methodology and Order of Merit of Radionuclide Study of Bone

Why	What	How	Yea--Nay
Mass lesions			
Primary	^{99m}Tc phosphate complex	static	++++
Metastatic	^{99m}Tc phosphate complex	static	++++
Infection			
Osteomyelitis	^{99m}Tc phosphate complex	static	++++
Arthritis	^{99m}Tc phosphate complex	static	++
Trauma			+++
Vascular			
Aseptic			
necrosis	^{99m}Tc phosphate complex	static	+++
Idiopathic			
Paget's	^{99m}Tc phosphate complex	static	++++

Table 5-2. More About What

Radiopharmaceuticals	Dose (mCi)	Physical Half-life (hr)	Energy Peak (keV)
^{99m}Tc Sn-polyphosphate	10–20	6	140
^{99m}Tc Sn-diphosphonate	10–20	6	140
^{99m}Tc Sn-pyrophosphate	10–20	6	140
^{18}F	1–5	1.8	511
^{85}Sr	0.1	64 days	513
^{87m}Sr	1–3	2.8	388

Table 5-3. More About How

Why	Preparation	Administration	Time Between Administration and Exam (hr)	Number of Exams	Time for Each Exam (min)	Time for Total Study (min)	Patient's Position	Instrument
Mass lesions Primary		IV	1–4	1	45–90	45–90	supine	camera or scanner
Metastatic	hydration after nuclide, voiding before scan	IV	1–4	1	45–90	45–90	supine	camera or scanner
Infection Osteomyelitis		IV	1–4	1	45–90	45–90	supine	camera or scanner
Arthritis		IV	1–4	1	45–90	45–90	supine	camera or scanner
Trauma		IV	1–4	1	45–90	45–90	supine	camera or scanner
Vascular		IV	1–4	1	45–90	45–90	supine	camera or scanner

BIBLIOGRAPHY

GENERAL

Bauer GC: Clinical uses of radioactive isotopes in orthopedics. Cornell Vet LVIII:149–175, 1968

Bauer GCH: Diagnosis of skeletal system disease. In Blahd WH (ed): Nuclear Medicine. New York, McGraw–Hill, 1971, pp 453–470

Bell EG: Nuclear medicine and skeletal disease. Hosp Prac 7(8): 49–60, 1972

Charkes ND: Bone scanning: principles, technique, and interpretation. Radiol Clin North Am 8(2):259–270, 1970

Charkes ND: Bone scanning, in Diagnosis of skeletal system disease. In Blahd WH (ed): Nuclear Medicine. New York, McGraw–Hill, 1971, pp 470–483

Charkes ND et al.: Interpretation of the normal ^{99m}Tc polyphosphate rectilinear bone scan. Radiology 107:563–570, 1973

Charkes ND, Sklaroff DM: The osseous system. In Freeman LM, Johnson PM (eds): Clinical Scintillation Scanning. Hagerstown, Harper & Row, 1969, pp 326–383

Greenberg EJ et al.: Effects of radiation therapy on bone lesions as measured by ^{47}Ca and ^{85}Sr local kinetics. J Nucl Med 13(10):747–751, 1972

James AE, Squire LF: Bone and bone marrow. In Nuclear Radiology. Philadelphia, WB Saunders, 1973, pp 124–137

Larson SM, Johnson GS: Interpretation of the ^{67}Ga photoscan. J Nucl Med 14(4):208–214, 1973

Moon NF: The skeleton. In Wagner HN Jr (ed): Principles of Nuclear Medicine. Philadelphia, WB Saunders, 1968, pp 703–721

PHARMACOLOGY

Ackerhalt RE et al.: A comparative study of three
99mTc-labeled phosphorous compounds and 18F-fluoride for
skeletal imaging (abstr). J Nucl Med 14(6):375, 1973

Bell EG et al.: Evaluation of 99m-Tc-polyphosphate bone
scanning for neoplastic skeletal disease. J Nucl Med
13(6):413, 1972

Blau M et al.: Fluorine-18: a new isotope for bone
scanning. J Nucl Med 3:332, 1962

Blau M et al.: 18F-fluoride for bone imaging. Semin Nucl
Med 2(1):31–37, 1972

Castronovo FP Jr: Letter: Pharmaceutical toxicity as a
function of biodegradability. J Nucl Med 14(9):719, 1973

Chervu LR et al.: Fluorotec: a new bone seeker. Radiology
107:435–437, 1973

DeLand FH et al.: Cellular location of 99mTc-polyphosphate
(abstr). J Nucl Med 14(6):390, 1973

Jones AE et al.: Clinical evaluation of orally administered
fluorine 18 for bone scanning. Radiology 107:129–131, 1973

King AG et al.: Polyphosphates: a chemical analysis of
average chain length and the relationship to bone
deposition in rats. J Nucl Med 14(9):695–698, 1973

O'Mara RE, Subramanian G: Experimental agents for
skeletal imaging. Semin Nucl Med 2(1):38–49, 1972

Pendergrass HP et al.: The clinical use of 99mTc-diphospho-
nate (HEDSPA). Radiology 107:557–562, 1973

Subramanian G, McAfee JG: A new complex of 99mTc for
skeletal imaging. Radiology 99:192–196, 1971

Subramanian G et al.: 99mTc-labeled polyphosphate as a
skeletal imaging agent. Radiology 102:701–704, 1972

Subramanian G et al.: 99mTc-MDP (methylene diphosphonate): a superior agent for skeletal imaging (abstr). J Nucl
Med 14(8):640, 1973

Yano Y et al.: Technetium-99m-labeled stannous ethane-
1-hydroxy-11-diphosphonate: a new bone scanning agent.
J Nucl Med 14(2):73–78, 1973

TUMOR

Charkes ND, Sklaroff DM: Early diagnosis of metastatic
bone cancer by photoscanning with strontium-85. J Nucl
Med 5:168–179, 1964

Charkes ND, Sklaroff DM: The radioactive strontium
photoscan as a diagnostic aid in primary and metastatic
cancer in bone. Radiol Clin North Am 3(3):499–509 1965

Charkes ND et al.: Detection of metastatic cancer to bone
by scintiscanning with strontium 87m. Am J Roentgenol
Radium Ther Nucl Med 91:1121–1127, 1964

DeNardo GL et al.: 85Sr bone scan in neoplastic disease.
Semin Nucl Med 2(1):18–30, 1972

Galasko CSB: Letter: False positives and negatives with
87mSr. J Nucl Med 12(3):142, 1971

Gerson BD et al.: Patterns of localization of 85strontium in
osteosarcoma: a correlative study using gross autoradiogra-
phy. J Bone Joint Surg 54:817–827, 1972

Greenberg EJ et al.: Bone scanning for metastatic cancer
with radioactive isotopes. Med Clin North Am 50:701–710,
1966

Greenberg EJ et al.: Detection of neoplastic bone lesions
by quantitative scanning and radiography. J Nucl Med
9:613–620, 1968

Harmer CL et al.: The value of fluorine-18 for scanning
bone tumors. Clin Radiol 20:204–212, 1969

Helson L et al.: F18 radioisotope scanning of metastatic
bone lesions in children with neuroblastoma. Am J
Roentgenol Radium Ther Nucl Med 115:191–199, 1972

Legge DA et al.: Radioisotope scanning of metastatic
lesions of bone. Mayo Clin Proc 45:755–761, 1970

Okuyama S et al.: Prospects of 67Ga scanning in bone
neoplasms. Radiology 107:123–128, 1973

Roy RR et al.: 18Fluorine total body scans in patients with
carcinoma of the prostate. Br J Urol 43:58–64, 1971

Samuels LD: Diagnosis of malignant bone disease with
strontium-87m scans. Can Med Assoc J 104:411–413, 1971

Sanders TP, Kuhl DE: Selective uptake of radionuclides,
as a basis for tumor detection. Radiol Clin North Am
7(2):257–264, 1969

Silberstein EB et al.: Imaging of bone metastases with
99mTc-Sn-EHDP (diphosphonate), 18F, and skeletal
radiography. Radiology 107:551–555, 1973

Sklaroff DM, Charkes ND: Bone metastases from breast
cancer at the time of radical mastectomy. Surg Gynecol
Obstet 127:763–768, 1968

Wellman HN et al.: Evaluation of bone malignancy with
99mTc-Sn-EHDP compared with Na18F (abstr). J Nucl Med
14(6):464, 1973

INFECTIONS, TRAUMA, AND OTHER DISEASES

Bauer GC, Smith EM: 85Sr scintimetry in osteoarthritis of
the knee. J Nucl Med 10(3):109–116, 1969

Charkes ND et al.: Bone pain in multiple myeloma: studies
with radioactive 87mSr. Arch Intern Med 130:53–58, 1972

Chaudhuri TK et al.: Positive 87mSr bone scan in a case of
hypertrophic pulmonary osteoarthropathy. J Nucl Med
13(1):120–121, 1972

Fellander M, Lindberg L: Clinical use of radiostrontium in
evaluation of spondylolitis. J Bone Joint Surg 48A:1585,
1966

Gates GF: Detection of premature craniosynostosis with
18F (abstr). J Nucl Med 14(6):397, 1973

Harbert JC, Ashburn WL: Radiostrontium bone scanning in
Hodgkin's disease. Cancer 22:58–63, 1968

Ngan H et al.: Bone changes in adult acute leukemia. Br J
Radiol 41:66–68, 1968

Rubin P et al.: The effects of intra-articular 198Au
instillations on articular cartilage. Radiology 103:685–690,
1972

Serafini A et al.: Paget's disease: a method of evaluation
of response to therapy using the anger scintillation camera
on-line to a computer (abstr). J Nucl Med 14(6):449, 1973

Shirazi PH et al.: Paget's disease of bone: bone scanning
experience with 80 cases (abstr). J Nucl Med 14(6):450,
1973

Sonnemaker RE et al.: 87mSr scintiphotography of the
sacro-iliac joints: a new criterion for the diagnosis of
ankylosing spondylitis (abstr). J Nucl Med 13(6):467, 1972

Staheli LT et al.: Sr87m scanning: early diagnosis of bone
and joint infections in children. JAMA 221:1159–1160, 1972

Stevenson JS et al.: 99mTc-polyphosphate bone imaging—
a quantitative method for assessing bone healing (abstr).
J Nucl Med 14(6):457, 1973

Waxman AD et al.: Bone scanning in the drug abuse patient: early detection of hematogenous osteomyelitis. J Nucl Med 14(9):647–650, 1973

Wellman HN et al.: The bone scan and radiograph in the evaluation of Paget's disease (abstr). J Nucl Med 14(6):464, 1973

EXTRAOSSEOUS

Chaudhuri TK et al.: Abnormal deposition of radiostrontium in lungs. Chest 61:190–192, 1972

Chaudhuri TK et al.: Uptake of ^{87m}Sr by liver metastasis from carcinoma of colon. J Nucl Med 14(5):293–294, 1973

Dalinka MK et al.: Metastatic extraosseous osteosarcoma to the liver: a case demonstrated by ^{85}Sr and ^{99m}Tc-colloid scanning. J Nucl Med 12(11):754–755, 1971

Grames GM, Jansen C: The abnormal bone scan in cerebral infarction. J Nucl Med 14(12):941–943, 1973

Griep RJ: Scanning soft tissue calcification with radio-strontium-85 (abstr). J Nucl Med 9(6):320, 1968

Holmes R: Detection of diffuse metastatic pulmonary calcification with radiostrontium (abstr). J Nucl Med 11(6):327, 1970

Moinuddin M et al.: ^{85}Sr lung scan in a case of pulmonary ossification. J Nucl Med 13(2):174–176, 1972

O'Mara RE et al.: ^{18}F uptake within metastatic osteosarcoma of the liver. Radiology 100:113–114, 1971

Ray GR et al.: Localization of strontium 85 in soft tissue infected by Aspergillus Niger. Radiology 101:119–124, 1971

Schall GL et al.: Uptake of ^{85}Sr by an osteosarcoma metastatic to lung. J Nucl Med 12(3):131–133, 1971

Shirvazi PH et al.: Extraosseous osteogenic sarcoma of the small bowel demonstrated by ^{18}F scanning. J Nucl Med 14(5):295–296, 1973

Except for matters religious, almost all quotable quotes or pithy proverbs can be attributed to either Shakespeare or Franklin. Thus it can be assumed that one of those soothsayers gave us: "Ignorance is bliss." Although improbable, could they have had pulmonary embolism in mind?

Less than 20 years ago everyone knew everything about pulmonary embolism. Embolism was synonymous with an event. The victim was invariably postoperative. She probably had not been ambulatory but was making an uneventful recovery. And then, it happened! While on the bedpan, or attempting to sit up, or getting out of bed, or sneezing, or whatever, she gasped, clutched her chest, and died. Or she gasped, clutched her chest, went into shock but survived, only to exhibit chest pain, dyspnea, and hemophthisis. Laboratory positives of elevated bilirubin and lactic dehydrogenase were obtained. X rays revealed several classic patterns: The "Westermark sign" (hyperaeration secondary to oligemia, secondary to an occluding embolism in a major vessel) or the "Hampton's hump" (a discrete abnormal density usually abutting a pleural fissure that wasn't really an embolism at all but evidence of infarction). And finally, the EKG, spewing tape all over the floor, squiggled out (on very rare occasions) right ventricular hypertrophy. "There you are, dear student," said the grand rounds man, "pulmonary embolism!"

Those were the days, my friend. It was all so neat, tidy, and simple. And as usual, some spoilsports couldn't leave it alone. Sly reports began to infiltrate the literature that pulmonary embolism was probably the most common acute disease in hospital practice, exceeding even pneumonia and emphysema in incidence. Then the dam broke, and everyone got into the act. One extensive series of angiographically proven cases of embolism revealed that dyspnea as a

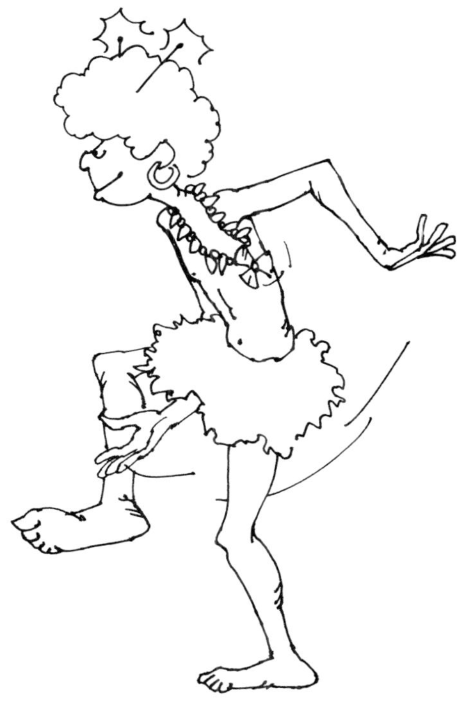

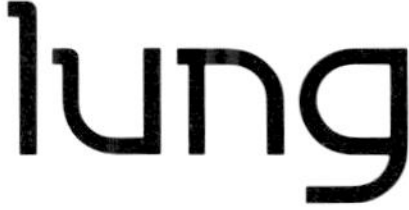

chapter b

lung

symptom was present in only 46% of cases and hemophthisis in only 29%. Another headline screamed that classic laboratory changes could be validated in only 18% of confirmed cases. Even the radiologist admitted that his pronouncements lacked any omniscient ring when referring to this problem. It became evident that embolism and infarction, so often used synonymously, were obviously different and that no definitive clinical pattern was necessarily present in embolism. Indeed, if the size and nature of the original thrombus was such as to produce massive occlusion, a catastrophic event existed. But, if the size and nature of the thrombi were such that multiple microemboli ensued, which undoubtedly was the rule, the clinical pattern had no specificity. This was particularly true if there was spontaneous resolution of the embolic event without infarction.

Undoubtedly, much of the previous "bliss" was founded on the misconception that emboli always led to infarction. Chest pain, previously taken to be the signature of embolism, is totally dependent on infarction. Pulmonary vessels contain no pain receptors. Only when the parietal pleura is involved, a consequence of infarction, does chest pain arise. So, too, the infarctive, not the embolic, event is responsible for the more specific of the multiple roentgen signs "suggestive of Westermark's sign or Hampton's hump." If all of this be true that emboli may possibly not have a specific clinical picture, nor develop specific laboratory values, nor produce specific x-ray patterns, how do we detect its presence and frequency? That sounds like a job for the man in the basement telephone booth—Super Nuclear Man!

Pulmonary emboli, by definition, obstruct pulmonary vessels. Perfusion is altered. If the obstructive vessels are relatively large, the obstruction can be identified by pulmonary angiography. If, however, the obstructive site is more distal in the vascular tree, *i.e.,* arteriolar or part of the capillary network, then even pulmonary angiography may fail to identify the lesion. But perfusion can be investigated in another way. If small, labeled particles are injected into the venous system, and their size carefully controlled so that they can perfuse the vascular tree to the arteriolar–capillary level, a picture of their distribution can be obtained. This picture would be bilaterally symmetric in contour, outline, and degree of activity. If however, a preexistant embolization existed so

that a segment or segments of the perfusion tree were embarrassed, the injection of labeled particles would not perfuse those areas, and the resultant picture would lack symmetry of contour, outline, and activity. Voila! Lung scanning!

Historically, lung scanning was conceptualized and developed as a technique to investigate pulmonary perfusion for regional defects. Time and experience has sophisticated and expanded on this original concept, and although the major indication is still the differential diagnosis of embolism, other applications exist. Deficiencies in perfusion pattern were quickly recognized as being nonspecific. Almost any pulmonary abnormality was associated with some alteration in perfusion. For the scan to be clinically meaningful and not just an exercise in distinguishing normal from abnormal, separation of the patterns of deficit, if possible, was essential. To this end, a second technique was introduced —ventilatory scanning.

It is necessary to carefully distinguish between the perfusion and ventilatory study. The common, garden-variety examination performed wherever a scanning beachhead exists is the perfusion technique using IV-injected macro-aggregated particles tagged with an appropriate radionuclide. The ventilatory technique is less widely performed but is coming up quickly on the outside. It measures regional ventilation by the inhalation of a radioactive gas or microparticle to obtain a host of both physiologic and morphologic measurements and determinations. If computer techniques are available and phthisiologists are on hand, many of the alphabet studies (*e.g.,* VC, MEV, FEV, IVC, TV, RUD, V:Q) usually reserved for the pulmonary function laboratory can be derived. Scans obtained at different phases of the respiratory cycle permit reasonable judgments of the integrity of the airways. An image immediately following the introduction of the gas depicts the distribution pattern on inspiration. Breathing is then restricted to a closed system so that the radioactive gas may be redistributed in situations in which major airway obstruction exists, reflecting the status of the bronchiolar–alveolar intercommunication system, such as the pores of Kohn. Once equilibrium has been reached, usually in 1–2 min, images are made sequentially of the wash-out phase. Breathing room air in and expiring the radioactive gas out into a trap permits a series of pictures documenting

the time and symmetry of the clearance.
Often small airway obstructions can be identified
by the delay or asymmetry of the wash-out
pattern.

WHAT

perfusion

Perfusion studies are usually performed with
radioactive labeled particles. The sizes and
number of particles are critical to the success of
the study and to the safety of the patient. The
thought of voluntarily producing some several
hundred thousand emboli in someone's lungs is
"breathtaking." To ensure that this dyspnea is
merely symbolic and not actual requires careful
use of these particles. It has been determined
that in man the arteriolar bed numbers some
300 million units and the capillary bed some
280 billion. The particle used in scanning is
adjusted in size from approximately 10μ–50μ.
(Capillary size is approximately 7μ–10μ.) The
average scanning dose contains some 800
thousand particles. This combination of size and
number results in the embolization of approximately 400 thousand arterioles (the particles
greater than 20μ in size) and approximately 400
thousand capillaries (the particles less than 20μ
in size). Thus a huge safety factor exists. When
these criteria are satisfied, an extraction
efficiency of 90+% is achieved on the first lung
pass-through. However, it has been determined
that even in the unlikely event of a right-to-left
cardiac shunt, with the particles by-passing the
pulmonary bed and reaching the cerebral
circulation, the standard dose presents no
hazard.

Having established acceptable criteria of
number and size, one last consideration had to
be satisfied. The particle has to be degradable.
The iatrogenic embolization has to be short-
lived. Ideally, the condition should exist only as
long as it is necessary to obtain the desired
studies. Aggregated human serum albumin meets
all of these criteria. It can be prepared in such a
manner as to guarantee particulate size range,
and it is cleared from the lungs with a half time
of 4–6 hours. Clearing is accomplished primarily
by the inherent fragility of the particle; pulsation
of the vessel on the entrapped particle results
in its ultimate fragmentation to sizes below 5μ,
the fragments being carried off to be cleared by
the reticuloendothelial system.

Until recently, the particles were tagged
with ^{131}I. This nuclide, while satisfactory for
performance of the study, has certain characteristics less desirable than those of other tracers.
Its half-life of approximately 8 days results in a
limitation of administered dose, which in turn
increases examination time. Thyroid accumulation occurs unless blocking medication is given
—a not insurmountable obstacle, but neverthe-
less, an additional nuisance. Additionally, its
gamma energy is less efficient if the camera is
the scanning instrument. Again, the breech was
filled by the radiopharmacologist. Kits are now
available to permit simple preparation of ^{99m}Tc
macroaggregated human serum albumin. This
agent has replaced the old standard ^{131}I macro-
aggregated human serum albumin since it
permits considerably larger scanning doses,
dramatically reducing the study time.

Other combinations are utilized and have
enthusiastic adherents. Microspheres of albumin
rather than the aggregated type guarantee a
more uniform particle size. The characteristics
of ^{99m}Tc iron hydroxide are suitable although its
retention time within the lung has been estimated
to be up to 1 year. A complex of ^{87m}Sr–Ca
phosphate has been suggested when combined
liver–lung scans are indicated.

ventilation

Decisions, decisions, decisions. A request for a
ventilatory study requires one basic choice—to
utilize gas or particulate matter. The usual pros
and cons of each must be examined and a
determination made. It is probably fair to state
that at this time, gas is more widely employed.
It is the more physiologic agent for the purpose
and permits wider latitudes of investigation.
However, it is more difficult to handle both on
administration and collection. Additionally,
because of its dynamic characteristics, only the
gamma camera can be used to capture its
pattern and then in only one projection. Inhaled
particulate matter distributes along the airways
and can be scanned slowly and in multiple views.
However, particle size is critical to success.
Localization within the tracheobronchial tree is
size dependent, larger particles lodge in the
larger airways. Since the purpose of this
technique is almost exclusively for the detection
of large airway obstruction, false positive studies
are not uncommon, resulting from unappreciated
and unanticipated microparticulate size vari-

ations. The procedure of administration is longer than that with gas and may be too tedious for many patients.

If gas is chosen, xenon (^{133}Xe) is almost the only agent available at this time. Nitrogen (^{13}N) and oxygen (^{15}O) have been utilized, but they are not suitable for routine and general use. Xenon 127 may eventually replace its cousin, but at this moment ^{133}Xe is it. This gas lends itself to physiologic study because even though it has a relatively long physical half-life (5.3 days) it has an almost negligible biologic half-life. Its inert characteristics result in almost immediate clearance from the lungs with respiration. Its gamma energy is slightly lower than ideal for imaging (81 keV), but all in all it is a useful agent.

If radioaerosol inhalation is the decision, ^{99m}Tc-tagged albumin particles are subjected to nebulizing techniques to produce a size range in the order of 0.5μ–10μ. Recently, ultrasonic devices have been introduced which produce an aerosol of appropriate size that can be administered more quickly. If the particle size exceeds 10μ it will deposit itself in the upper airways, *i.e.,* the nose, mouth, and pharynx. Only the small units reach the alveoli. It is estimated that 90% of the inhaled particles do not become localized and are exhaled.

HOW

perfusion

The determination of regional perfusion is as simple as any scanning test can be. Unfortunately, the patients requiring this study may be the sickest of the entire scanning population. Therefore, closer coordination between the clinical and nuclear divisions is mandatory to achieve maximum efficiency. The actual procedure consists of the introduction of the labeled particles by an IV puncture. Usually, the patient is supine, although some prefer to introduce half of the dose with the patient supine and the second half prone. Imaging is initiated immediately. A minimum of four views is desired. The clinical state of the patient often governs the length of the study and the views obtained. If a dual-headed rectilinear instrument is available, permitting the four views—anterior, posterior, right and left lateral—to be obtained in two

imaging periods, the time of study is approximately 30 min (Fig. 6-1). If only one view is possible at a time either with a single-headed rectilinear or gamma camera then the total study time may reach an hour. Often in the critical patient, a recumbent posture is difficult or impossible. In these situations the camera is far more versatile, permitting study in any position. Often continuous oxygen or some other supportive measure is required. These need not seriously interfere with the performance of the study. With sufficient patience in both explanation and reassurance even the most critical and anxious patient can usually be studied.

ventilation

Pictorial representation of regional ventilation is more difficult to obtain than its perfusion cousin. A specialized apparatus is required to keep the gas contained. The agent is introduced by having the patient take in a deep breath through a carefully sealed system and then continue to breathe into this system until all images, including the washout of all the gas from the lungs, have been obtained (Fig. 6-2). A modification of this approach is to introduce the gas dissolved in saline IV. An immediate image following injection gives a perfusion distribution: the gas quickly diffuses into the alveoli and the patient again breathes in a closed system. All subsequent scans are then of the ventilatory type.

The type of apparatus employed is a function of the Rube Goldberg in man. Tubing, valves, nose clips, mouth pieces, spirometers, filters, traps, collection bags, shielding material, etc. are packaged into "the thing." It must be capable of permitting simple delivery of the active gas and of then capturing the exhalation. The gas is eventually evacuated into the atmosphere through a variety of techniques, the most common being some type of venting system.

If microspheres are employed, they too require a special breathing apparatus.

The ventilatory study is not appropriate for the acutely ill since patient cooperation is mandatory. For all others it can be accomplished in 5–10 min. It is usually done in conjunction with and preceding a perfusion evaluation.

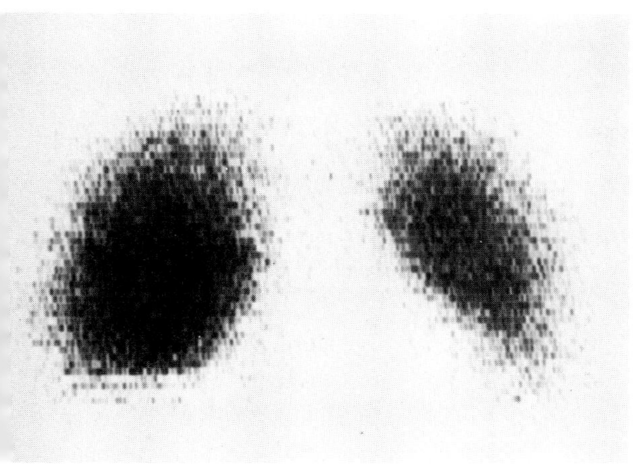
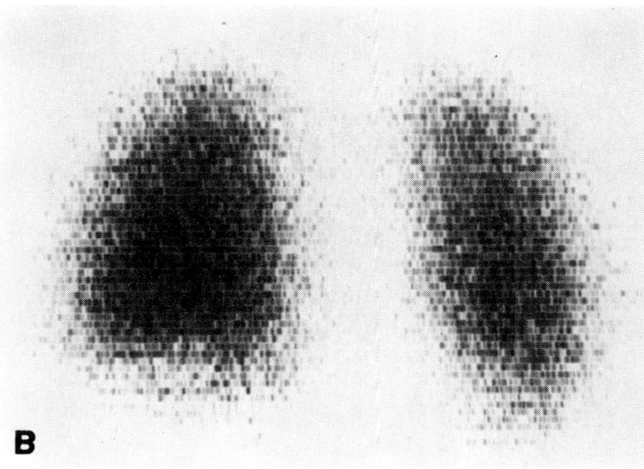

B

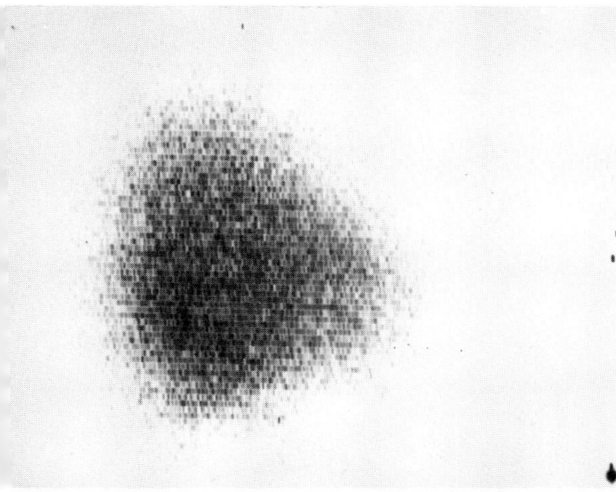
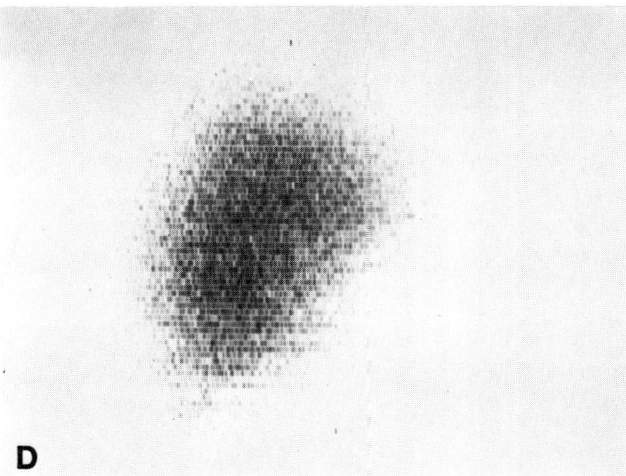

D

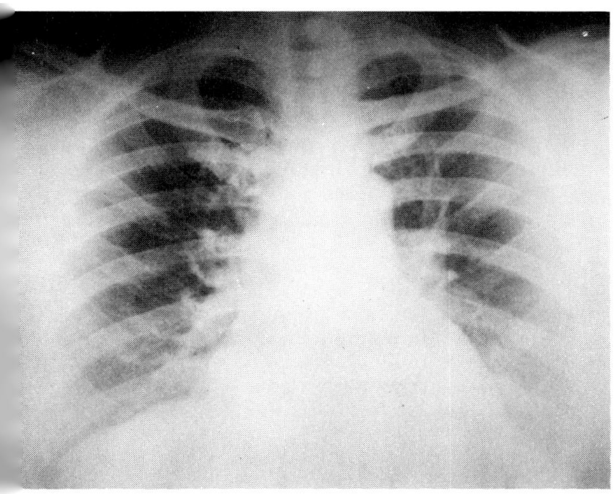

Fig. 6-1. Normal pulmonary perfusion

A. Anterior. Each lung is seen with the space between them representing the cardiac silhouette. This contour varies and affects the visualized left lung base. In this case the left cardiac segment is prominent and obscures the base of the left lung. Activity is uniform throughout.

B. Posterior. The lung bases are best seen in this view. The right is usually slightly higher than the left because of the higher normal right diaphragm. Often the most dependent portions of the bases are unsharp secondary to diaphragmatic motion. The levels of the apices are identical.

C and D. Right and left lateral. Often there is an impression on the anterior aspect of the left lung from the heart. The right lung presents with convex margins.

E. X ray. No pulmonary disease

WHY

embolism–infarction

Perfusion lung scanning is the ideal procedure to confirm or deny a differential diagnosis that includes embolism–infarction. As has been discussed, the informational bits that lead to the suspicion are highly variable. The scan is particularly valuable when the chest x ray is negative. It must be clearly understood that the scan depicts only perfusion, and the etiology of defects cannot be deduced from the scan alone. Thus, any major parenchymal or mediastinal disorder visualized by a positive x-ray image can be expected to have a comparable, positive scan image (Figs. 6-3 and 6-4), but there are diseases in which the x ray is normal and the scan identifies a perfusion deficit. This combination of x-ray negative–scan positive is highly suggestive of embolism if embolism was initially suspected (Fig. 6-5). Embolism, however, is not the only explanation for the negative–positive combination. A similar pattern can be obtained in acute bronchial asthma. The bronchospasm

Fig. 6-3. Right lower lobe pneumonia ▶
A. X ray. There is a consolidative process in the lower right lung.
B. Perfusion scan. In the posterior view a large perfusion defect corresponds to the consolidative process. No other perfusion changes are present.

Fig. 6-4. Sulcus tumor (right lung) ▶
    A. X ray. Original interpretation was concerned with atypical linear densities in each lung base. No apical pathology was described.
B and C. Anterior and posterior perfusion scans. Perfusion was preserved bilaterally except for the right apex. The apex activity was lower than the left. Review of the chest x ray now suggested a right apical mass.
    D. X ray. Laminograph of the right apex confirms a mass (arrows) and explains the absence of apical perfusion.

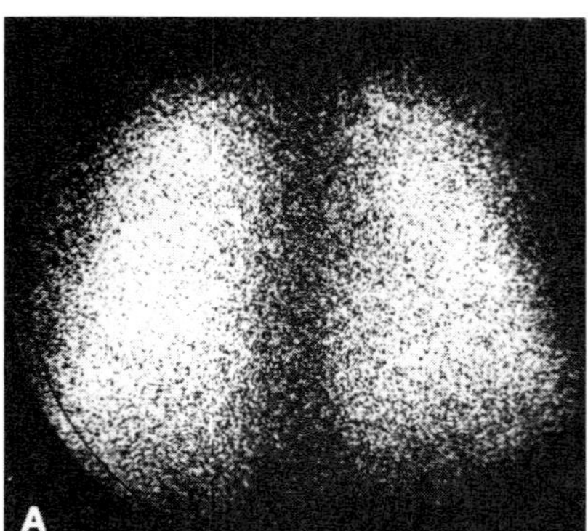
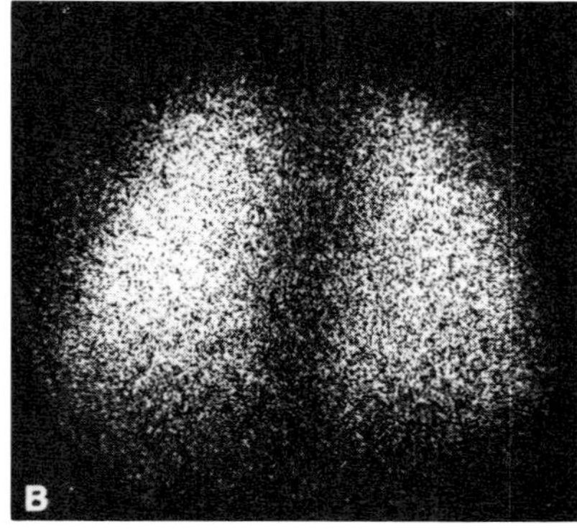
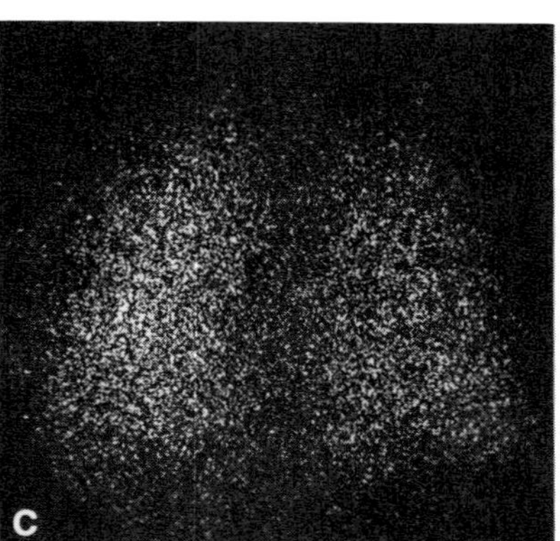

Fig. 6-2. Normal pulmonary ventilation
A. Scan, 0–30 sec. The patient is seated with his back to the camera. A deep inhalation of air and ^{133}Xe is taken, and the breath is held. Activity is equally distributed throughout both lungs.
B. Scan, 120–150 sec. Following a period of normal breathing in the closed ^{133}Xe system, inhalation of room air is initiated with exhalation still into the closed system. The ^{133}Xe is "washed out." Activity begins to diminish. The decrease is uniform throughout the lung and bilaterally symmetric.
C. Scan, 150–180 sec. Wash-out is almost complete.

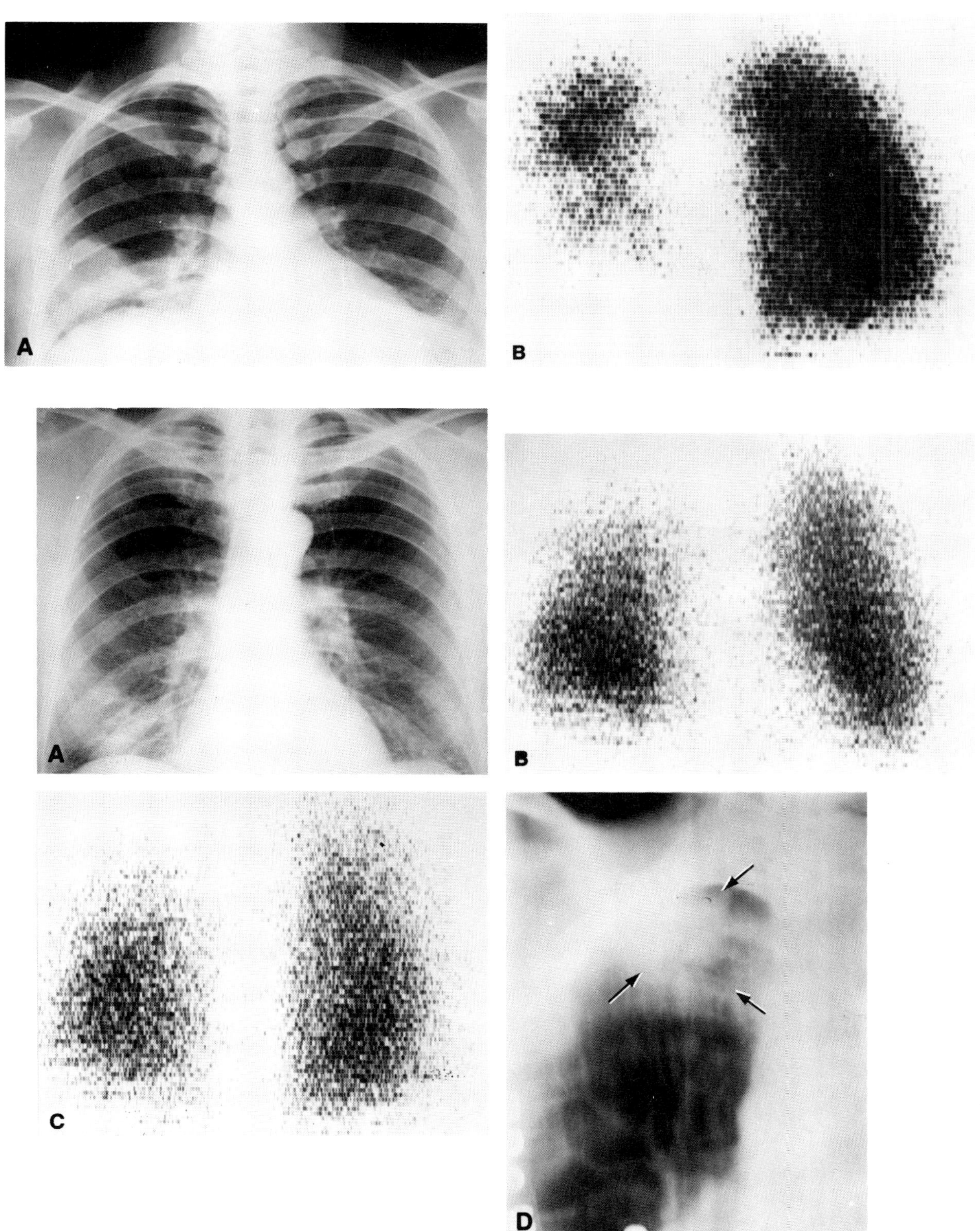

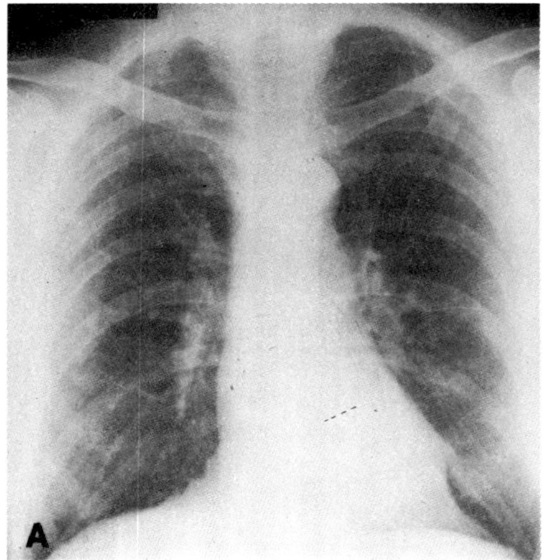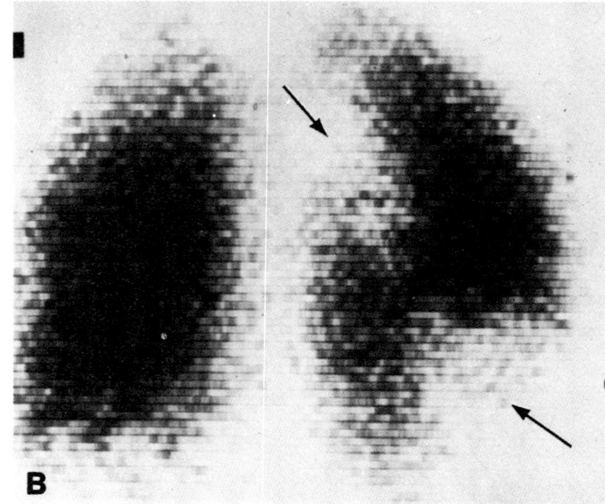

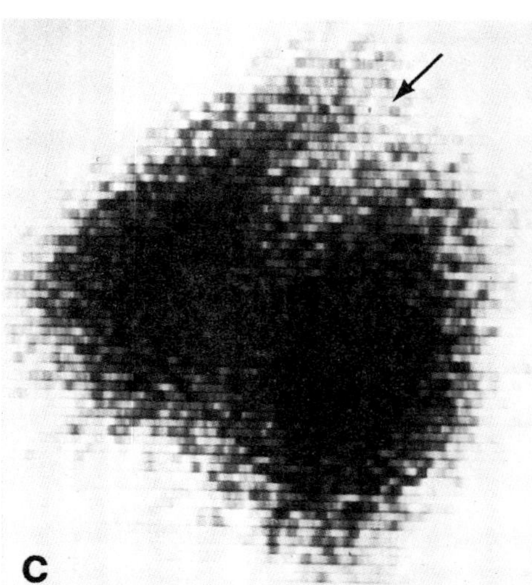

Fig. 6-5. Pulmonary embolism

A. X ray. No gross cardiac or pulmonary pathology. The patient was admitted because of an acute left lower extremity thrombophlebitis. There were no symptoms of embolism. Perfusion scan was routinely performed because of the phlebitis.

B and C. Posterior **(B)** and left lateral **(C)** perfusion scan. Perfusion defects (arrows) are present in the apical posterior segment of the upper left lobe and the lateral basilar segment of the left lower lobe.

D. Perfusion scan, 2 weeks later. Perfusion is restored.

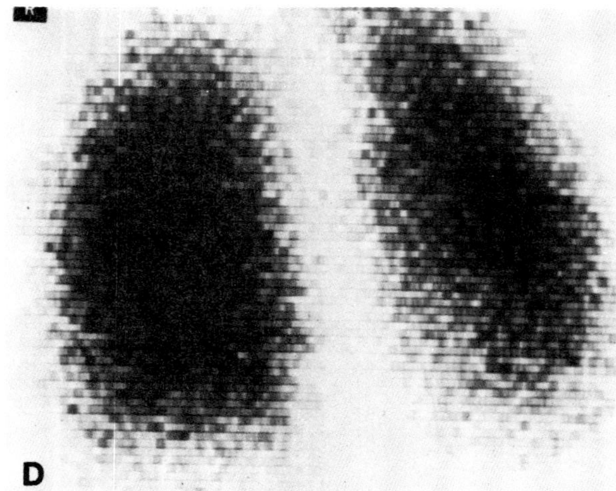

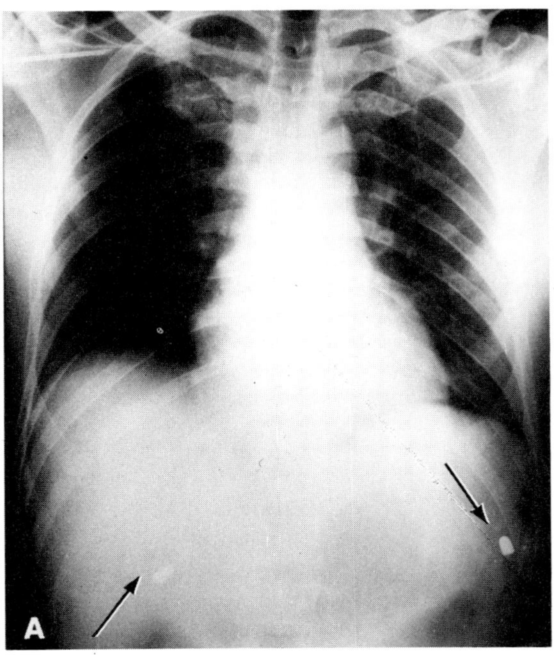

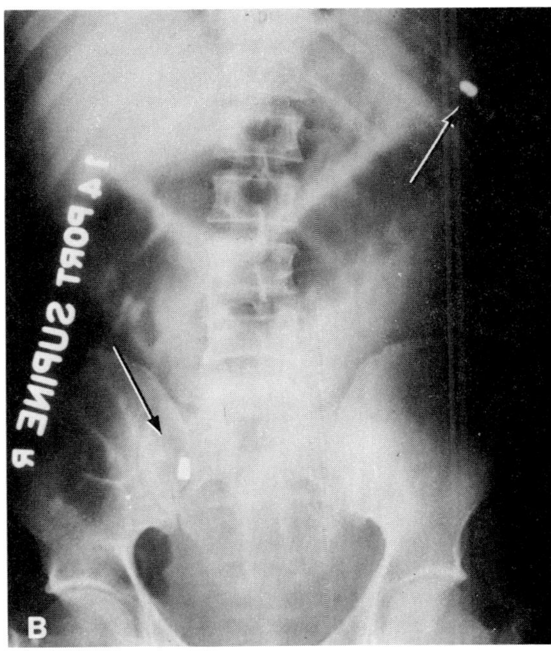

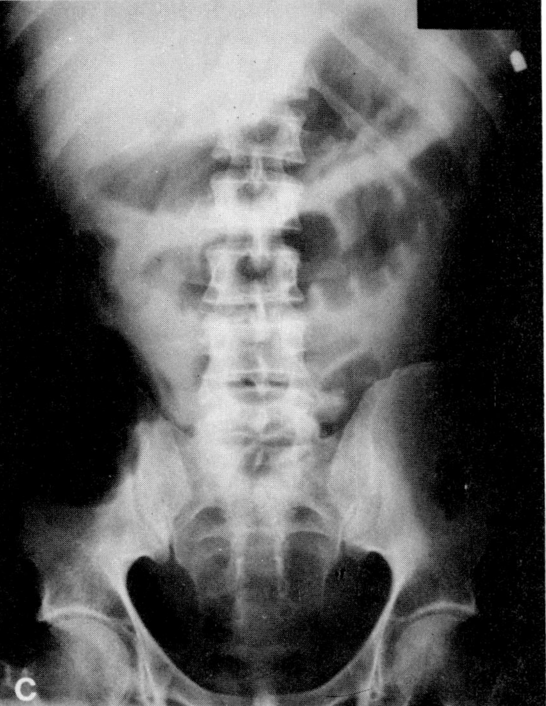

Fig. 6-6. Bullet embolism. Immediately following multiple gunshot wounds to the abdomen, an acute abdominal x-ray series was initiated.

A. Supine chest, 1st exposure. Bullets (arrows) are present in both the upper left and right abdominal quadrants.

B. Supine abdomen, 2nd exposure, 3–4 min after **A.** There is a significant change in position of the right bullet. The left is unchanged (arrows).

C. Supine abdomen, 3rd exposure, 10 min later. The right bullet is no longer apparent. The left is unchanged.

D. Chest x ray, 2 hours later. The left bullet has been removed surgically. The right bullet has migrated and embolized a pulmonary artery to the left upper lobe.

E. Perfusion scan, anterior. No obvious perfusion changes.

F. Perfusion scan, left lateral. There is a discrete defect (arrows) in the perfusion of the anterior segment of the left upper lobe supplied by the bullet—embolized pulmonary artery. In the anterior view the deficit is masked by "shine thru" activity from the posterior segments.

(continued)

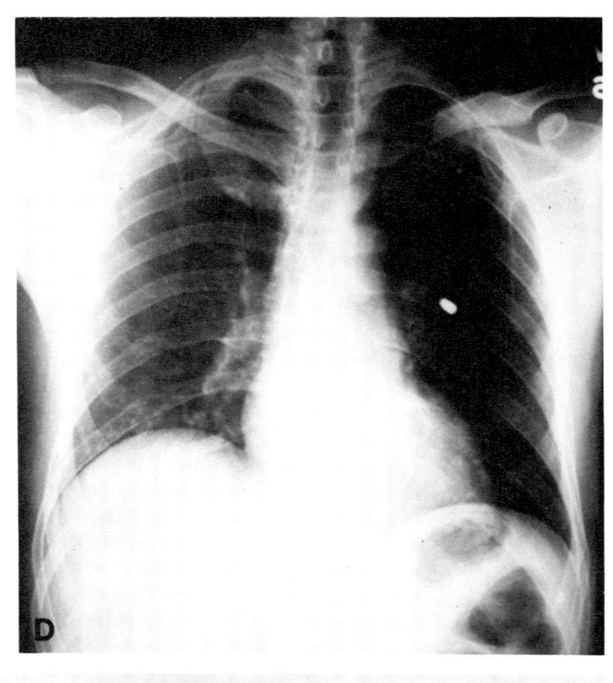

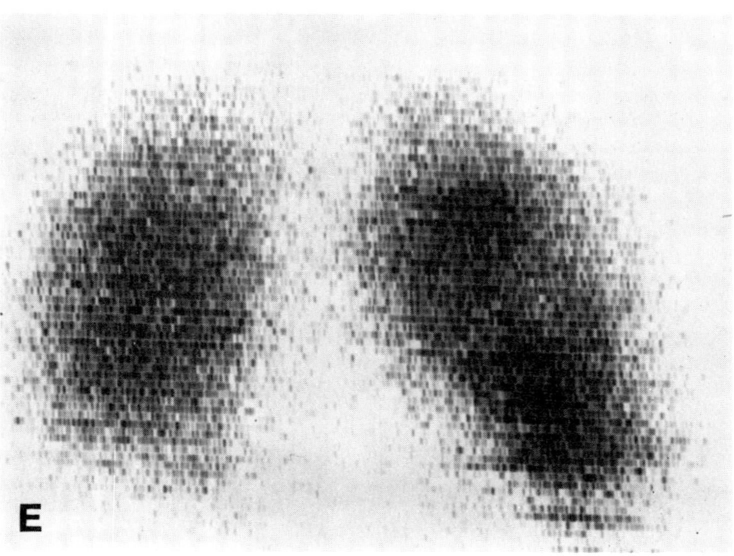

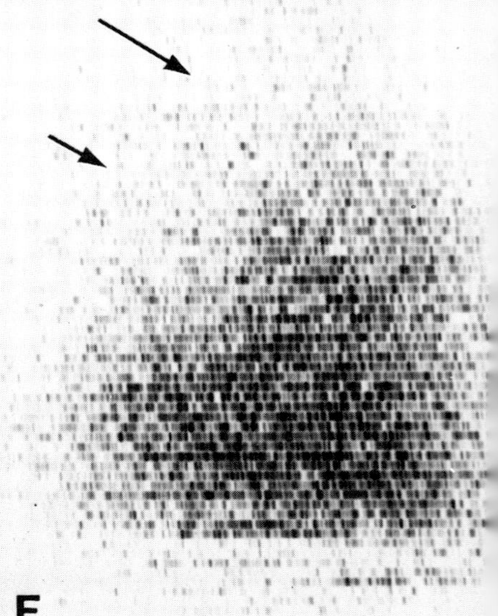

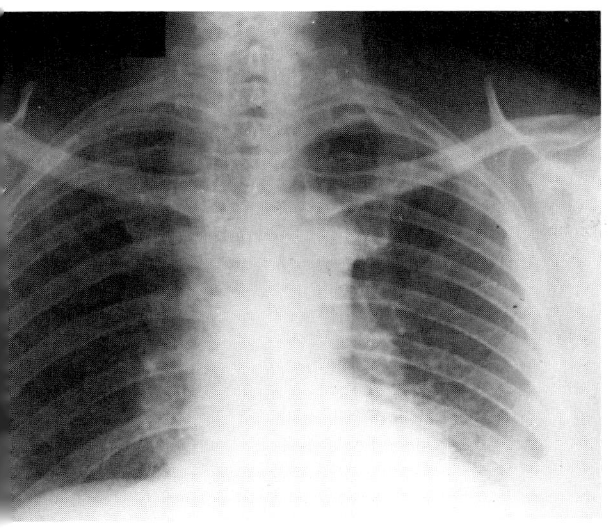
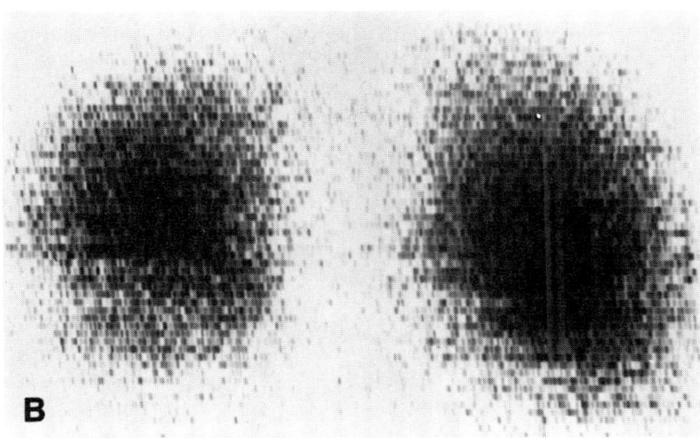
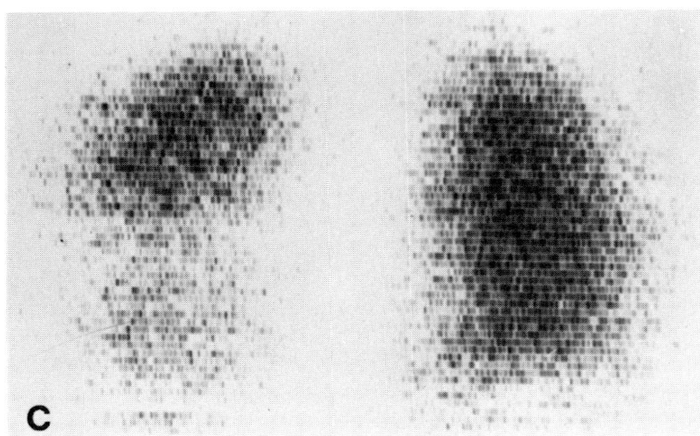
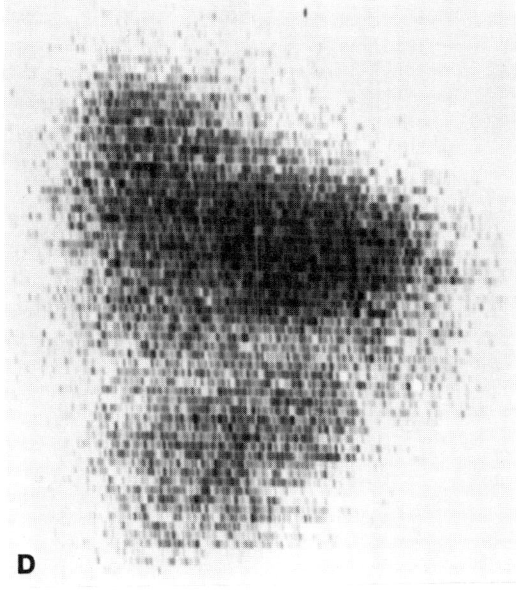
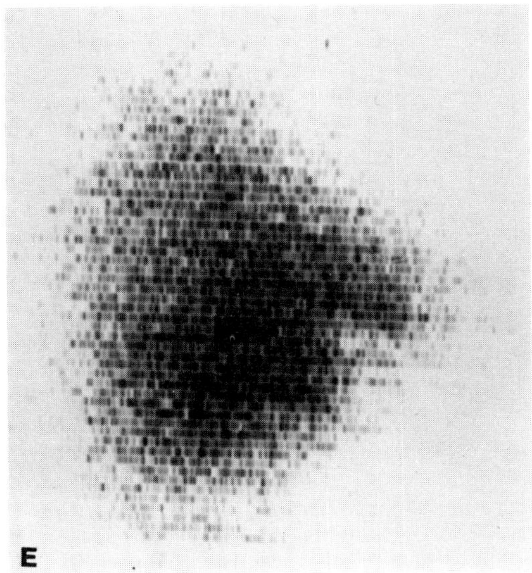

Fig. 6-7. Pulmonary embolism (right middle and lower lobes)

A. X ray. The left lower lung region is less well aerated than is the normal-appearing right base. The left diaphragm and left costophrenic angle are less well defined than on the right.

B. Perfusion scan, anterior. Minimal decrease in right lower lobe perfusion

C. Perfusion scan, posterior. Marked loss of perfusion of the inferior half of the right lung

D. Perfusion scan, right lateral. Areas of decreased activity in right middle and lower lobes

E. Perfusion scan, left lateral. Questionable focal defect in lingular segment of upper lobe

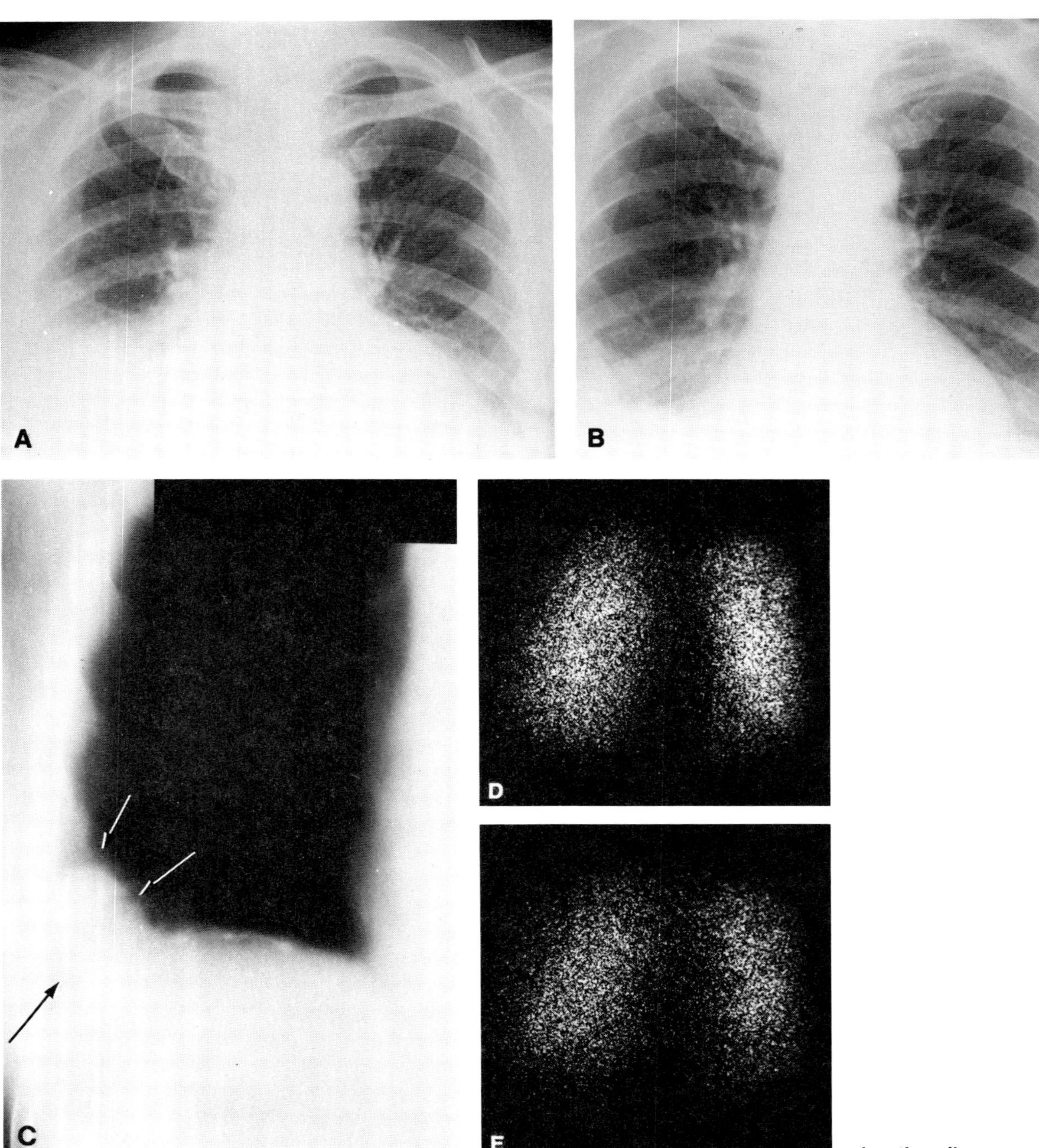

(continued)

Fig. 6-8. Pulmonary embolism with infarction.
Diagnosis: Embolism—left lower lobe, infarct—right lower lobe

- **A.** X ray. An ill-defined abnormal density obscures the right lung base suggesting consolidation and effusion. There is minimal effusion in the left lung base.
- **B.** X ray, 10 days later. The right base changes are now more discrete and ovoid in contour. The left base is clear.
- **C.** X ray, laminographic section. The right lower lobe lesion is discrete and homogeneous (arrows). Additionally, pleural calcification is identified. Questionable tumor; questionable organizing infarct.
- **D and E.** Ventilation scan. Wash-in and wash-out images are within normal limits.
- **F.** Perfusion scan, posterior. There is no significant change in right lower lobe perfusion, but a surprising gross loss in left lower lobe.
- **G.** Perfusion scan, left lateral. Almost the entire lower lobe is affected (arrow).

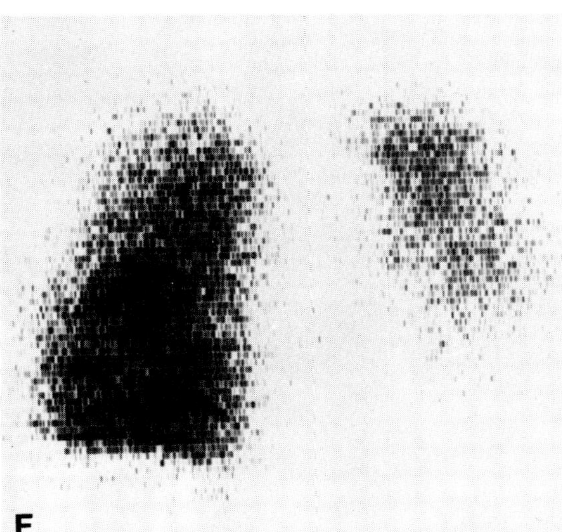

F

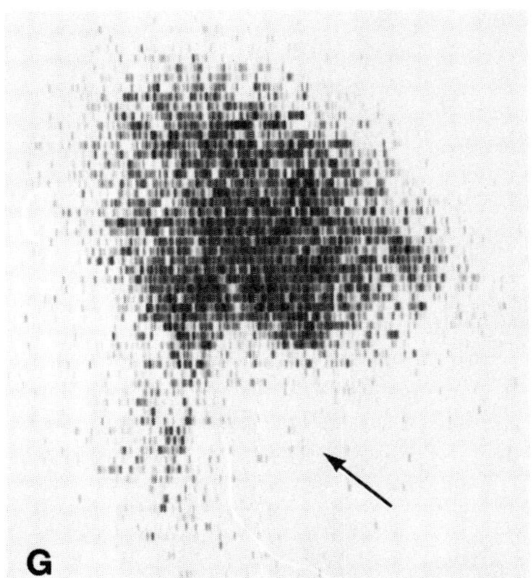

G

quickly leads to vasospasm, which is reflected on scanning as perfusion deficits. The x ray may be normal. These patients, however, do not usually present a clinical diagnostic dilemma.

Other combinations may suggest embolism as the etiology of obvious deficit. Embolism or infarction is a disorder of fixed anatomic geography. A lung segment is affected by the condition. Therefore, the consequent perfusion deficit will be anatomically consistent with a vascular distribution. The area of involvement will usually be discrete (Fig. 6-6). Additionally, the exciting event will frequently result in more than one site of insult. The thrombi responsible may occur as a shower so that multiple areas are involved. Not uncommonly when the x ray is positive for a nonspecific change the scan will not only depict this area as one of deficit, but will also demonstrate other sites of deficit not suspected on x ray. This combination of single positive (x ray) and multiple positive (scan) is also highly suggestive of embolism (Fig. 6-7).

In those cases in which there is an x-ray lesion and the scan lesion is limited to that location alone, the diagnosis may be no clearer than before the scan was made. It is hoped, in this example, that the x-ray abnormality is sufficiently specific as to permit diagnosis on its pattern alone. A common example of such a finding is consolidation consistent with pneumonia. However, many x-ray positive lesions are nonspecific, *e.g.*, a linear density or pleural effusion. In this situation, a ventilatory study may improve the differentiation since a negative scan suggests that the perfusion defect is purely vascular and probably embolic. If, however, the ventilatory scan is also abnormal, nothing has changed. Although the lesion may be obstruction (such as atelectasis) producing ventilatory defect, embolism will also produce eventual airway obstruction. So a pattern of abnormal x ray with abnormal perfusion and normal ventilation probably equals embolism–infarction (Fig. 6-8). When the pattern is abnormal: abnormal: abnormal, contrast angiography may be necessary for diagnosis. It should again be stressed that even angiography may prove fallible if the embolization has occurred at the arteriolar–capillary level and not in a major vessel.

Serial perfusion scanning is of value both for initial diagnosis and to assess the affects of therapy and aid in determining prognosis. It is not unusual to evaluate a scan with an ischemic

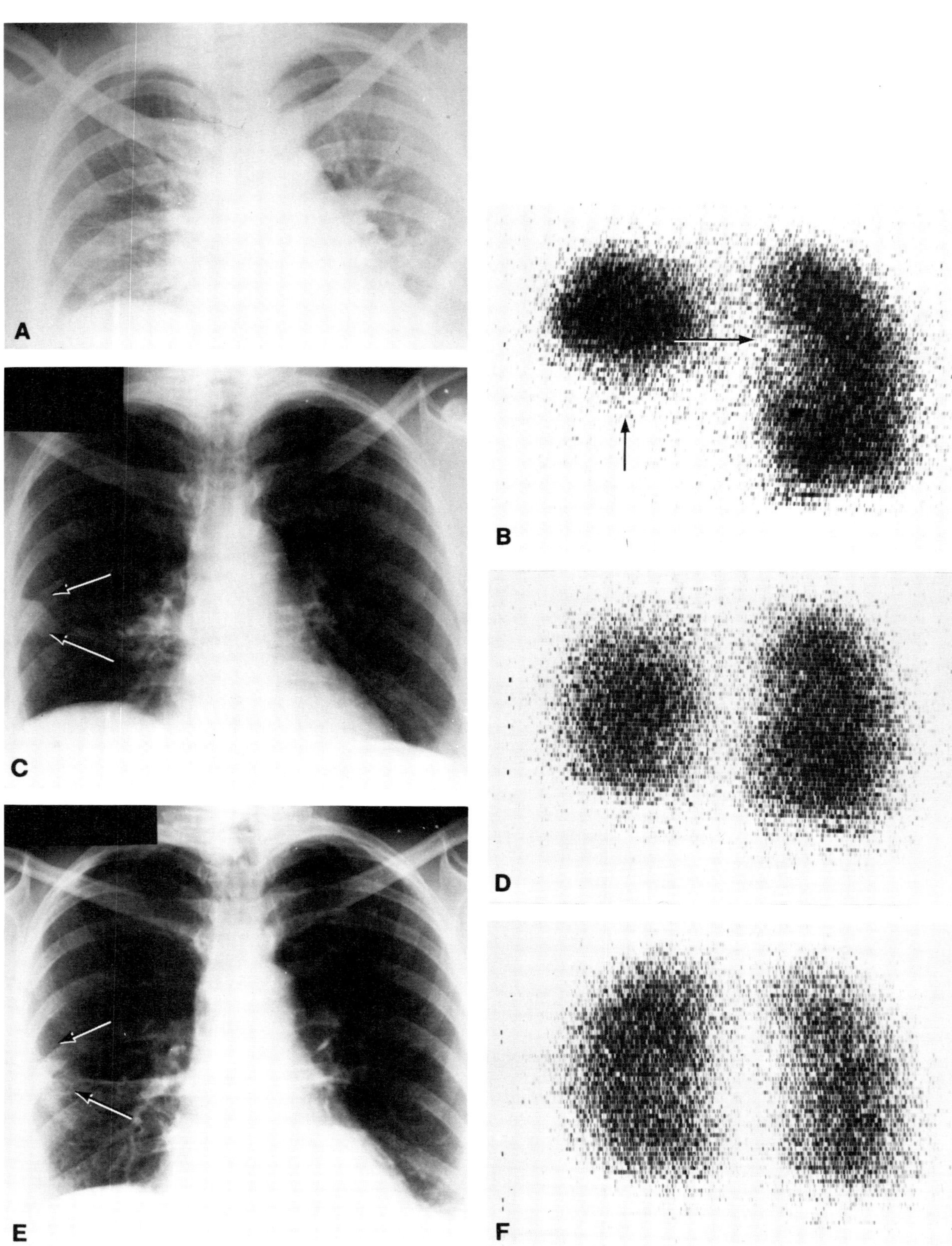

**Fig. 6-9. Pulmonary emboli with infarction and
cavitation**
  A. X ray (11/26/73). Bilateral hilar prominence,
  vascular congestion, and minimal elevation of the
  right hemidiaphragm
  B. Perfusion scan (11/26/73). Massive perfusion
  defect (arrow) involving the right middle and
  lower lobes and a smaller deficit (arrow) in a
  segment of the left upper lobe
  C. X ray (12/11/73). Congestive changes have
  resolved. A triangular density (arrows) abuts the
  pleural surfaces of the interlobar fissure and
  lateral chest wall.
  D. Perfusion scan (12/11/73). The left upper lobe
  defect is completely resolved; the right middle
  lower lobe changes are almost completely
  resolved.
  E. X ray (1/2/74). The right lateral midlung defect is
  no longer homogeneous. A lucent central change
  is now present (arrows).
  F. Perfusion scan (1/2/74). Complete resolution with
  satisfactory bilateral perfusion

defect(s) in a patient suffering from emphysema.
Is the ischemic zone secondary to a newly
acquired embolism or does it reflect the chronic
obstructive lung disease? The ischemia of
embolism–infarction, as a rule, is a dynamic,
changing phenomenon. Within 3–5 days some
change should occur in the scan pattern. If
there have been no new or additional insults,
the original defect will be significantly reduced
in volume or even resolved. If embolic showers
have continued, new or greater volumes of
perfusion deficit will be recognized. On the other
hand, the ischemia of emphysema is static.
Thus, when reviewed with the original the
second scan may permit a valid differential
judgment as to the cause of the lesions. The
serial approach also documents the efficacy
of therapy. The appearance of new lesions
demonstrates that management has been
ineffectual and more-dramatic measures may be
indicated (Fig. 6-9). If improvement is noted, as
is the usual rule unless the patient has serious
preexisting cardiopulmonary disease or is very
elderly, repetitive studies at 3- to 5-day intervals
should be performed until either there is
complete resolution, commonly in 1–2 weeks, or
until the pattern remains constant on two
successive studies in a clinically well patient.
Often a residual defect will remain. It is most
helpful to have such documentation available
for comparison at some future date. It is not
uncommon for a patient who has suffered one
embolic event to have repetitive episodes. A
scan at the time of a suspected recurrent acute
problem depicting a focal ischemic area cannot
be differentiated from the residual infarctive
defect of a preceding insult. The availability of
the old study for comparison with the new
permits definitive judgment as to the significance of the defect (Fig. 6-10).

chronic obstructive lung disease

Ischemia produces defects in perfusion scans.
Ischemia probably produces defects in ventilatory scans. It is the "probably" that makes the
difference. Embolic–infarctive disease always
causes ischemia, whereas chronic obstructive
lung disease (COLD) probably always causes
ischemia (Fig. 6-11). It is the "probably" that
makes the difference. The "difference" is whether
or not perfusion scanning or ventilatory scanning,
or both, are of any significant value in studying
lung pathologies other than embolic events. Are

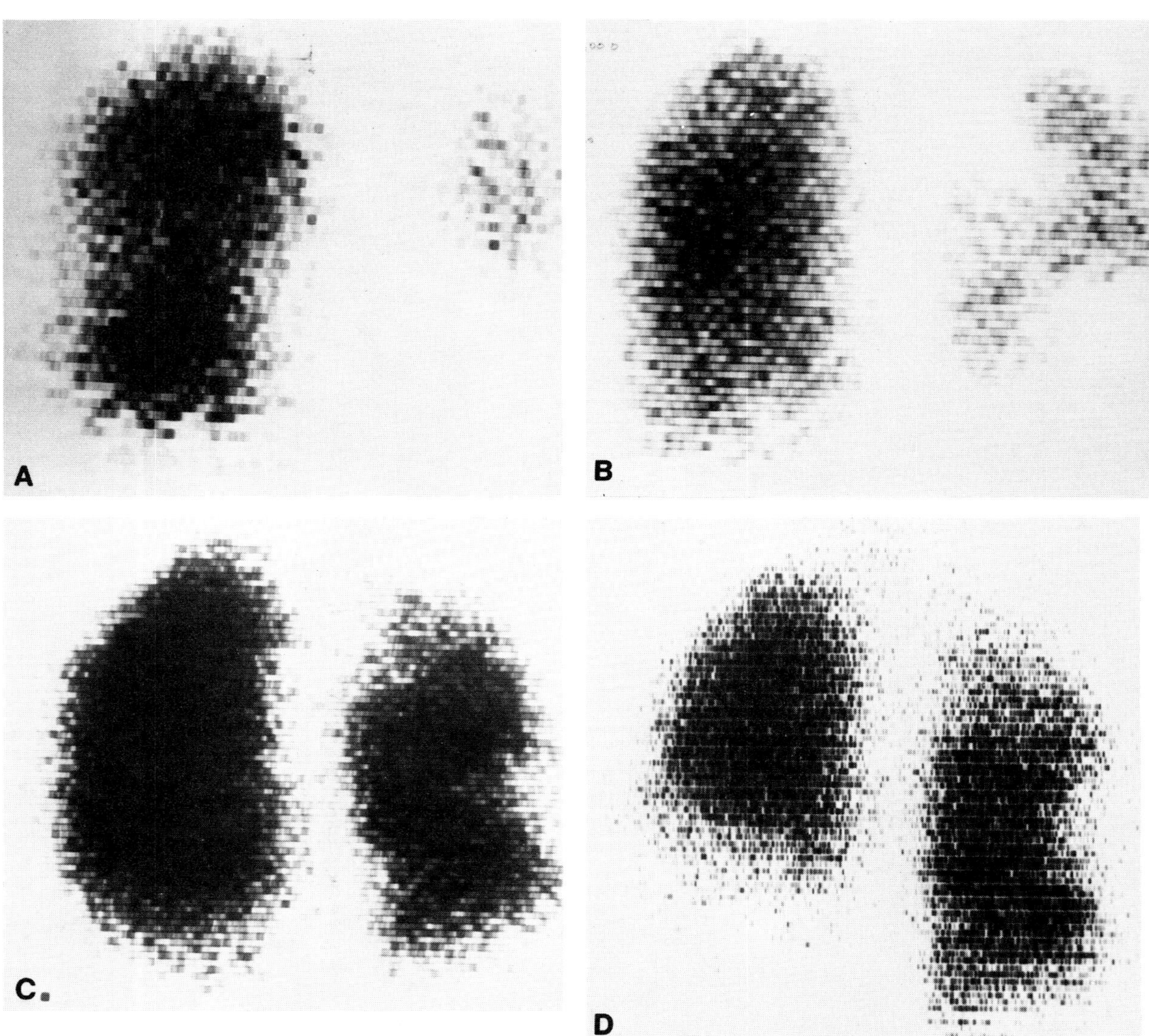

Fig. 6-10. Pulmonary emboli with residual defects and recurrence
A. Perfusion scan (5/12/67). The posterior perfusion image identifies almost
complete loss of left lung perfusion and a defect at the lateral margin of the
right lung.
B. Perfusion scan (5/29/67). Posterior image suggests improvement of left lung
perfusion and complete resolution of right lung changes.
C. Perfusion scan (9/5/67). Posterior image 4 months later indicates a normal
perfusion of the right lung but residual defects in the left apex and lateral margin.
D. Perfusion scan (9/21/71). Posterior image 4 years later suggests a large defect
in right lower lobe perfusion, but no new changes in the left.

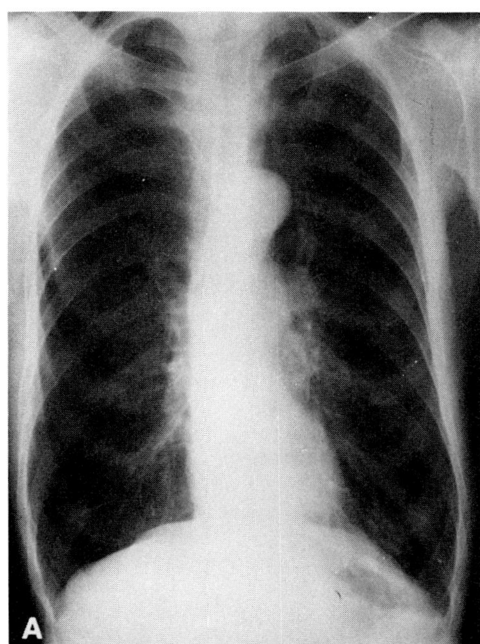

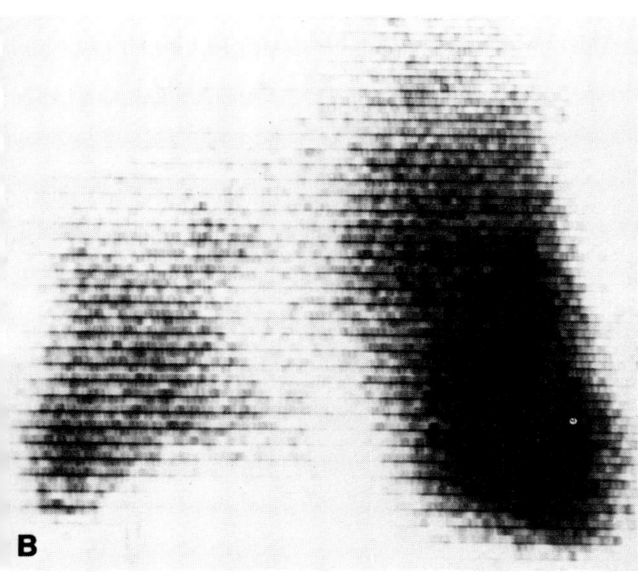

Fig. 6-11. Chronic obstructive lung disease
A. X ray. There is bilateral pulmonary hyperaeration. The diaphragms are depressed and scalloped. No bulla are recognized.
B. Perfusion scan. There is almost complete absence of right upper lobe perfusion and grossly impaired right middle and lower lobe perfusion. The left upper lobe is also affected.

the many varieties of COLD, *e.g.,* emphysema, asthma, bronchitis, bronchiectasis, and their related 57 cousins—α-1-antitrypsin deficiencies, cystic fibrosis—areas for scanning investigation? (Fig. 6-12) If the studies are performed, particularly the ventilatory, with computer potential so that function can be analysed, the answer is probably yes. If, on the other hand, as we have said many times earlier, we deal primarily with the potentials of the community hospital facility, which at least now does not routinely possess such sophisticated machinery, the answer is probably maybe.

Routine is the key condition in the debate. There are many situations in which COLD patients are studied with benefit. (Does many equal routine?) For instance, the patient with chronic emphysema and a negative chest x ray who is suspected of having suffered from an embolic episode has been mentioned earlier. Although the defects of emphysema do not follow the same anatomic pattern supposedly so readily recognized in embolism, the distinction may be difficult to make with certainty. The perfusion scan showing sites of ischemia is by itself nondiagnostic, but if an accompanying ventilatory scan is negative, then the diagnosis of embolism can be made with reasonable certainty. It is conceivable that the initial held breath inspiratory view could be normal in emphysema even if later "wash-out" images are abnormal. If, however, the ventilatory study is positive—which is far more common—then the immediate differential is still uncertain. As has also been previously noted, serial perfusion scanning alone usually permits retrospective diagnosis because of the static pattern of emphysema and the changing pattern of embolism.

Another case in point is the wheezing patient who has no previous history of asthma and who may have embolism. There have been reports of wheezing as a physical sign accompanying an embolic episode. Both perfusion and ventilatory studies may aid in the differential. Acute asthma produces the most bizarre of all defect patterns on both perfusion and ventilatory scan. Thus, a severe double positive pattern contrasted to a perfusion positive with a less-severe ventilatory positive or even ventilatory negative probably means asthma in the former and embolism in the latter. Distinction is also improved by rescanning following the administration of vasodilaters. The asthmatic wheezer will demonstrate some

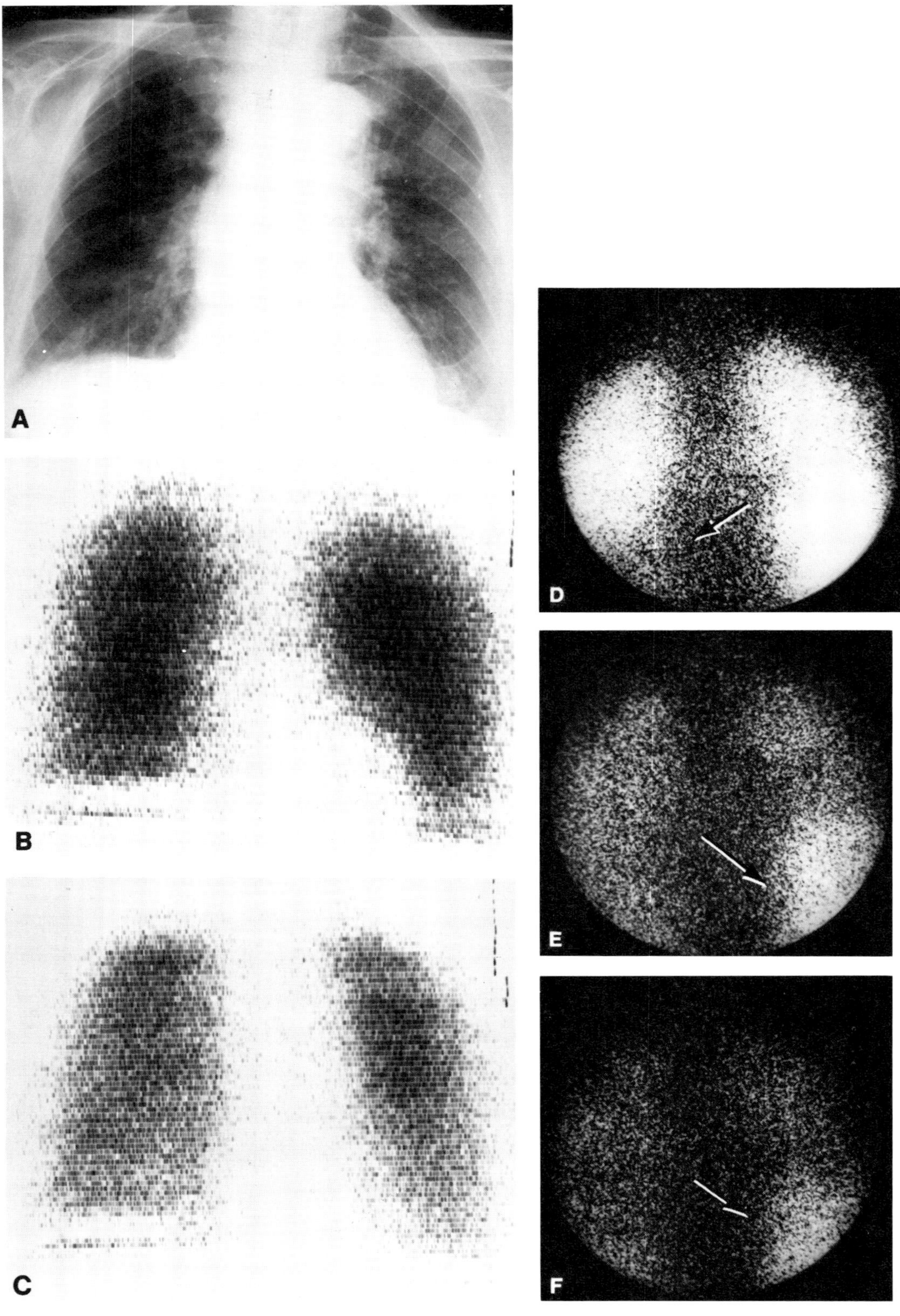

response; the embolic wheezer will still flunk
his scan.

Thus, except in the differential diagnosis
from embolism the routine applicability of
ventilatory scanning when computerized function
studies are excluded is still questionable. The
clinical status of these patients is usually
defined by history and physical findings, x ray,
and laboratory studies. Pictorial documentation
by scanning, as a rule, does not add a significant
parameter to their management.

tumor

Here, too, the role of scanning has questionable
primary significance. If a lung mass is clearly
identified and is clearly malignant, the contribution of the perfusion scan alone is dubious. If
a mass is clearly identified but not clearly
malignant, the scan may contribute inferentially
to the differential diagnosis. Almost any parenchymal defect visualized by x ray will have a
corresponding perfusion defect. However,
certain malignant neoplasms produce a
perfusion defect far in excess of that which
would be anticipated from their size alone. Total
loss of perfusion can be noted in a lung in which
only a relatively small lesion is seen on films
(Fig. 6-13). The mechanism is not completely

established. In some cases it is a direct
consequence of encroachment or invasion of
the pulmonary artery by the tumor or nodes.
Another hypothesis that has been offered is
reflex hypoperfusion secondary to the regional
hypoxia. Regardless of the mechanism, a
relatively innocuous-appearing x-ray lesion with
a disproportionate perfusion defect may well
indicate a malignant process.

Although hardly a common dilemma,
occasional tumor problems may mask as other
pulmonary pathologies. Occasionally, the mask
resembles embolism, and the original perfusion
study may continue the charade. However, the
follow-up scan or serial studies demonstrate no
improvement. This is unusual, and when a major
perfusion deficit remains constant with time,
i.e., 1–2 weeks, consideration of neoplasm as
the etiology of the perfusion defect is warranted
(Fig. 6-14).

Occasionally, the addition of a ventilatory
study will also improve the zero-in time. The
demonstration of a bronchial obstruction along
with the other changes adds another bit of data
to solve the diagnostic puzzle (Fig. 6-15).

Of far greater value would be the detection
of a malignant tumor before it was x ray obvious.
To this end and for similar detection elsewhere,
an endless search exists for a "tumor-seeking"
radiopharmaceutical. The indications for such
an agent and its value requires no description—
it would have to rival the philosophers' touch
stone sought for by alchemists. Although such
nuclides have been identified, they are not too
good. Not only do they have the ability to
concentrate more actively in neoplastic than in
normal tissue, they also unfortunately do the
same in inflammatory tissue. Thus, positive
accumulation does not differentiate tumor from
inflammation. They are not tumor specific but
probably reflect only higher cellular and
metabolic activity. But all is not lost. These
agents can often be used effectively. Of the
group, which includes ^{67}Ga, ^{67}Cu bleomycin,
^{111}In bleomycin, and ^{197}Hg chlormerodrin,
perhaps ^{67}Ga has received the most attention.
Clinical situations arise in which there is a
strong presumption that a hidden primary
neoplasm exists, or nodal biopsy establishes the
existence of a primary but its site is unknown.
In these cases, the use of a tumor-seeking
radionuclide could be of value since if a positive
accumulation site were localized all necessary
diagnostic guns could be trained on that

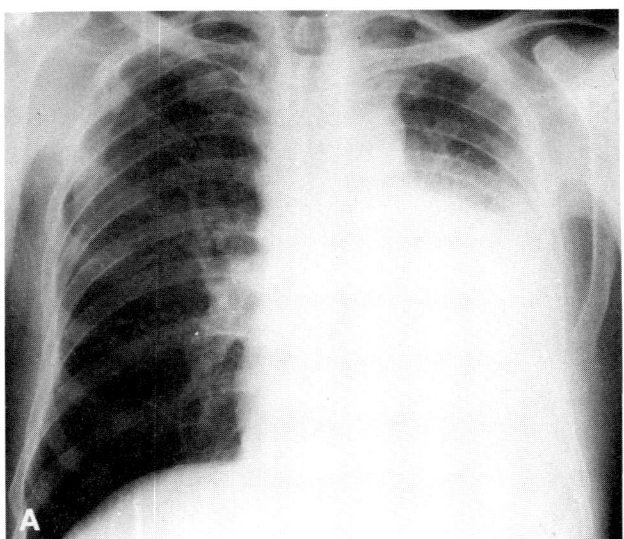

Fig. 6-13. Epidermoid carcinoma left lung

    A. X ray. The inferior half of the left hemithorax is obscured by a homogeneous density. The upper left lung appears to ventilate satisfactorily.

B and C. Perfusion scans. Anterior **(B)** and posterior **(C)** images show complete absence of left lung perfusion—far in excess of the x ray lesion.

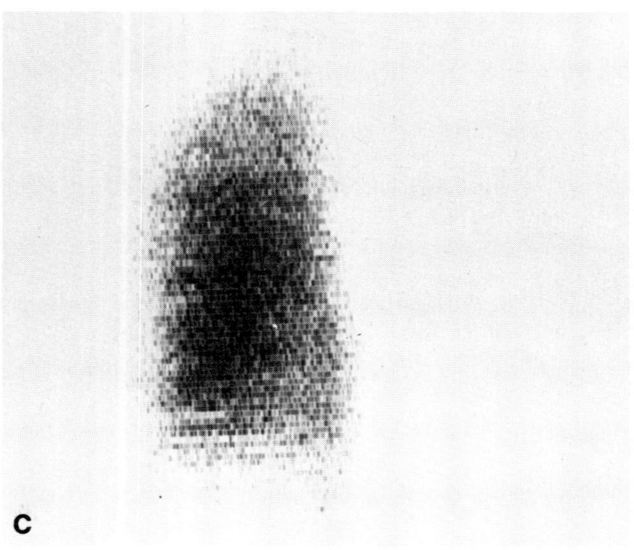

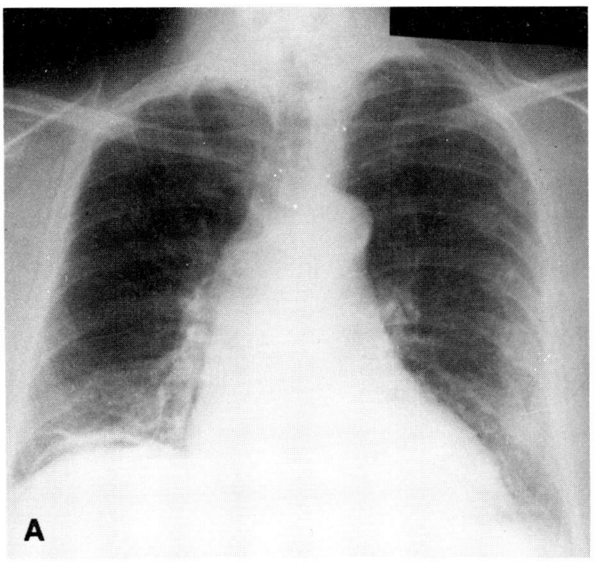

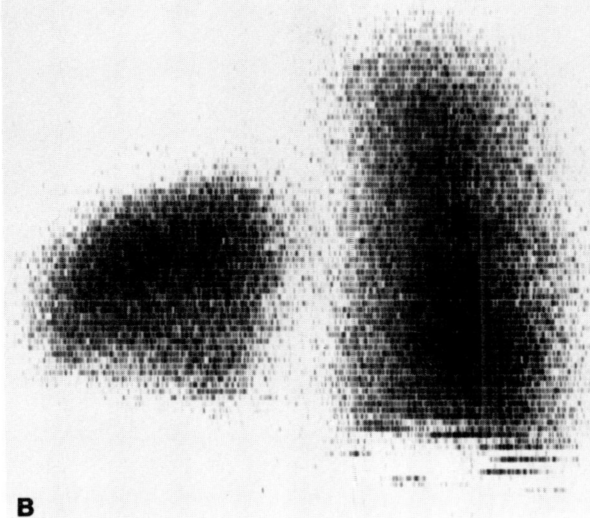

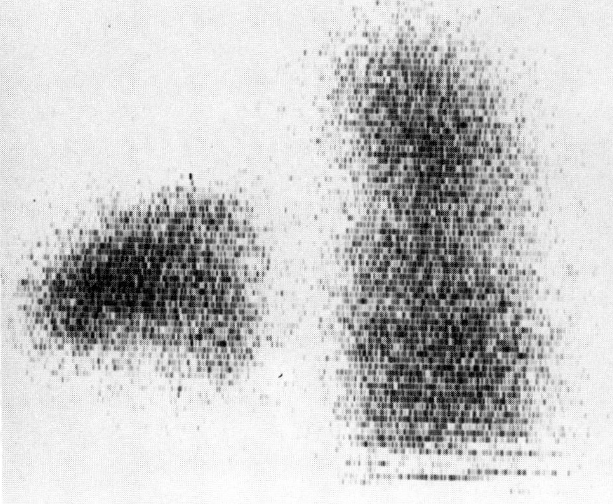

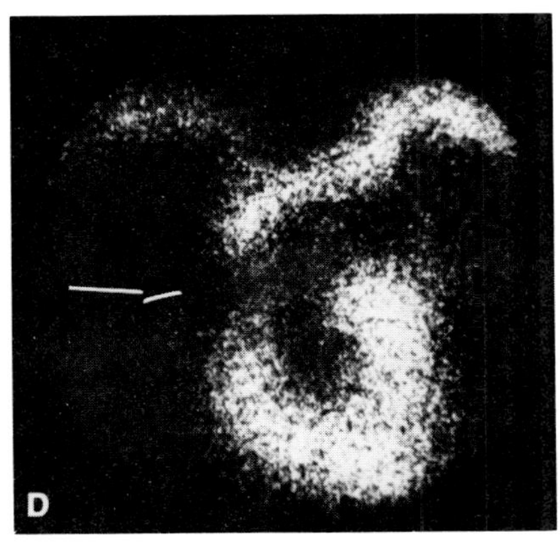

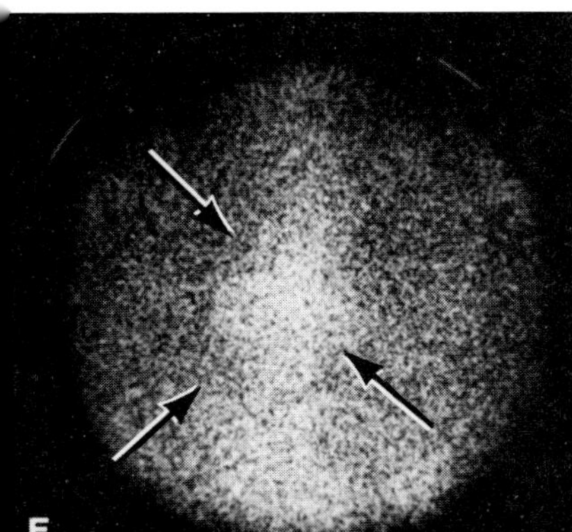

Fig. 6-14. Squamous cell carcinoma right lung

A. X ray. The admitting complaint was severe right lower chest pain and dyspnea. The only unusual finding s an atypical curvilinear density in the right supradiaphragmatic region and minimal elevation of the right diaphragm.

B. Perfusion scan. There is a nonperfusion of the right upper lobe and possibly a lower lobe defect.

C. Perfusion scan, 1 week later. No significant improvement in the right lung perfusion. A questionable marginal defect was noted at the left midlung margin. The nonchanging pattern suggested possible tumor.

D. Mediastinal flow. A defect in the superior vena cava is present (arrow).

E. ^{67}Ga scan. An abnormal accumulation in the region of the right hilum was identified (arrows).

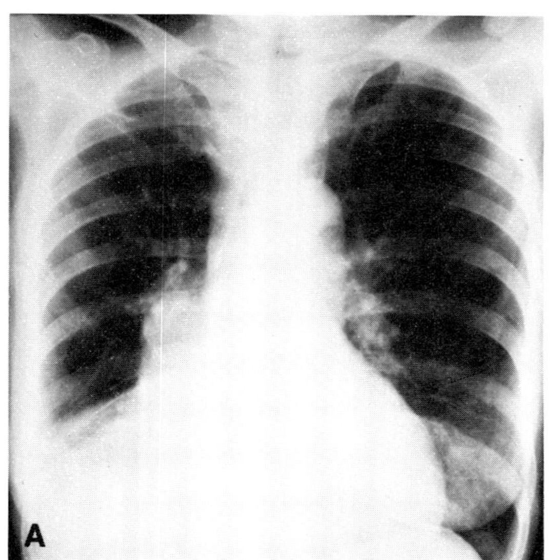

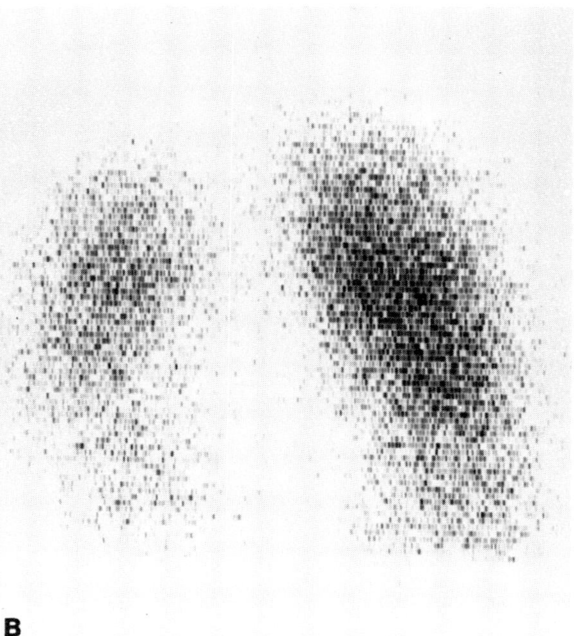

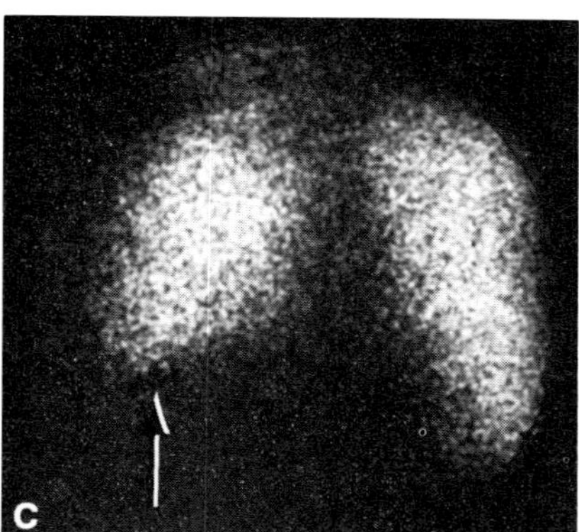

Fig. 6-15. Epidermoid carcinoma right lung
A. X ray. The right lung base is hypoventilated by a nonhomogeneous zone of increased density. There is an increased prominence in the right hilar area.
B. Perfusion scan. The entire right lung is hypoperfused. Although the base demonstrates the major deficit, changes are more extensive than anticipated from x-ray findings.
C. Ventilation scan. Complete obstruction of the right lower lobe (arrow)

location. This is in contradistinction to the daily seek (and often patient destroy) missions to define the primary when there is no existing clue as to its state of origin. Multiple series have been reported in which the localization accuracy of ^{67}Ga in pulmonary neoplasm exceeds 90% (the same localization occurs if there is tuberculosis, sarcoid, or pneumoconiosis). Thus, in the suspect patient with a negative chest x ray, a positive lung scan would focus attention to the positive site to identify its nature (Fig. 6-16). If, however, such a lung scan were normal, there would be good reason to look elsewhere.

Occasionally, even with obviously positive chest x rays, the differential diagnosis could be enhanced with a positive scan. These are lesser problems, but when there is considerable pleural effusion it is helpful to know whether the abnormal density is only fluid or whether something is being hidden by the fluid (Fig. 6-17).

Other indications for lung scanning exist, but their relative importance is minor compared to those already discussed. Isolated situations arise in which scanning techniques provide diagnostic aid, but for the most part these problems are better solved by other means.

congenital anomalies

Shunts. An unsuspected right-to-left cardiac shunt may first be appreciated when a perfusion scan is performed, usually for some other reason. The shunt's existence is discovered by the distribution of aggregates beyond the pulmonary arteriole–capillary network. Good brain and kidney scans are obtained by this route, but it is not suggested for routine use.

Pulmonary Artery Agenesis. This relatively uncommon anomaly yields a most dramatic scan. The involved side is totally without perfusion. The differential diagnosis of massive defects of this kind include only major vessel embolization, malignant neoplasm, and extensive consolidative processes. In each, the patient is either very ill or the x rays are very positive, or both. In pulmonary artery agenesis the patient may be completely asymptomatic. The x ray may identify an asymmetric hilar prominence which on cursory inspection may suggest that the side of the existing and obvious pulmonary artery is abnormal. Additionally, the lung of agenesis may appear to be the more normal of the two since it may be more lucent due to the absence of vessel markings. However, closer analysis usually suggests the true etiology, or at least suggests that a perfusion scan be done. The dilemma is then resolved (Fig. 6-18).

cardiovascular disease

Pulmonary Effusion. Effusion of any etiology (usually secondary to left heart failure) will affect the perfusion scan if it is of any significant volume. Often the degree of effusion is inadequately appreciated on conventional x rays, particularly if it is of the infrapulmonary type. With the patient supine, the effusion layers out posteriorly and forms a "water bed" between

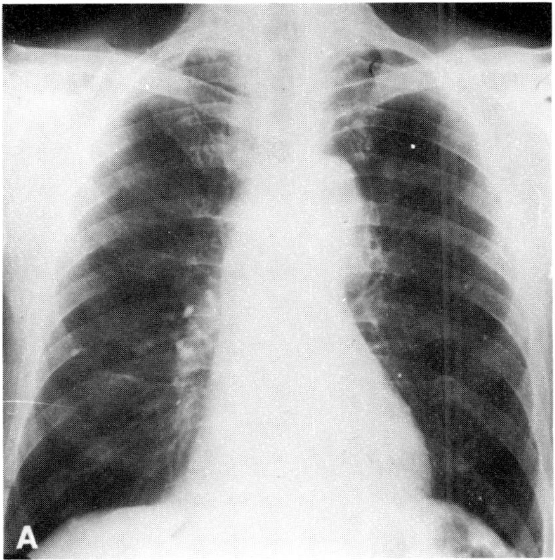

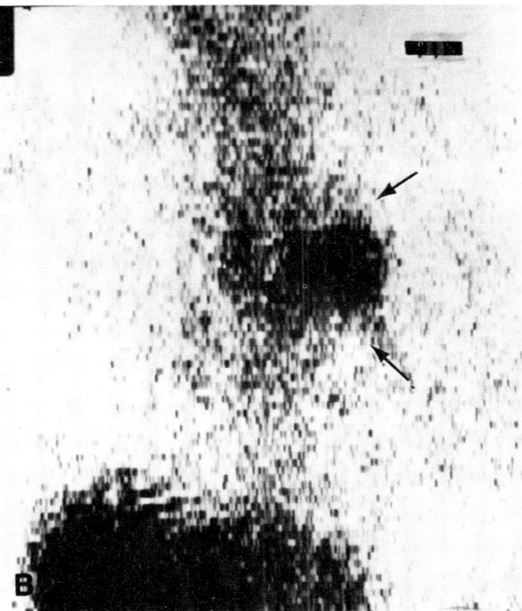

Fig. 6-16. Bronchogenic carcinoma. The patient was a 57-year-old male complaining of weight loss, malaise, and a questionable episode of hemoptysis. He was a heavy cigarette user.
A. X ray. Chest film is essentially normal for detectable pulmonary pathology.
B. Scan. 72 hours following a tracer dose of ^{67}Ga citrate a grossly abnormal accumulation of activity (arrows) is present in the left hilar region. (The lower right activity is normal liver accumulation.)
(Courtesy of D. Charkes, Temple University Hospital, Philadelphia, Pa.)

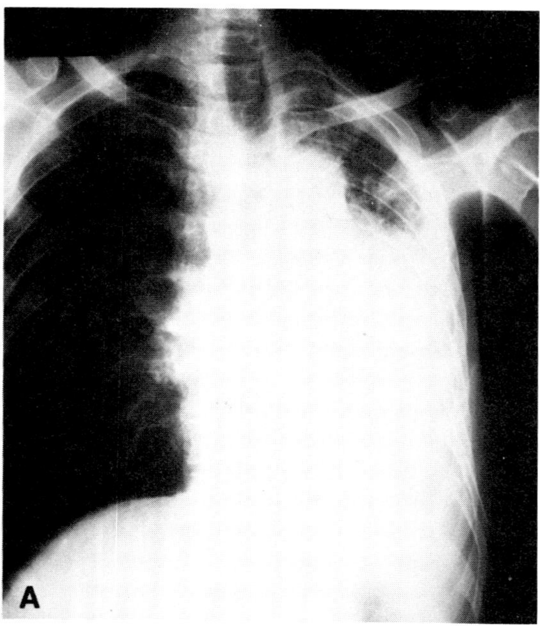

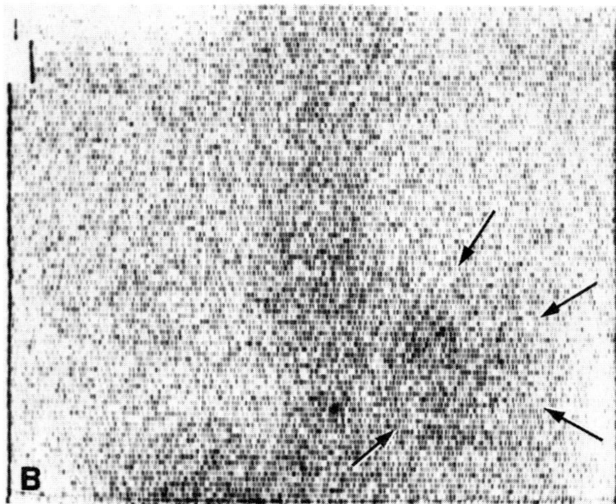

Fig. 6-17. Bronchogenic carcinoma with pleural effusion
A. X ray. Massive left pleural effusion. There is also a probable mediastinal shift to the left.
B. Scan. 72 hours following the administration of ^{67}Ga citrate there is abnormal localization (arrows) in the left lung base.

Fig. 6-18. Right pulmonary artery agenesis
A. X ray. Chest x ray of 9-year-old patient for elective tonsillectomy identifies a prominent left pulmonary artery and a decrease of vessel markings on the right.
B. Perfusion scan. Following ^{131}I MAA there is complete absence of right lung perfusion.
C. Flow scan, 4–6 sec. There is a complete absence of right pulmonary artery perfusion. The left artery and left lung perfuse well.
(Courtesy of E. Sloane, Tri-County Osteopathic Hospital, Springfield, Pa.)

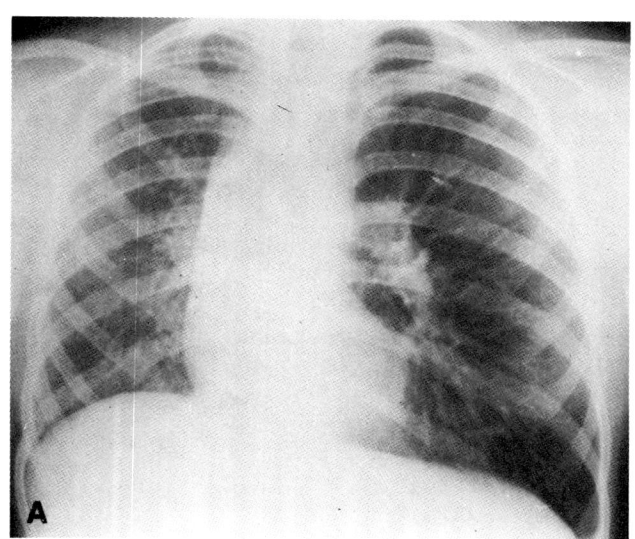

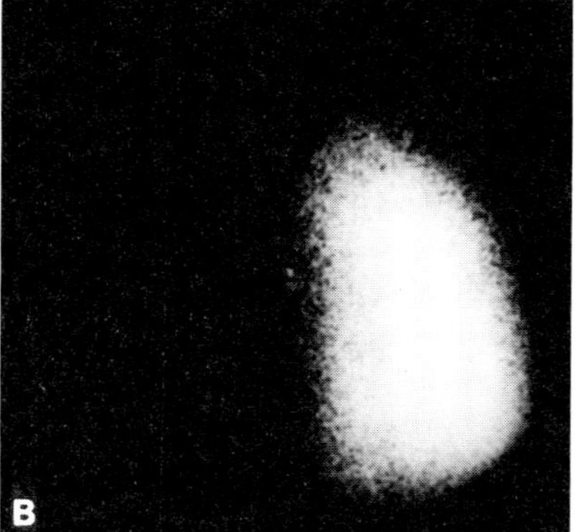

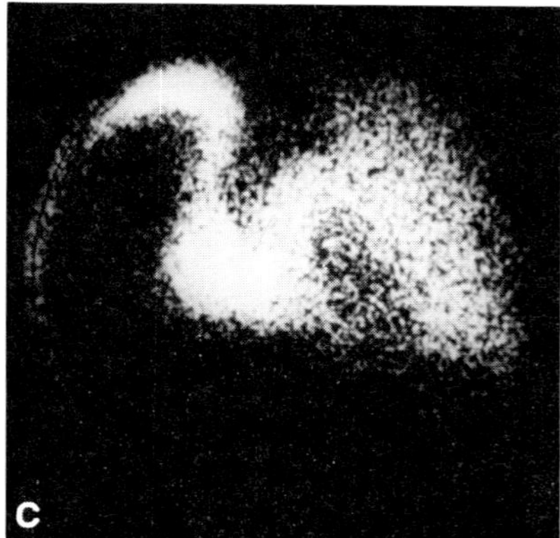

Fig. 6-19. Right pleural effusion
A. X ray. The right hemidiaphragm is unsharp. Each costophrenic angle is blunted.
B. Perfusion scan, anterior supine. No gross perfusion deficit of either lung
C. Perfusion scan, posterior supine. Significant apparent loss of the entire right lung

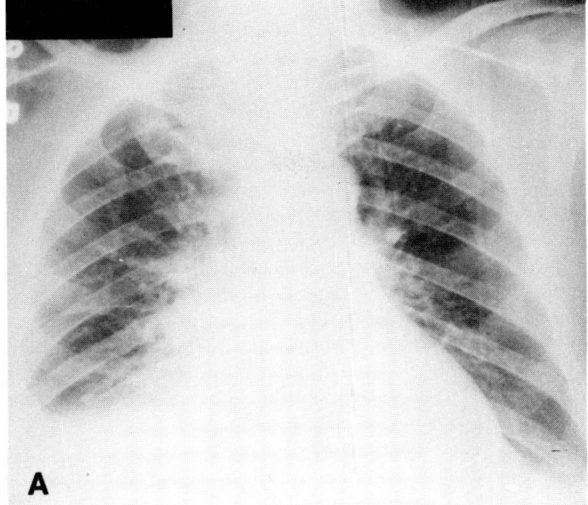

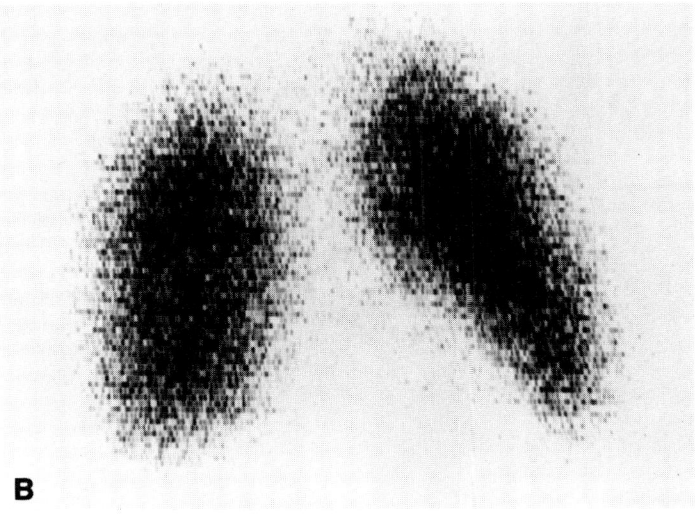

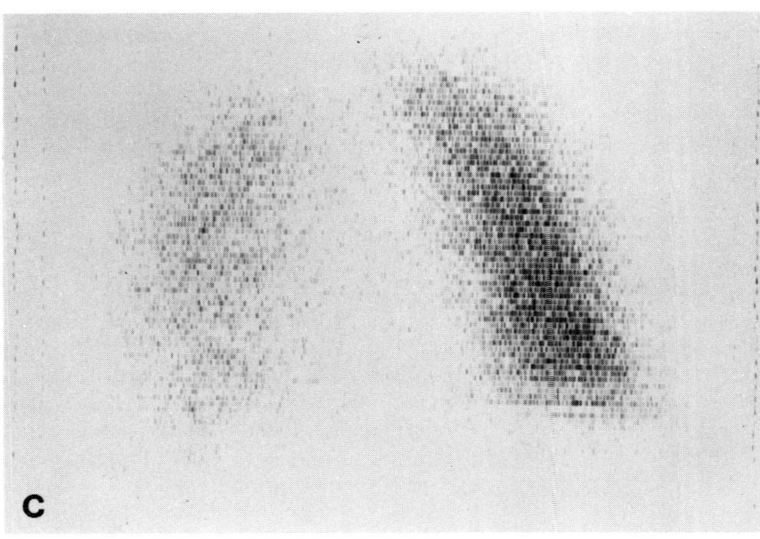

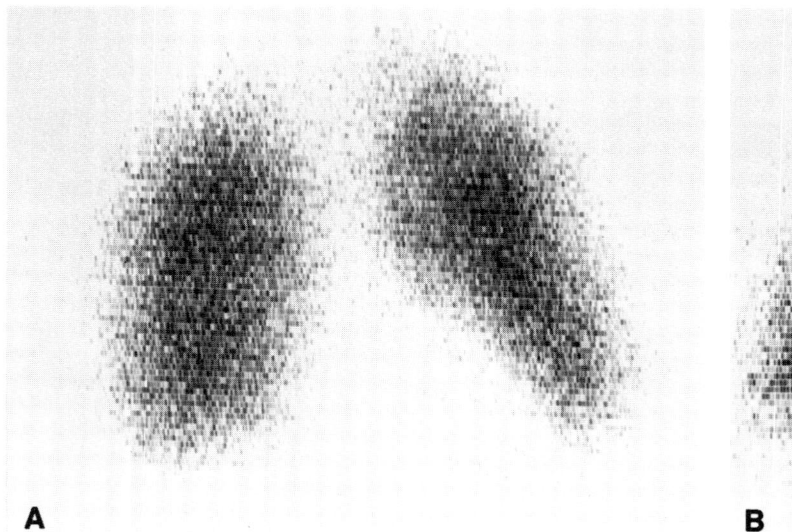

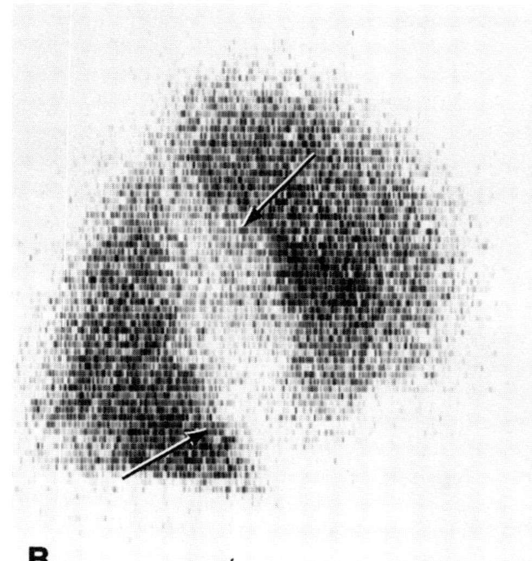

A

B

Fig. 6-20. Pleural fluid in the left interlobar fissure— fissure sign
A. Anterior perfusion scan. No evidence of abnormal perfusion
B. Left lateral perfusion scan. Patient lying on his left side. The oblique band of absent activity (arrows) corresponds to the interlobar fissure— widened by the presence of fluid.

the lung and the under table probe when dual image scanning is performed. This insulating wafer becomes a gamma filter and the apparent intensity of perfusion over the entire lung is diminished. This decrease is dramatic by comparison if the effusion is greater on one side than on the other or unilateral. The apparently normal perfusion of the same lung in the supine or anterior view establishes its etiology (Fig. 6-19).

Another common finding secondary to effusion is the "fissure sign," usually appearing in the lateral view and usually in the patient's down-side as a band of absent perfusion corresponding to a major interlobar fissure (Fig. 6-20). Initially, and perhaps still as a differential consideration, this configuration was thought to be secondary to microemboli with secondary infarction abutting the pleural surface of the fissure. However, unless the effusion is loculated, a postural change will mobilize the "defect" so that this zone of lucency can

usually be "cured" by repeating the scan with the patient in another position.

Congestive Failure. When there is interstitial pulmonary edema the perfusion pattern is best described as ugly. There are no discrete defects of embolization. There are no massive zones of anoxia. There is just a diffuse, nonfocal deficit, undoubtedly secondary to increased interstitial pressures that increase the intervascular pressures with subsequent increased resistance to blood flow. Although the findings are fairly characteristic, the perfusion scan is hardly the most-sophisticated technique to establish this diagnosis. Usually studies are performed on these patients because embolism is suspected.

Mitral Valvular Disease. Any mechanism that affects the left outflow tract will ultimately affect the pulmonary vascular distribution pattern, and mitral valvular disease is perhaps the most common etiologic culprit. Pulmonary hypertension develops, and—eventually—preferential shunting of blood to the upper lobes occurs. This shunting pattern may be more easily appreciated on perfusion scanning than on x ray. Normally, the blood volume (and thus the scan activity) is greater in the lung bases. Shunting reverses distribution of blood, and the scan reflects this change with a pattern of increased apical, as opposed to basilar, activity. Again, scanning is not the best way to diagnose mitral stenosis.

Subdiaphragmatic Abscess. Right-sided abscess formation may be detectable by a combination liver–lung scan. This has been described more fully with the studies of the liver because technically the disorder is intraabdominal and thus extrapulmonary (see chapter 2). Suffice it to say here that simultaneous imaging of the liver and lung identifies a separation between the normally opposing organs which represents the interposition of fluid.

Table 6-1. Indications, Pharmaceuticals, Methodology and Order of Merit of Radionuclide Study of Lung

Why	What	How	Yea–Nay
Perfusion			
Embolism–Infarction	^{99m}Tc human	static	++++
Mass lesions	serum albumin	static	++++
Subdiaphragmatic abscess (rt.)	microspheres	static	+++
Miscellaneous	or		
Congenital shunts	macroaggregated	static	+++
Pulmonary artery agenesis	human serum	static	++++
Pulmonary effusion	albumin	static	+++
Congestive failure	(MAHSA)	static	++
Ventilation			
Chronic obstructive disease	^{133}Xe	dynamic	++++
Perfusion and Ventilation			
Embolism–infection	^{133}Xe–^{99m}Tc MAHSA	dynamic-static	++++
Chronic obstructive disease	^{133}Xe–^{99m}Tc MAHSA	dynamic-static	++++

Table 6-2. More About What

Radiopharma-ceutical	Dose (mCi)	Physical Half-life	Energy Peak (keV)
^{99m}Tc human serum albumin (as macro-aggregates)	1–3	6 hr	140
^{99m}Tc human serum albumin (as micro-spheres)	1–3	6 hr	140
^{131}I human serum albumin (as macro-aggregates)	0.3	8.05 days	364
^{99m}Tc iron hydroxide	1–3	6 hr	140
^{133}Xe (as gas or dis-solved in saline)	5–10	5.3 days	81

Why	Prepa-ration	Adminis-tration	Time Be-tween Adminis-tration and Exam	Num-ber of Exams	Time for Each Exam (min)	Time for Total Study (min)	Pa-tient's Posi-tion	Instru-ment
Embolism or Infarction	Chest x ray (Lugol's $I_2 \bar{c}$ 131I)	IV	immed	1	20–45	20–45	recum-bent or sitting	camera or scanner
Mass lesions	chest x ray (Lugol's $I_2 \bar{c}$ 131I)	IV	immed	1	20–45	20–45	recum-bent or sitting	camera or scanner
Subdiaphrag-matic ab-scess (rt side)	chest x ray liver scan	IV	immed	1	20–30	20–30	supine and rt lateral	camera or scanner
Miscella-neous	chest x ray (Lugol's $I_2 \bar{c}$ 131I)	IV	immed	1	20–45	20–45	recum-bent or sitting	camera or scanner
Chronic ob-structive	chest x ray	IV or inhala-tion	immed	1	5–10	5–10	sitting	camera

BIBLIOGRAPHY

GENERAL

DeLand FH, Wagner HN: Lung. In Atlas of Nuclear Medicine, Vol II, Lung and Heart. Philadelphia, WB Saunders, 1970, pp 3–215

James AE, Squire LF: The lung. In Nuclear Radiology. Philadelphia, WB Saunders, 1973, pp 1–47

Jones RH et al.: Lung scanning in pediatrics. In James AE, Wagner HN, Cooke RE (eds): Pediatric Nuclear Medicine. Philadelphia, WB Saunders, 1974, pp 180–203

Poe ND, Taplin GV: Pulmonary function and disease. In Blahd WH (ed): Nuclear Medicine. New York, McGraw–Hill, 1971, pp 313–349

Potchen EJ, Evens RG: The physiologic factors affecting regional ventilation and perfusion. Semin Nucl Med 1(2): 153–160, 1971

Quinn JL, Koch DF: The lung. In Freeman LM, Johnson PM (eds): Clinical Scintillation Scanning. Hagerstown, Harper & Row, 1969, pp 304–325

PHARMACOLOGY

Chaudhuri TK et al.: A new radiopharmaceutical for combined lung-liver scan—preliminary experiment in animals (abstr). J Nucl Med 14(6):346–347, 1973

Hoffer PB et al.: Improved xenon images with 127Xe. J Nucl Med 14(3):172–174, 1973

Monroe LA et al.: Evaluation of an improved 99mTc-stannous aggregated albumin preparation for lung imaging. J Nucl Med 15(3):192–194, 1974

Pena HG et al.: Retention and disappearance of 59Fe-iron hydroxide particles in rhesus monkeys' lungs (abstr). J Nucl Med 14(6):437, 1973

Raynaud C et al.: Lung cancer diagnosis with 67Cu: preliminary results. J Nucl Med 14(12):947–950, 1973

Robinowitz M et al.: Fatal reactions following 99mTc-ferrous hydroxide lung scans (abstr). J Nucl Med 14(6):445–446, 1973

Taplin GV, MacDonald NS: Radiochemistry of macro-aggregated albumin and newer lung scanning agents. Semin Nucl Med 1(2):132–152, 1971

Watts RS: Iron hydroxide particle retention in primate lungs. J Nucl Med 15(7):616–619, 1974

PERFUSION

Allen DR et al.: Critical assessment of changes in pulmonary circulation following injection of lung-scanning agent (MAA) (abstr). J Nucl Med 14(6):375–376, 1973

Apau RL et al.: Bloodless lung due to bronchial obstruction. J Nucl Med 13(7):561–562, 1972

Isawa T et al.: Pulmonary perfusion changes after experimental unilateral bronchial occlusion and their clinical implications. Radiology 99:355–360, 1971

James AE Jr et al.: The fissure sign: its multiple causes. Am J Roentgenol Radium Ther Nucl Med 111:492–500, 1971

Johnson PM: The role of lung scanning in pulmonary embolism. Semin Nucl Med 1(2):161–184, 1971

Milstein DM et al.: Pulmonary scintiphotography in the fat embolism syndrome (abstr). J Nucl Med 15(6):517, 1974

Moser KM et al.: Differentiation of pulmonary vascular from parenchymal diseases by ventilation-perfusion scintiphotography. Ann Int Med 75:597–605, 1971

Partlow WF, McCormack KR: Changes in lung scan pattern related to free fluid and cardiac position. J Nucl Med 12(1):2–4, 1971

Quinn JL III: Perfusion scanning in chronic obstructive lung disease. Semin Nucl Med 1(2):185–194, 1971

Sasahara AA et al.: Problems in the diagnosis and management of pulmonary embolism. Semin Nucl Med 1(2):122–131, 1971

Shtasel P: Reappraisal of pulmonary embolic-infarctive pathology. JAOA 69:561–572, 1970

Yang CS et al.: Cardiovascular dynamic perfusion study in lung perfusion scan with ^{99m}Tc-MAA (abstr). J Nucl Med 15(6):545, 1974

VENTILATION

Dittrich FA et al.: Early recognition of chronic airway disease by the ^{133}Xe lung scan. JAMA 220:1120–1122, 1972

Inkley SR, MacIntyre WJ: Measurement of regional area gas exchange by perfusion and clearance of ^{133}Xe from the lung. J Nucl Med 14(7):490–495, 1973

Inkley SR et al.: ^{133}Xe in preoperative assessment of patients with bronchogenic carcinoma (abstr). J Nucl Med 14(6):410, 1973

Ishii Y et al.: Comparative studies between ventilation and perfusion distribution in lung (abstr). J Nucl Med 14(6):411, 1973

Jacobstein JG, Quinn JL III: ^{133}Xe ventilation scanning immediately following the ^{99m}Tc perfusion scan (abstr). J Nucl Med 14(6):412, 1973

Jones RH et al.: Evaluation of ^{133}Xe techniques for measurement of regional ventilation. J Nucl Med 15(7):598–604, 1974

Lin MS et al.: Small-particle radioaerosol for inhalation lung scintigraphy (abstr). J Nucl Med 14(8):630, 1973

Loken MK et al.: Dual-camera studies of pulmonary function with computer processing of data (abstr). J Nucl Med 14(6):422–423, 1973

Miller DP et al.: Improved system for administration of ^{133}Xe in pulmonary ventilation scintiphotography (abstr). J Nucl Med 14(6):475, 1973

Rogers WL et al.: Sensitivity for detecting ventilation defect wtih ^{133}Xe and an Anger camera (abstr). J Nucl Med 14(6):447–448, 1973

Secker–Walker RH et al.: A simple ^{133}Xe delivery system for studies of regional ventilation. J Nucl Med 15(4):288–290, 1974

Serino TV et al.: Differential vital capacity determinations with radioactive xenon. J Nucl Med 15(7):625–629, 1974

Siemsen JK, Telfer N: Regional ventilation studies at different lung volumes (abstr). J Nucl Med 14(6):453, 1973

Taplin GV et al.: Potential value and high efficiency of dry aerosols for lung imaging (abstr). J Nucl Med 15(6):537, 1974

Treves S et al.: Radionuclide evaluation of regional lung function in children. J Nucl Med 15(7):582–587, 1974

TUMOR

Dige–Petersen H et al.: ^{67}Ga-scintigraphy in non-malignant lung disease. Scand J Resp Dis 53:314–319, 1972

Farrer PA et al.: Radionuclide imaging of intrathoracic mass-lesions using ^{197}HgCl$_2$ and ^{99m}Tc macroaggregated human serum albumin (abstr). J Nucl Med 15(6):490, 1974

Grebe SF et al.: Value of radiogallium studies in chest disease (abstr). J Nucl Med 15(6):497, 1974

Grove RB et al.: Clinical evaluation of radiolabeled bleomycin (bleo) for tumor detection. J Nucl Med 15(6):386–390, 1974

Jereb M et al.: Radionuclear selenite (^{75}Se) for scintigraphic demonstration of lung cancer and metastases in mediastinum: preliminary report. Scand J Resp Dis 53:331–337, 1972

Kinoshita F et al.: Scintiscanning of pulmonary diseases with ^{67}Ga-citrate. J Nucl Med 15(4):227–233, 1974

Maynard CD, Cowan RJ: Role of the scan in bronchogenic carcinoma. Semin Nucl Med 1(2):195–205, 1971

McCormack KR et al.: Serial pulmonary perfusion scanning in radiation therapy for bronchogenic carcinoma. J Nucl Med 12(12):800–803, 1971

Nolan NG: Use of ^{133}xenon in localization of x-ray-occult sputum-positive lung cancer. J Nucl Med 15(6):520, 1974

Raynaud C et al.: Lung cancer diagnosis with ^{67}Cu: preliminary results. J Nucl Med 14(12):947–950, 1973

Van der Schoot JB et al.: ^{67}Gallium scintigraphy in lung disease. Thorax 27:546, 1972

CHRONIC OBSTRUCTIVE LUNG DISEASE

Busse W et al.: Prolonged retention of radioactivity following perfusion lung scan in asthmatic patients. J Nucl Med 14(11):837–839, 1973

Fallat RJ et al.: ^{133}Xe ventilatory studies in antitrypsin deficiency. J Nucl Med 14(1):5–13, 1973

McKusick KA et al.: Measurement of regional lung function in the early detection of chronic obstructive lung disease (abstr). J Nucl Med 14(6):427, 1973

Piepsz A et al.: Scintigraphic study of pulmonary blood flow distribution in cystic fibrosis. J Nucl Med 14(6):326–330, 1973

Quinn JL III: Perfusion scanning in chronic obstructive lung disease. Semin Nucl Med 1(2):185–194, 1971

RETICULOENDOTHELIAL SYSTEM UPTAKE

Gillespie PJ et al.: High concentration of ^{99m}Tc-sulfur colloid found during routine liver scan in lungs of patient with advanced breast cancer. J Nucl Med 14(9):711–712, 1973

Keyes JW Jr et al.: Evaluation of lung uptake of colloid during liver imaging (abstr). J Nucl Med 14(6):415, 1973

Keyes JW Jr et al.: An evaluation of lung uptake of colloid during liver imaging. J Nucl Med 14(9):687–691, 1973

Klingensmith WC III et al.: Lung uptake of ^{99m}Tc-sulfur colloid in organ transplantation. J Nucl Med 14(10):757–759, 1973

Klingensmith WC III, Ryerson TW: Lung uptake of ^{99m}Tc-sulfur colloid. J Nucl Med 14(4):201–203, 1973

Quinones JD: Localization of technetium-sulfur colloid after RES stimulation (abstr). J Nucl Med 14(6):443, 1973

MISCELLANEOUS

Berke RA et al.: Radiation dose to breast-feeding child after mother has ^{99m}Tc-MAA lung scan. J Nucl Med 14(1):51–52, 1973

Busse W et al: Prolonged retention of radioactivity following perfusion lung scan in asthmatic patients. J Nucl Med 14(11):837–839, 1973

Fallat RJ et al.: Pulmonary deposition and clearance of ^{131}I-labeled oil after lymphography in man. Radiology 97:511–520, 1970

Fleming JS, Goddard BA: Regional lung volume measurement by transmission scintigraphy. J Nucl Med 15(7):605–609, 1974

McCartney WH et al.: Value of carcinoembryonic antigen (CEA) titer determination on bronchial washing specimens in the diagnosis of lung malignancy (abstr). J Nucl Med 14(6):424–425, 1973

McDonald GB et al.: Segmental pulmonary arteriography and lung scanning (abstr). J Nucl Med 14(8):631, 1973

Piepsz A et al.: Scintigraphic study of pulmonary blood flow distribution in cystic fibrosis. J Nucl Med 14(6):326–330, 1973

Prosin MA, Mishkin FS: Radionuclide diagnosis of pulmonary sequestration. J Nucl Med 15(7):636–638, 1974

Snyder RE, Overton TR: System for handling and dispensing ^{133}Xe. J Nucl Med 14(1):56–58, 1973

Soin JS et al.: Abnormalities of regional lung function in asymptomatic narcotic addicts (abstr). J Nucl Med 14(6):455–456, 1973

Tetalman MR et al.: Efficacy of emergency lung scans (abstr). J Nucl Med 14(6):460, 1973

If the fraternity of nuclear medicine men were ever to adapt a uniform its emblem must be a thyroid gland emblazoned on a sea of ^{131}I. No other organ and no other nuclide in combination approach the historic legacy owed this dynamic duo to the birth of this specialty. For many years, it was the sole raison d'etre. Like the rare astrologic wonder of the ideal alignment of the moons of Jupiter (or some such other magical moment) the symbiosis of the thyroid and a radioisotope of iodine which was available and acceptable was the miraculous key that opened the medical door for the nuclear huckster. The thyroid has as its major function the extraction of inorganic iodine from the plasma, its organification to hormone triiodothyronine and tetraiodothyronine (thyroxin), and its subsequent release back into the circulation.

Iodine 131 became the first available nuclide for human testing because it is treated by the gland like stable ^{127}I. Thus, the birth of the tracer! When a known amount of ^{131}I was administered, the percentage extracted by the thyroid in a given period of time (its uptake) could easily be quantitated. The determination was made even easier by the superficial location of the gland and the gamma energy of the nuclide, which was readily captured and measured by existing instruments. Experience quickly provided a range of uptake, initially set by agreement at 24 hours, which would be equated to normal, hypofunction, and hyperfunction. (Experience also quickly identified a plethora of traps for the unwary which will be discussed shortly.) And throughout the literature a new litany could be identified. "The BMR is dead! Long live the ^{131}I uptake!"

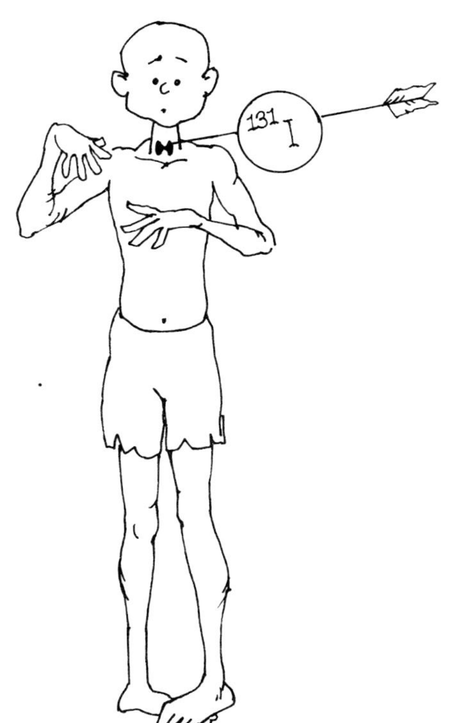

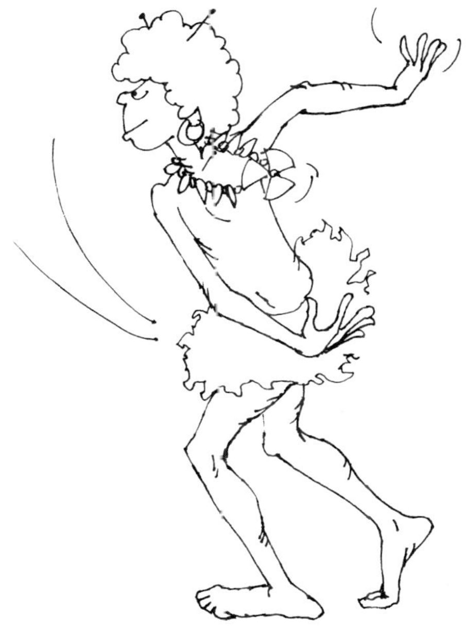

chapter 7

thyroid

Actually, the extracted nuclide was stored before excretion. With proper instrumentation the storage distribution could be mapped. Initially, this imaging was accomplished by laborious point counts over the gland, but Yankee ingenuity eventually yielded a picture, and then image scanning was born. At first the picture was a carbonized impression produced by a mechanical tapper. This was followed by electric sparking on carbonized paper, which was in turn followed by a black and white representation on film that resembled an x ray but was more properly the result of a gamma ray. Today, for them that want it, color images are also possible. The nuclear rocket was launched—a technique exploded across the diagnostic horizon which could both measure the extraction ability of a gland (which could be equated to function) and provide a pictorial representation of gross anatomy and morphology. But that was only the beginning, folks, for yet another plus was to ensue: the specificity of uptake and storage could be utilized to deliver quantifiable (well, almost) doses of irradiation to the gland for therapeutic effects. This constituted a three-way parlay—function, morphology, and therapy—in one plain brown-wrapped package, an accomplishment as yet unequalled in any other organ system. That, brothers and sisters, is called a real "Break through!".

WHAT

After extensive investigation, it has been concluded that only 3 of the 20-odd isotopes of iodine have routine medical adaptability. Iodine 131 is still the most widely employed, but as mentioned many times in earlier chapters, what was great then (circa 1940) ain't now. The half-life of ^{131}I (8 days) is too long to permit any but microcurie doses, which in turn diminishes image quality and speed of study, and its peak energy (364 keV), which is less than ideal for present instrumentation, particularly the gamma camera, account for the fall of ^{131}I from grace. Although advocated by some with excellent documentation, ^{125}I has a half-life far too long (60 days) and a gamma energy far too low (less than 40 keV) for general acceptance in *in vivo* testing. Both qualities are, however, exploited for *in vitro* determinations. Unquestionably, the tracer with the mostest is ^{123}I, with a beautiful half-life of 13.3 hours and an efficient gamma

peak of 158 keV. Unfortunately, it is cyclotron-produced, which for our purposes can be translated into high cost. Additionally, it is prone to contamination with ^{124}I, which impairs its goodness. But these problems can be conquered.

Technetium 99m in the pertechnetate form has a metabolic pathway similar to that of iodine. It is extracted but not organified by the thyroid. Thus, it can be used as a function study, albeit with difficulty, and can also be used as a scanning agent. Although neither potential is universally employed, the use of this nuclide as a scanning agent is becoming more and more prevalent. Its physical properties lend themselves well to camera imaging. Detail is excellent and scans can be obtained within a half-hour of IV administration.

HOW

Unlike all other organ systems, after some 30-odd years of experience thyroid function studies have remained equal in importance with imaging. Where in other systems the isotopic contribution to function is almost exclusively a research exercise, isotopic testing of the thyroid has almost replaced all other methods of evaluation. Many of the acceptable procedures have the additional advantage of being *in vitro,* which obviates the dubious hazard of introducing radioactive substances into the patient. The various procedures can thus be characterized and discussed as either *in vitro* or *in vivo.*

in vitro

An historic review of all of the techniques expounded, attempted, and ultimately discarded to measure trapped hormones in the saliva, urine, sweat, and even lactating milk would add intolerable confusion to what already has eventuated as barely tolerable confusion. The name, rank, and number of those currently invoked will be discussed shortly. All are initiated by a sample of the patient's blood.

in vivo

In vivo determinations can be divided into function and imaging studies. Imaging is the simpler of the two to identify, so it will come first.

Routine Imaging. If the nuclide employed is an
isotope of iodine, it is usually administered
orally or as a capsule or liquid with the patient
being asked to return in several hours and again
in 24 hours. (It is remarkable how few patients
are prewarned that a second visit is necessary.)
Occasionally, with ^{123}I, imaging is done in 6
hours. If the rectilinear scanner is used, the
patient is supine. Generally, the neck is hyper-
extended to bring the gland closer to the crystal.
The instrument moves backward and forward
across the neck and occasionally across the
upper mediastinum. Except for the mild
discomfort of the scanning position, there
should be no other patient complaints, except if
there is glandular tenderness, since physical
examination with palpation must be done. The
average thyroid can be imaged in about 15 min.

When ^{99m}Tc pertechnetate is the scanning
agent it is common to utilize the gamma camera
as the scanning instrument. Images can be
obtained in approximately ½ hour following IV
administration. Patient position is more flexible,
either a seated or recumbent position being
acceptable. This combination also permits
images in other than straight anterior views.
Oblique projections are readily obtained, and
these often prove most helpful, particularly in
the evaluation of nodules. Total examination
time is similar to that of the rectilinear method,
approximately 15 min (Fig. 7-1).

Special Imaging. Following a routine scan the
pattern may present some special and additional
problems that require further clarification. This
occurs primarily in nodular disease. It is often
beneficial in attempting to define the type and
mechanism of the nodule to rescan following IM
administration of thyroid-stimulating hormone
(TSH) or after several days of triiodothyronine
(T_3) administration or both. Usually if ^{131}I is the
original scanning agent, these specialized
procedures should be deferred approximately
2 weeks to permit major clearance of the initial
dose. Except for the administration of T_3 (the
technique varies, 75–100 µg/day for 3–7 days—
check with your laboratory) or the injection of
TSH (1–3 daily doses IM 5–10 units—check with
your laboratory) the scanning procedure is
identical with the original.

Function
UPTAKE. This is the common and routine
evaluation for the glandular functional status. It

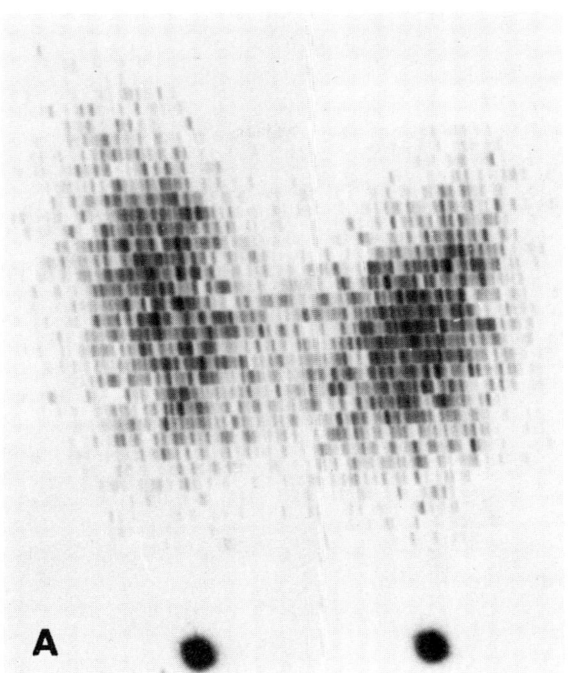

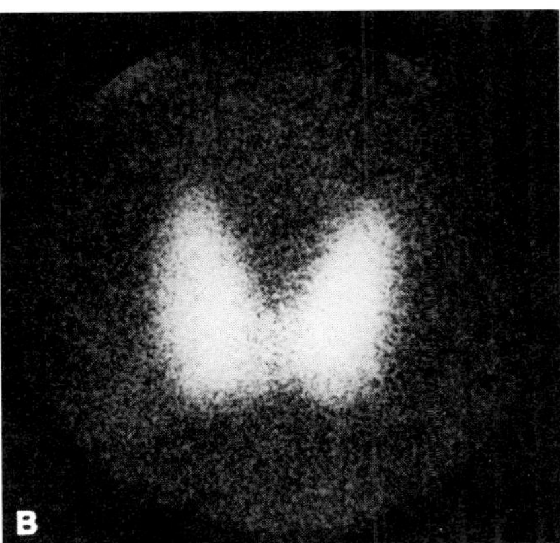

Fig. 7-1. Normal thyroid
A. Rectilinear scan, 24 hours, ^{131}I. There may be
normal variation in gross size and contour, but the
lobes are essentially symmetric. The distribution
of activity is uniform, and the entire gland is above
the sternal inlet. (The two black dots identify each
sternoclavicular junction.)
B. Gamma camera, 30 min, ^{99m}TcO$_4$. Pattern similar
to that in **A.** A pinhole collimator is employed.
Landmarks are not as easily identified as in **A.** The
lobes are symmetric and the distribution of activity
uniform.

is almost universally performed 24 hours following the ingestion of a tracer dose. The patient should preferably be fasted approximately 2 hours prior to being fed. It is also common that an early evaluation be made. Customarily, this is done 2, 3, or 6 hours after feeding. (Some laboratories have discarded this immediate post-feeding uptake and have gone back to using only the 24-hour value.) Ascertain from your laboratory which technique is utilized so that the out-patient can be forewarned to make the necessary arrangements. The actual procedure is simple. A cylindrical instrument, the probe, is placed against the neck with the patient either sitting or supine for 2–5 min, during which time it is counting the accumulation of the nuclide.

SUPPRESSION. Occasionally, after all the tests have been tested there is still uncertainty as to whether or not hyperfunction exists. A 3- to 7-day administration of T_3 followed by another uptake evaluation will often clarify the status. Except for the premedication, from the patient's standpoint the study is identical with the original uptake, and no other instructions or explanations are necessary.

TSH STIMULATION. When hypofunction is established, it is occasionally of value to differentiate its etiology as to primarily pituitary or thyroid in origin. A recheck of uptake 24 hours following IM TSH may resolve the question.

WHY

masses—nodules

Any palpable abnormality in the thyroid deserves —yea demands—to be scanned. Theoretically, the image will identify the nodule(s) and establish their functioning status. They may function equally with the surrounding parenchyma or accumulate increased activity referable to the surrounding tissue or be nonfunctioning. When equal, they may not be visually detectable and are recognized only by localizing the palpable finding to the scan. They appear blacker than the background when excessive uptake is present and are whiter when nonfunctioning if the record is made on x-ray film. The opposite colors obtain with Polaroid, *i.e.,* absent uptake is black, excessive is white (Figs. 7-2 to 7-4). The

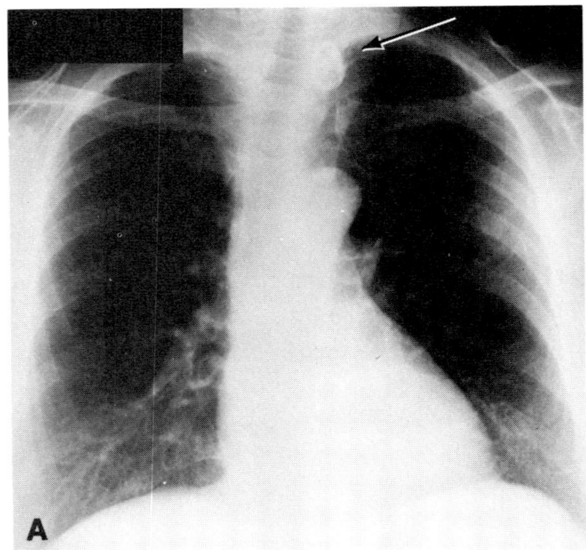

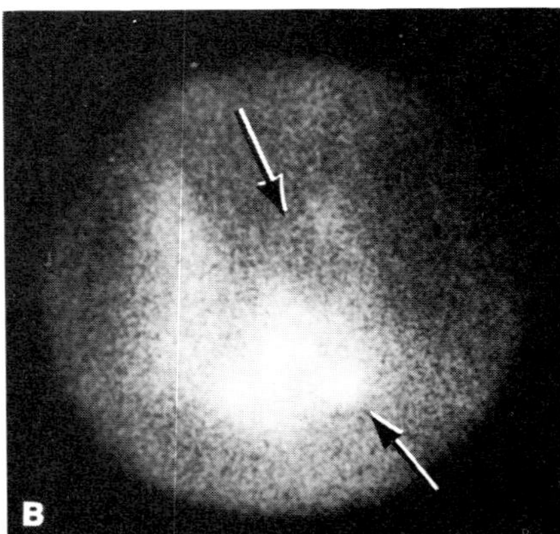

Fig. 7-2. Multinodular goiter with calcified adenoma
A. X ray. Just above the head of the left clavicle (arrow) there is a ring-shaped calcification.
B. Scan, $^{99m}TcO_4$. Discrete ovoid area devoid of activity (arrows) in the left upper pole corresponds to the calcification on the chest x ray. This is characterized as "cold." Also, in the base of the left lobe are several discrete areas of increased ("hot") activity. The total gland is enlarged.

Fig. 7-3. Multinodular goiter. 24 hours following tracer dose of ^{131}I the enlarged thyroid image reveals an absence of trapping in the inferior half of the left lobe. Immediately above this cold defect is a small discrete area of hyperfunction.

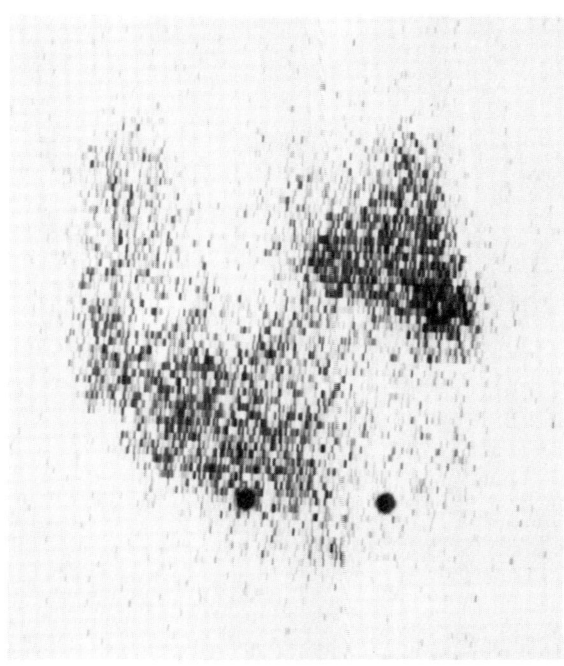

Fig. 7-4. Multinodular goiter
  A. Scan, [99m]TcO$_4$. 2 min following IV injection the thyroid can be identified. There appears to be increased trapping activity in the midportion of the right lobe and an area of absent activity in the midportion of the left lobe (arrows). The symmetric activity above the thyroid is in the submaxillary salivary glands.
  B. Scan, [99m]TcO$_4$. 30 min later and employing a pinhole collimator the hot and cold nodules are clearly identified (arrows).

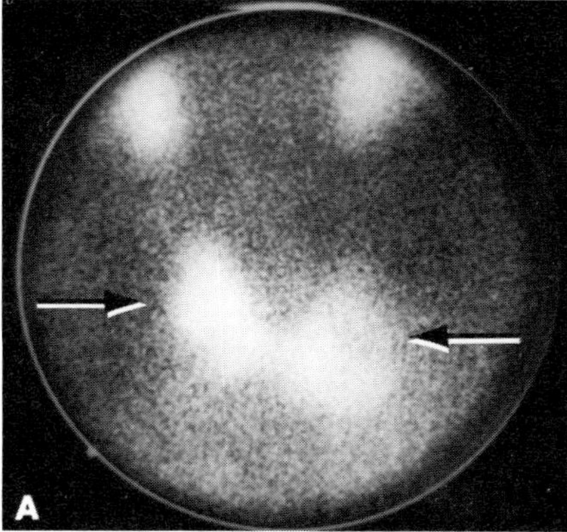
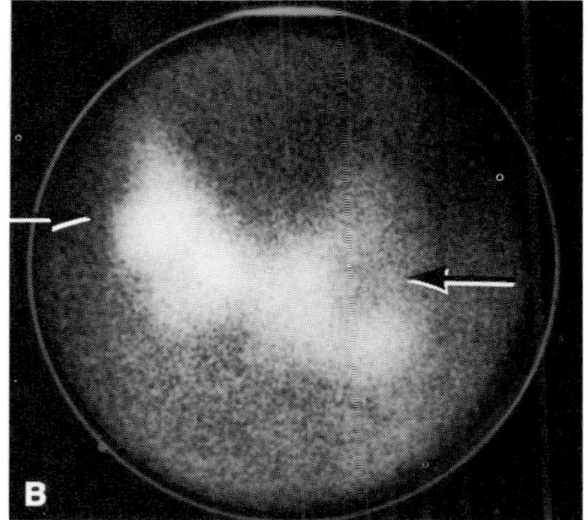

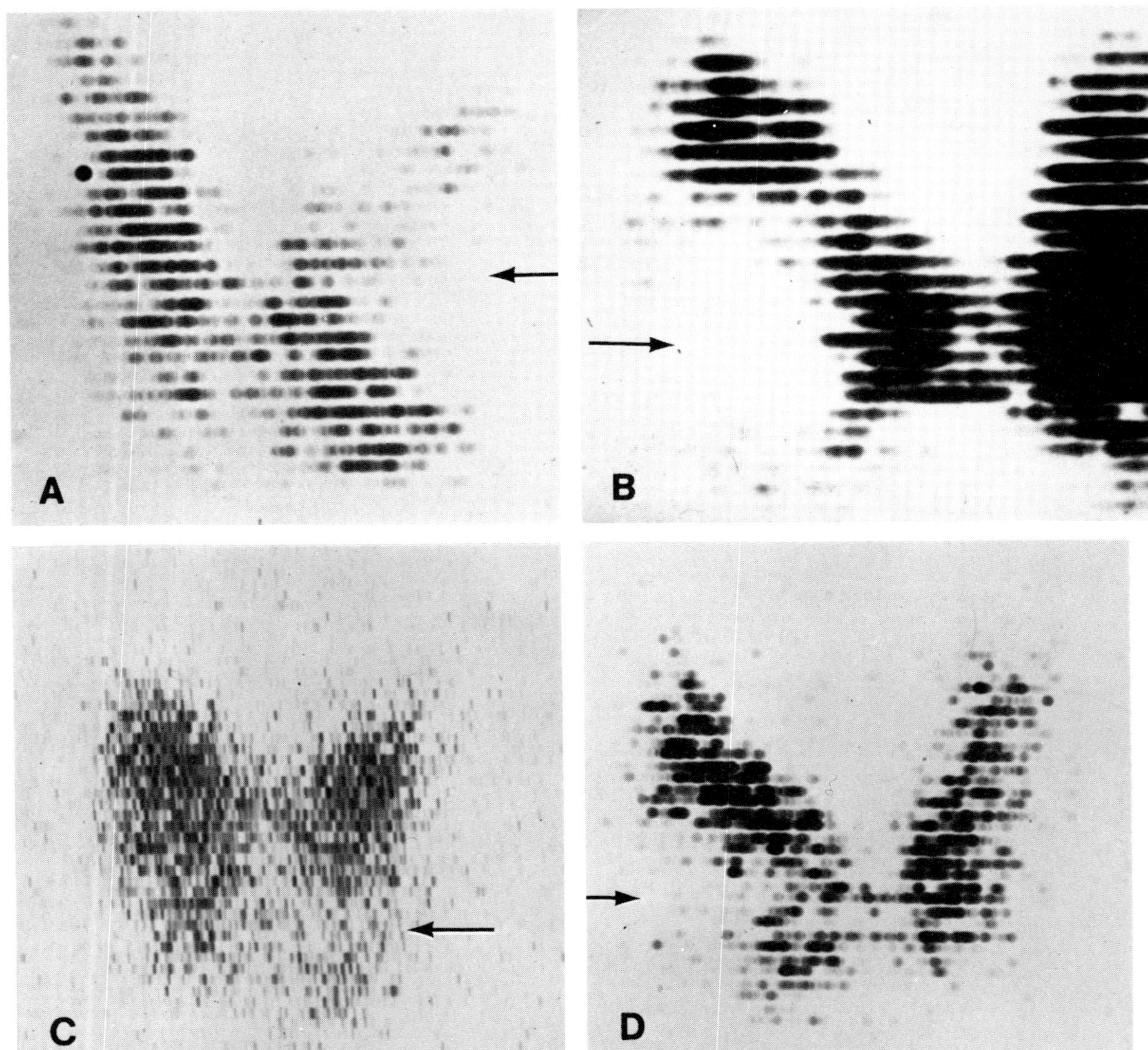

Fig. 7-5. Nodules
Diagnosis: Hemorrhage into a colloid cyst
A. 24 hour, ^{131}I. Large nontrapping defect left lobe (arrow).
Diagnosis: Follicular and papillary carcinoma
B. 24 hour, ^{131}I. Large nontrapping defect right lobe (arrow)
Diagnosis: Adenoma
C. 24 hour, ^{131}I. Small defect lower pole of left lobe (arrow)
Diagnosis: Follicular carcinoma
D. 24 hour, ^{131}I. Small right marginal defect (arrow)

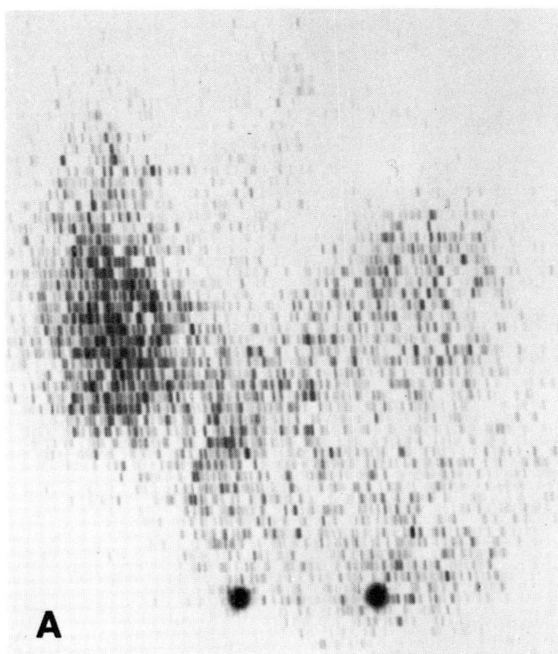

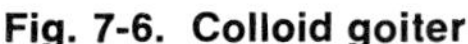

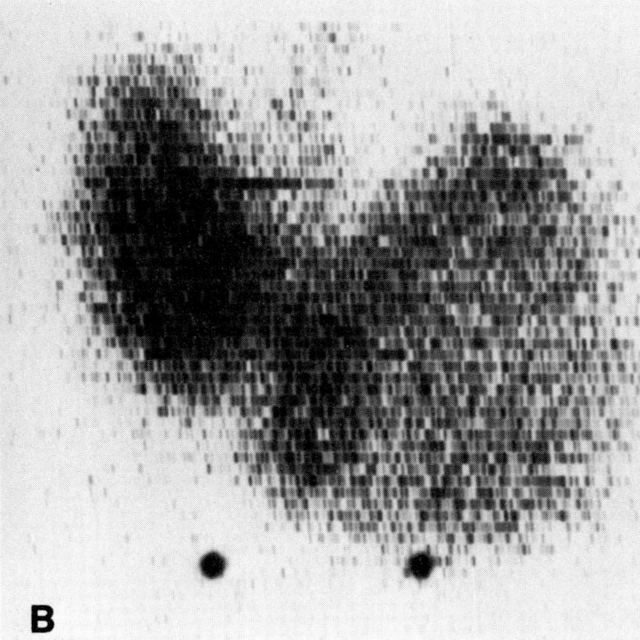

Fig. 7-6. Colloid goiter
A. 24 hour, [131]I. The left thyroid lobe is significantly enlarged, and its central area suggests a possible cold nodule.
B. Post-TSH, [131]I. Generalized improvement in uptake. The enlarged left lobe now demonstrates functional capability.

euphemism "hot" has been applied to the hyper-functioning nodule, "cold" to the nonfunctioning, and "warm" to the equal. Original judgments referable to these "temperatures" have not changed markedly over the years. If one has to have a nodule, a hot one is good, cold is bad, and the more nodules the better. These scanning generalities stem from evidence that malignant nodules are almost invariably nonfunctioning or cold. It has also been established that with only rare exception (and some will not even concede the exceptions) hyperfunctioning lesions are benign. Fortunately, only 1 in 5 single cold nodules proves to be malignant (Fig. 7-5). This 20% probability represents the worst combination of events, *i.e.,* a girl under 14 or a 20- to 30-year-old male. When there are multiple cold nodules, the probability decreases to 1 in 20 or less. Yet there is still no reliable technique for differentiating the bad cold from the good cold. Different modalities have been explored.

Rescanning after stimulatory thyroid uptake with TSH may occasionally improve the diagnostic potential if the cold nodule is more apparent than real. Occasionally, poor statistics result in an image that suggests an area of absent uptake which when stimulated proves to be merely poorly functioning (Fig. 7-6). This combination is helpful to separate the functioning from the truly nonfunctioning lesions. When the nodule is truly cold there is no enhancement and no differentiation (Fig. 7-7).

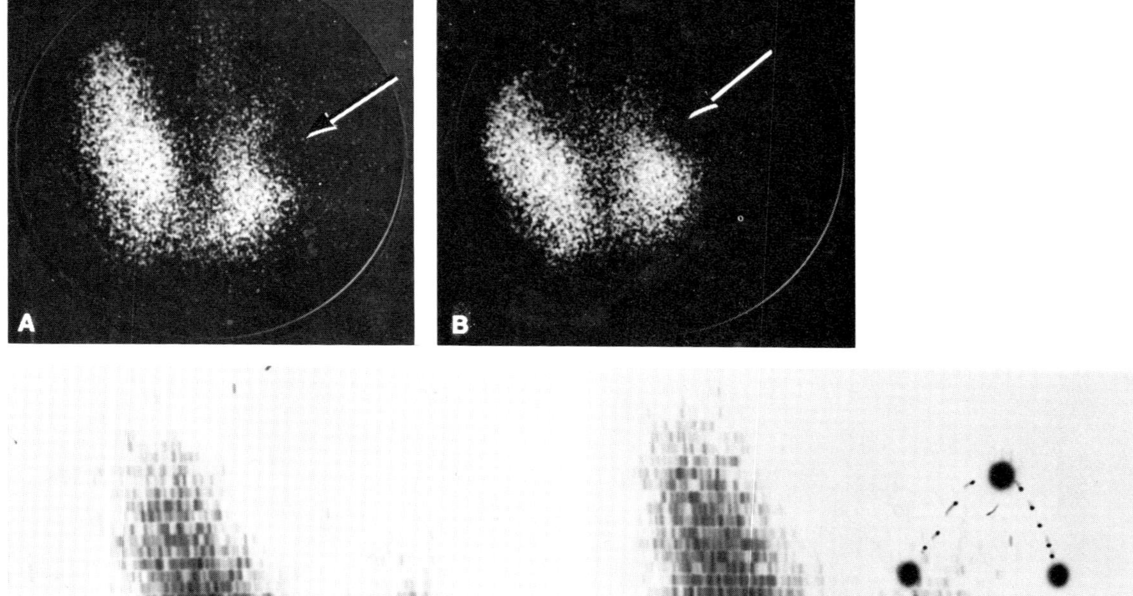

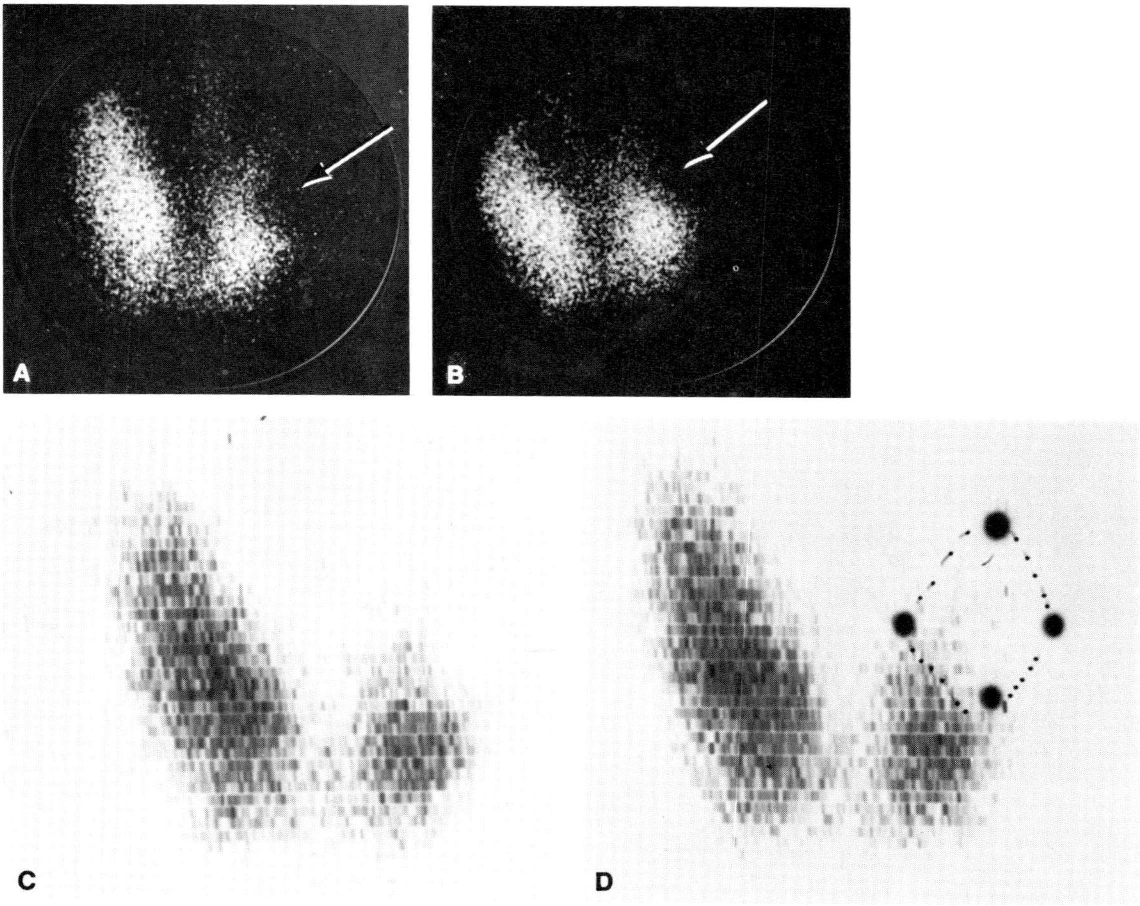

Fig. 7-7. Thyroid adenoma

A and B. 30 min, $^{99m}TcO_4$. Anterior **(A)** and left oblique **(B)** views identify a nonactive zone (arrow) in the upper pole of the left lobe. A firm nodule was palpated in this location.

C and D. Post-TSH, ^{131}I. Anterior views. The four black dots conform to the margins of the palpable mass. No improvement in uptake. The lesion is cold.

Fig. 7-8. Thyroid follicular adenoma (Hurthele cell variety). The patient was a 19-year-old female with a large palpable firm mass in the left lower anterior neck.

A. 24 hour, ^{131}I. Thyroid scan appears to be within normal limits. The dotted circle outlines the mass.

B. Perfusion scan, 14–16 sec, $^{99m}TcO_4$. The carotid arteries are just visualized.

C. Perfusion scan, 16–19 sec, $^{99m}TcO_4$. Early activity in the region of the thyroid. The left lobe appears enlarged and blends inferiorly with the left subclavian activity (arrow).

D. Perfusion scan, 2 min, $^{99m}TcO_4$. The right lobe of the thyroid is essentially normal. The left lobe is grossly enlarged and corresponds to the palpable mass in **A** (arrow).

Rescanning by serial perfusion methods with ^{99m}Tc pertechnetate will not improve the differential diagnostic potential if the lesion remains cold. Occasionally, the previously cold zone will light up when perfused, and this may improve judgment, particularly if there is any question as to whether the palpated lesion is or is not thyroid in origin (Figs. 7-8 and 7-9).

Ultrasonics offer some promise of separation but only of solid from cystic. Not all solid nodules, *e.g.,* adenomas, are malignant, but perhaps it's a start.

It is not uncommon to identify a hyperfunctioning nodule in a gland that looks peculiar.

Only the hot areas are seen, or if other portions of the gland are identified, they may show less than usual activity. This may be the pattern of the "autonomous" nodule, which suppresses uptake in the remainder of the organ. The diagnosis is tested by rescanning after administering 10 units of TSH. If there is suppression by the nodule, the scan image will change markedly (Fig. 7-10).

These examples are the easy cases. Many conditions exist in which the scan will appear free of nodules when in fact nodules exist. This occurs when either the nodular function equals the surrounding parenchymal activity so that there is no distinction or when the nodule's

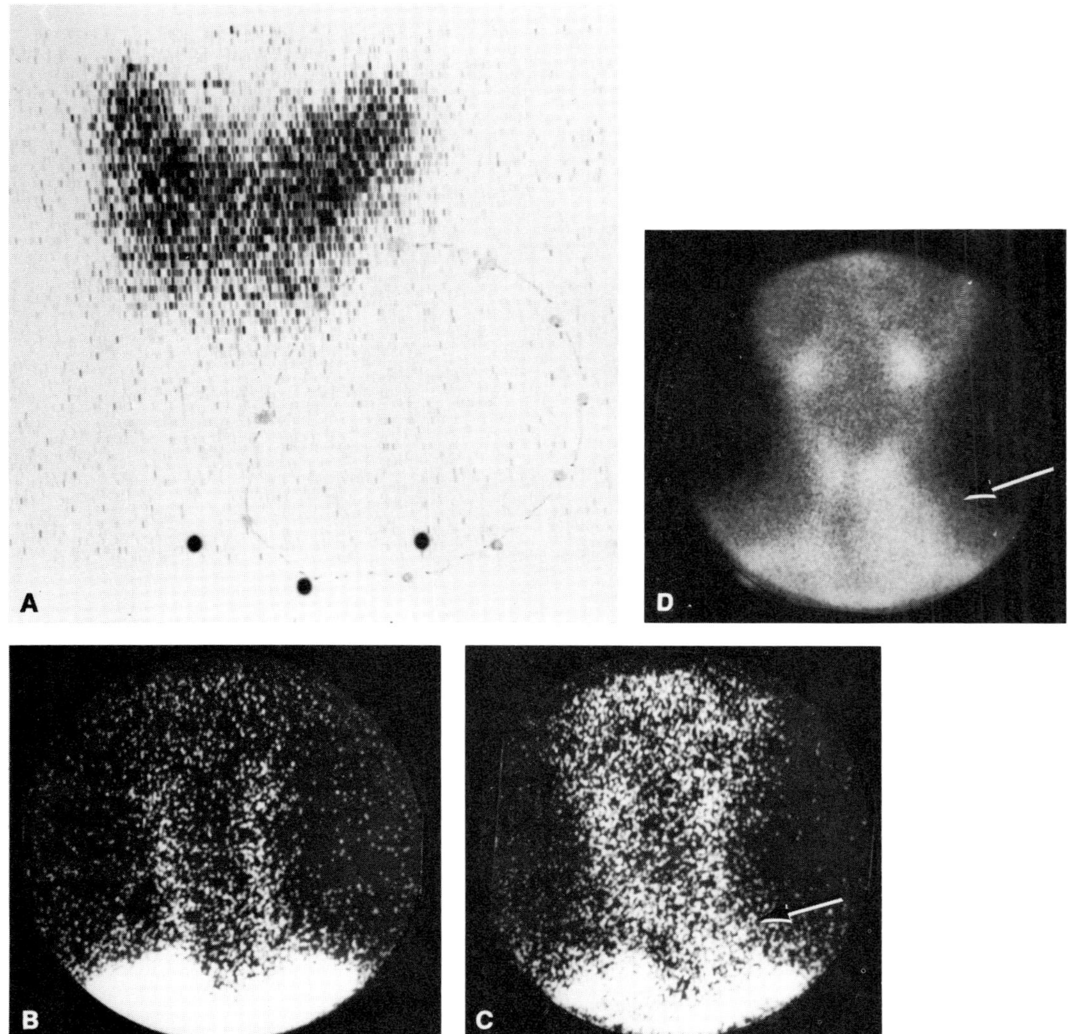

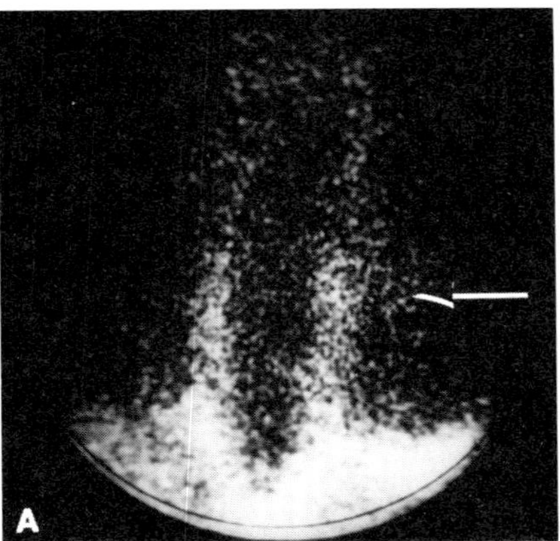
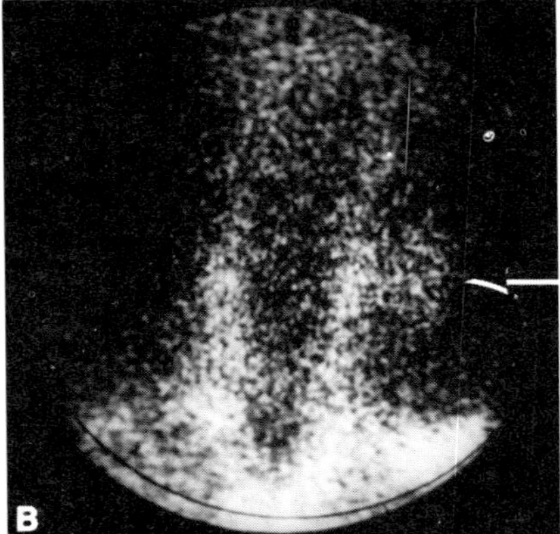
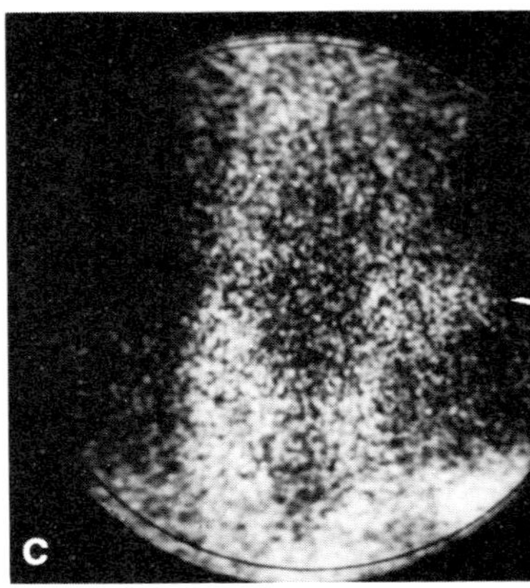
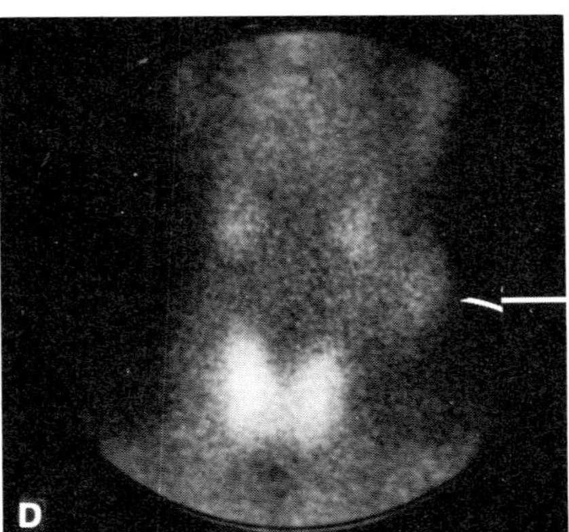

Fig. 7-9. Metastatic carcinoma—site unknown. The patient was a 74-year-old male with a palpable mass in the left lateral anterior neck, which could not be definitely separated from the thyroid.
A–D. Sequential flow scans, ^{99m}Tc. Serial images clearly identify the perfusion lesion to be extrathyroidal (arrows).

position is such that it fools the scanner. If, as an example, the nodule is a nonfunctioning type but is deep in the gland with normal tissue in front of it the activity from the functioning portion will be seen by the scanner. Even when this type of nodule is anterior, activity from behind it may shine through and obscure the lesion. Thus, it is imperative that a good physical palpation be performed at the time of the scan, preferably in the scanning position. Any palpable lesion must be marked in some way and correlated with the image. If a palpable lesion is not seen, it cannot be assumed that it is warm and therefore safe. It may be a nonfunctioning anterior nodule with a posterior "shine through" or a posterior defect with a superimposed functioning element. Oblique scans, if feasible, may help (lateral thyroid imaging is almost impossible because of the shoulders). Some have advocated tomographic scanning and this may resolve some of the difficulty, but as of yet it is hardly a routine procedure.

Despite a seemingly great number of exceptions, nodular scanning is a solid and valuable contribution to the understanding and management of these problems. No other technique is routinely available to supply *in vivo* functional data.

size, shape, and position

Thyroid imaging is often initiated by a routine chest x ray that suggests a widened superior mediastinal shadow, frequently with associated tracheal deviation. The most common cause for these changes is a substernally positioned thyroid (Fig. 7-11). Scanning confirms a thyroid etiology. If the gland is in normal position, it is imperative that the explanation for the widening be discovered since a mediastinal tumor may be present.

Any unexplained anterior neck mass should be investigated by thyroid scanning (Fig. 7-12). Ectopic implants are not remarkably uncommon (Figs. 7-13 and 7-14). Additionally, goiter

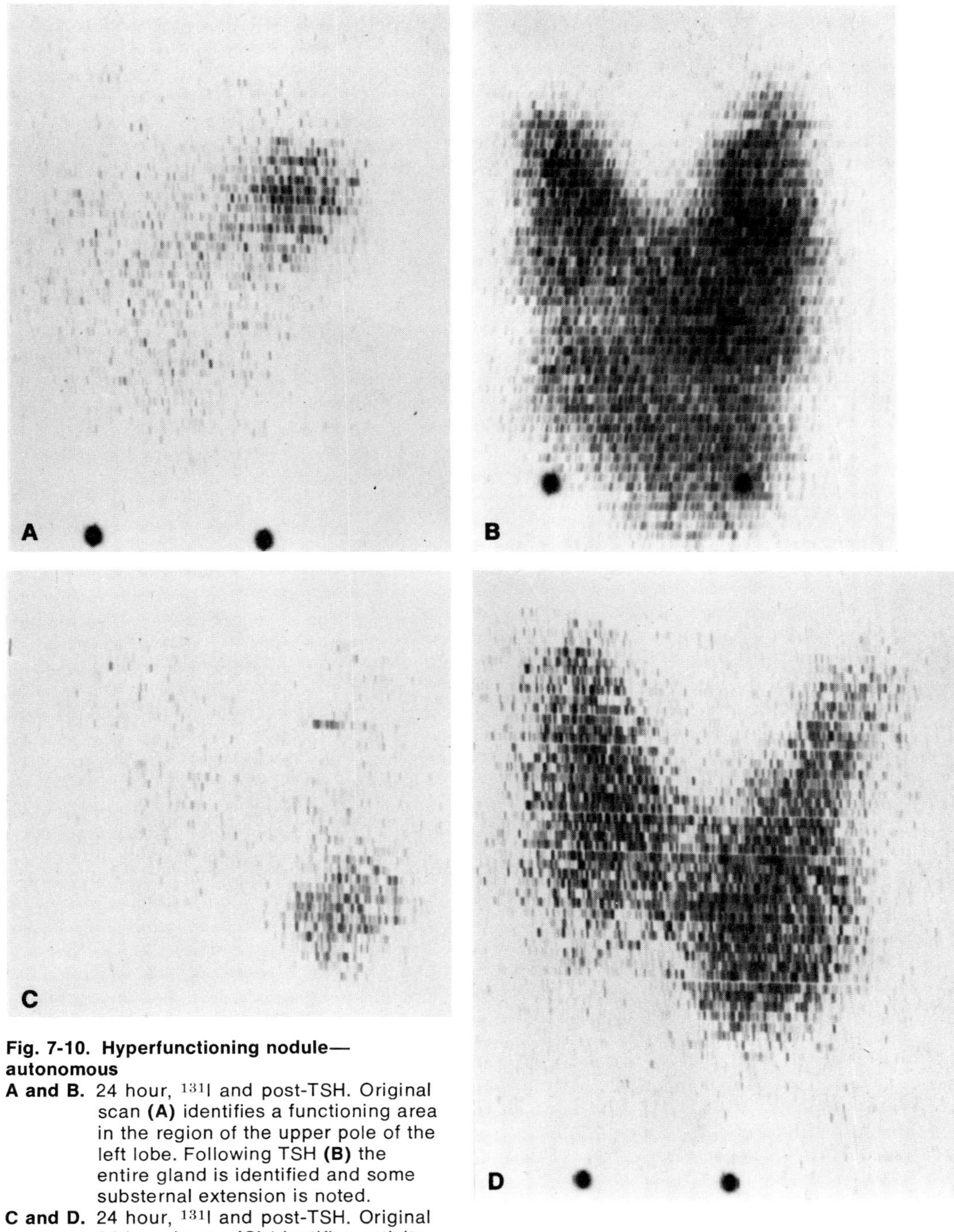

Fig. 7-10. Hyperfunctioning nodule—autonomous

A and B. 24 hour, ^{131}I and post-TSH. Original scan **(A)** identifies a functioning area in the region of the upper pole of the left lobe. Following TSH **(B)** the entire gland is identified and some substernal extension is noted.

C and D. 24 hour, ^{131}I and post-TSH. Original 24-hour image **(C)** identifies activity in the left lower pole. Remainder of the gland is barely perceived. Following TSH **(D)** the "suppressed" gland is visualized.

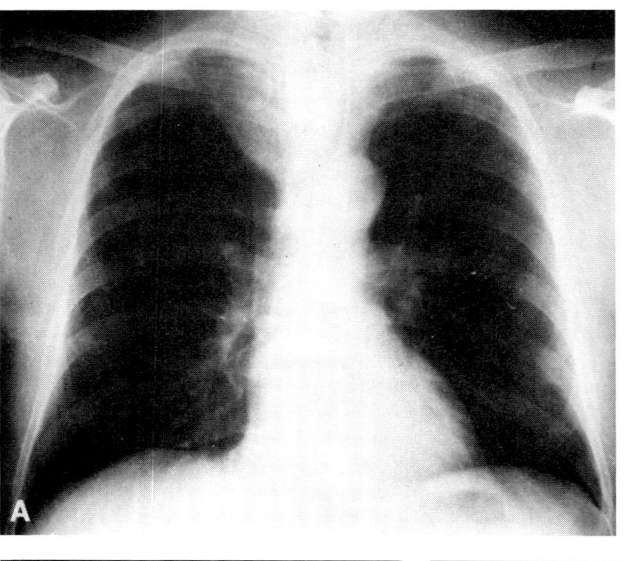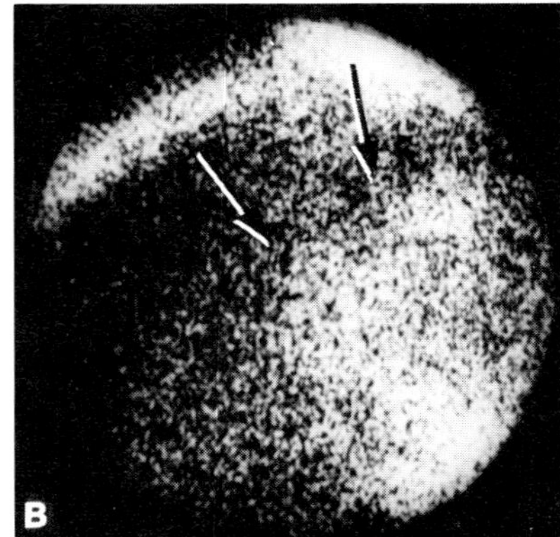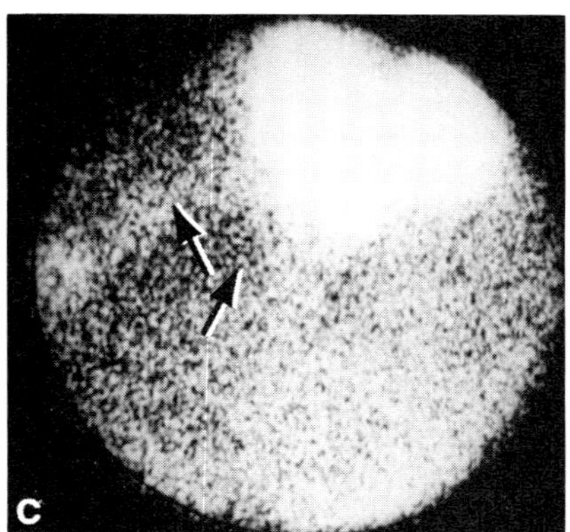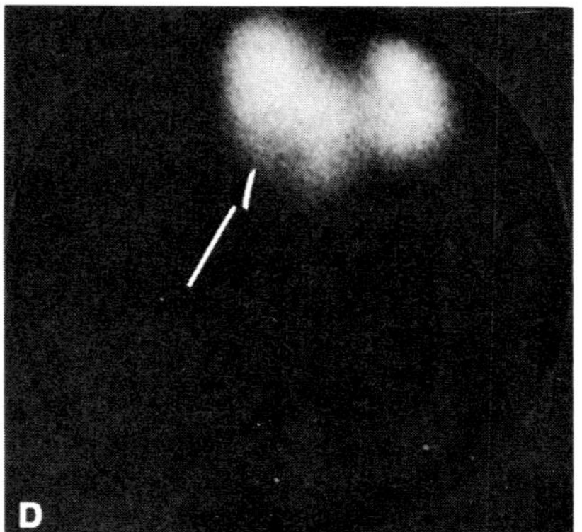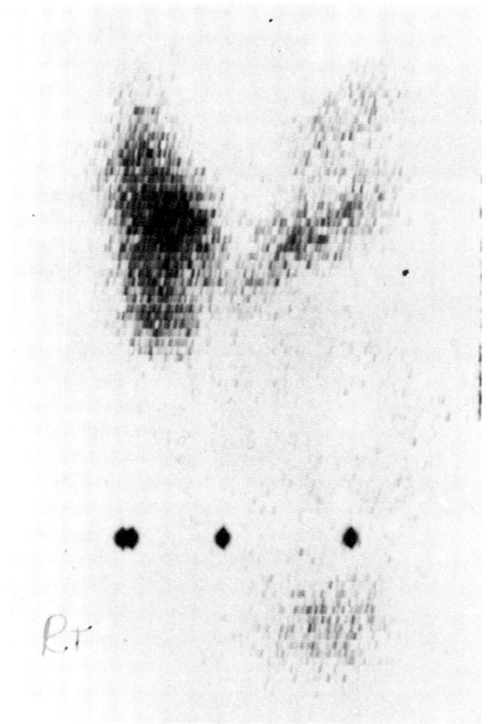

Fig. 7-11. Substernal thyroid

A. X ray. The chest x ray demonstrates a significant right superior mediastinal prominence that deviates the trachea to the left.

B. Sequential scan, 24–27 sec. Mediastinal flow study identifies the ascending aorta (arrow). There is no obvious structure to explain the mediastinal prominence.

C. Sequential scan, 45–50 sec. The thyroid is now clearly evident. The right lobe is enlarged and partially substernal. (Note the relationship of the inferior half of the lobe to the still faintly active right subclavian vein—arrows.)

D. Static scan, 5 min. The thyroid clearly explains the mediastinal changes. Additionally, a cold nodule is present at the inferior pole of the right lobe (arrow).

Fig. 7-13. Multinodular goiter with an ectopic thyroid nodule. Scan, 24-hour, [131]I. Nonhomogeneous distribution suggesting hyperfunctioning and nonfunctioning nodules. Additionally, there is an ectopic focus of activity just medial to the left sternoclavicular junction (arrow).

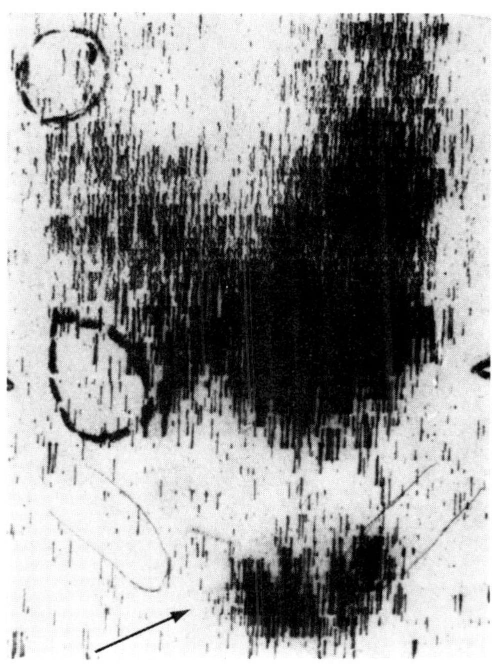

◀ **Fig. 7-12. Colloid goiter with substernal extension.** The patient presented with a huge, soft, ill-defined neck mass probably contiguous with the left thyroid lobe, which was average in size. The right lobe was palpably normal.

Scan, 24-hour, [131]I. The right lobe of the thyroid is within normal limits. The left lobe is huge, poorly functioning, and the lower pole extends deep into the mediastinum. (The two spaced black dots identify the sternal ends of the clavicle; the two close dots, the right side.)

Fig. 7-14. Subtotal thyroidectomy with ectopic thyroid tissue. Scan, 24-hour, [131]I. Left lobe is average in size. Right lobe is small with trapping only in upper pole. Considerable activity is present in ectopic sublingual thyroid tissue (arrow). (There was a history of antecedent right subtotal resection.)

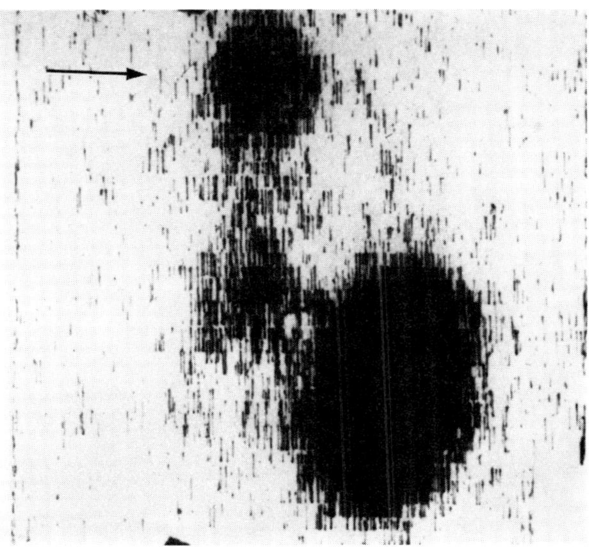

extensions may not always be appreciated, and it is consoling to know that "that thing" is capable of trapping iodine.

post operative

Following thyroid surgery for any cause it is advantageous to scan the neck. If the disease was nonmalignant and only a subtotal resection was performed, a postsurgical baseline image may be helpful if any problem recurs in the future and scanning is necessary. Although not essential it is occasionally valuable. If, however, the original pathology was malignant and a total thyroidectomy was performed, the need for postsurgical imaging is far more urgent. A total thyroidectomy is difficult to perform. More commonly than not the postoperative image will show that there is residual functioning gland despite the surgeon's protestations, "That's impossible!" (Fig. 7-15). Such data may affect subsequent management. If total ablation is desired, the mopping up with ^{131}I in therapeutic doses is initiated. The postoperative scan and the postoperative surgical record are frequently in disagreement—what was meant to be a complete is more often not. Only the scan can validate the postsurgical statement.

metastasis

When a diagnosis of thyroid carcinoma has been made and therapy initiated, it is valuable to determine whether or not metastasis has occurred. Usually, there must be complete extirpation of functioning neck thyroid, either by surgical or radiation means, in order to detect such changes. Whole body imaging in these situations occasionally identifies a metastatic focus (Fig. 7-16).

infection

The diagnosis of thyroiditis is rarely made by scanning alone. The classic acute and subacute problem with the tender neck and hyperthyroid symptoms is thought to be viral in origin and frequently exhibits no uptake of ^{131}I. With no uptake, there is obviously no scan. However, if the infection does not involve the entire gland, a unilateral nonfunctioning defect may localize the site of involvement. Documentation of the response to therapy is made possible by serial recheck. As the process subsides, function is restored (Fig. 7-17).

Hashimoto's thyroiditis is probably a disorder of the immune system. The glands are usually enlarged, and hypothyroid symptoms may be exhibited. Although not pathognomonic the scan may demonstrate a nonhomogeneous trapping pattern. No specific nodules are identified; it just looks like a poor study.

The problems of infection do not represent a big, big indication for imaging, but in some cases it is helpful.

function

In Vivo. Estimation of functional status has become the almost exclusive domain of the nuclear medicine man. Originally, the estimation was based on the percentage uptake of the ingested tracer dose in 24 hours. Although this is still a valuable and common determination, more reliance is now being placed on circulating hormonal levels. These studies are *in vitro* in nature and will be discussed shortly. Initially, a range of values was established which were to correlate with hypofunction, eufunction, or hyperfunction. Shortly into the mission it was realized that these values could not be considered as sharp boundaries since many clinical hyperthyroid patients exhibited uptakes in the euthyroid range. That was easily rationalized— the turnover rate in the toxic gland was so rapid that by 24 hours the peak was past. Therefore, test earlier. Thus the 2-, 3-, and 6-hour uptakes were added and values for these established. This helped. Then someone reported some high uptakes in obviously euthyroid individuals. Investigation showed that in edemic regions in which dietary iodine is low, the gland may be "starved" and may respond by excessive trapping.

On the other end, there were reports of no uptake or grossly depressed uptake being encountered in patients obviously not myxedematous. This yielded libraries of literature on all of the conditions that depress uptake: thyroid pharmaceuticals, iodine in any form, contrast x-ray media, cough expectorants, even topical application of iodinated antiseptics, certain hormones, etc., etc., etc. Thus, a whole checklist of no-nos, must be explored before a feeding dose is given.

And after all of the above, and many, many more besides have been built into the results, the conclusions are still based on inference. Uptake measures the thyroid's trapping mechanism, but it is usually the hormone production

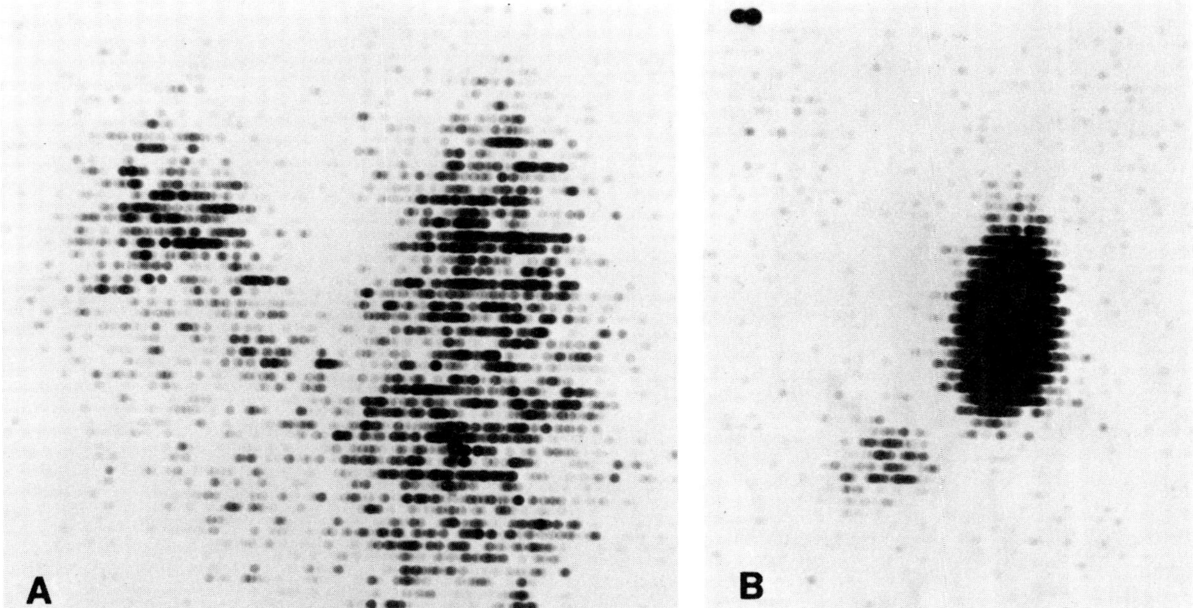

Fig. 7-15. Residual thyroid tissue following "total" thyroidectomy
A. Scan, 24-hour, [131]I. Thyroid is diffusely enlarged with nontrapping of a major portion of the right lobe. A total thyroidectomy was performed when frozen section identified the cold lesions to be follicular carcinoma.
B. Scan, (1 week postoperatively and following enhancement with TSH). Rescanning with ^{131}I demonstrates considerable residual functioning tissue.

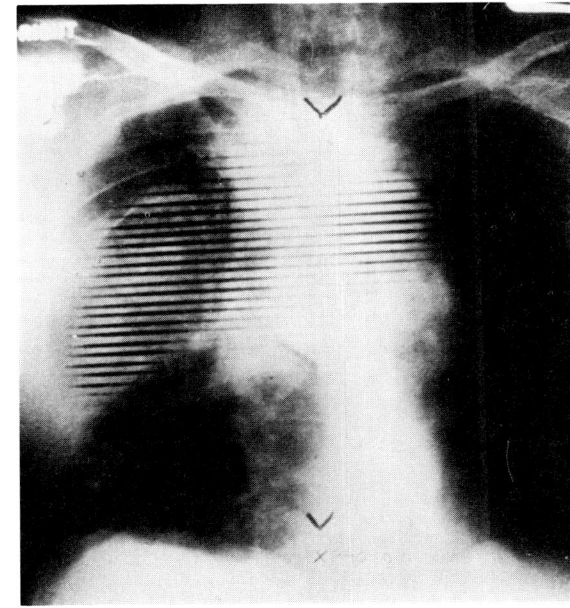

Fig. 7-16. Metastatic follicular carcinoma of the thyroid. Scan, 24-hour, [131]I. The scan is superimposed of the chest x ray of a patient complaining of severe right thoracic wall pain 3 years following diagnosis of follicular carcinoma of the thyroid. The linear strips represent ^{131}I uptake in the regions of bony metastasis.

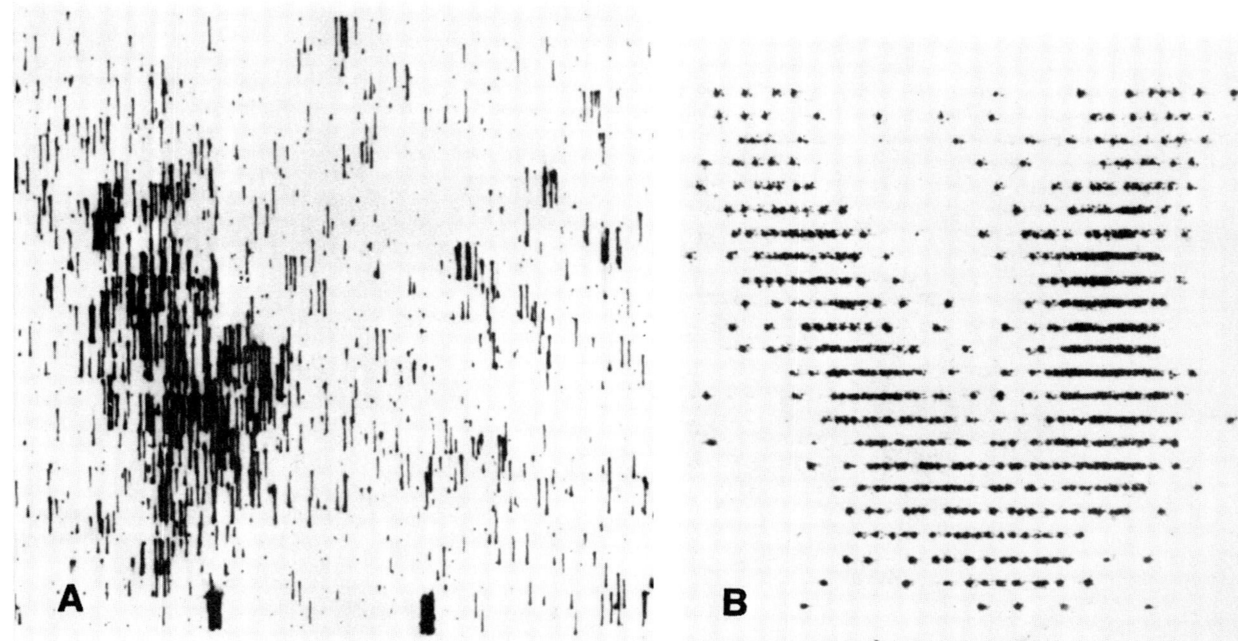

Fig. 7-17. Unilateral thyroiditis
A. Scan, 24-hour, ^{131}I. There is no uptake in the left lobe. The patient complained of left-sided neck pain.
B. Scan, 24-hour, ^{131}I. Recheck 3 months later identifies normal left lobe uptake. All previous symptoms had resolved.

and discharge function that result in those changes synonymous with hyperthyroidism and hypothyroidism. So, unless a thyroid scan is to be done, feeding the patient ^{131}I for uptake alone is no longer fashionable.

There is, of course, an exception. When there is clinical uncertainty as to whether a patient is or is not toxic and all other function studies are equally unclear (this does happen), an uptake followed by a T_3 suppression uptake is most useful. Patients whose thyroid is normal will exhibit a decrease in uptake by at least 50% of the original value after a 3- to 7-day course of T_3. This is the suppression invoked by the T_3. A toxic gland will not be suppressed. The technique, although infrequently necessary, does serve a most helpful function in those special cases.

Lastly, in patients suspected of secondary hypothyroidism, *e.g.*, the problem is primarily in the pituitary and results from low TSH elaboration, rechecking uptake after administering parenteral TSH will result in a significant rise in trapping. If the hypothyroid state is of thyroid origin, the TSH will not significantly affect the depressed uptake. Again, this is a less than daily differential problem, but when present it is answerable.

In Vitro. Within the past few years the *in vitro* function studies have spawned a virtual hormone jungle. To sell his product and make it distinctive from the next, each commercial radiopharmaceutical distributor has juggled the name and skewed the values so that a scorecard is required to keep the players straight. We shall describe the basic determinations available, offer an opinion on their relative merit, and provide a road map through the quagmire. Consultation should be had with the person in the basement to clarify which and what is being done and the particular range of values.

Although admittedly flirting with the hazards of oversimplification, the plethora of studies can only be sensibly rationalized by a general understanding of what they are attempting to measure and why.

The thyroid elaborates and discharges two hormones, thyroxin (T_4) and triiodothyronine

(T_3). In the plasma most (but not all) of the T_4 is bound to thyroxin-binding globulin (TBG) and thyroxin-binding prealbumin (TBPA). Approximately 0.03% of the total is "free," *i.e.,* unbound. It is this unbound fraction that is the active or metabolically determinate form. (Recent evidence suggests that even this free T_4 must first be converted to T_3 before it becomes metabolically significant.)

Direct measurement of the free T_4 fraction is possible but difficult. Measurement of the total circulating T_4, protein bound and free, is much simpler. If all things (in this case, the circulating TBG levels) were constant, estimating the serum T_4 would give indirect indication of thyroid function. Elevation would be presumptive evidence of hyperthyroidism, depression-hypo. But that would be too easy—all things just won't remain constant! Many factors influence the concentration of the binding proteins, and these in turn offer the total concentration of bound hormones. Increased estrogen levels as in pregnancy or where employing oral contraceptives (just one of many examples) will evidence increased TBG concentrations. Decreased concentration occurs when androgens or anabolic steroids are employed. In the former example the serum T_4 will be elevated, in the latter depressed, but in each the patient is euthyroid since the percentage of free T_4 has not been affected and remains constant.

Thus, it becomes imperative to separate the abnormal levels induced by true grandular functional change from those caused by extra-glandular influences.

To this end, a second determination can be utilized. This, too, is an indirect determination, the measurement of available binding sites within the circulatory TBG. When the T_4 level is elevated but the TBG concentration is normal there are fewer binding sites, but when the TBG concentration has been expanded the sites are increased. The vice-versa obtains with decreased T_4 or decreased TBG. Originally, this determination was performed by adding T_3 labeled with ^{131}I to a sample of the patient's whole blood and determining the amount of labeled T_3 that became bound. This technique was modified so as to substitute resin or charcoal for the patient's red blood cells. (These modifications account for the countless numbers of available commercial technique kits.) This estimation is generally known as the T_3 resin uptake, which must not be confused with techniques that directly measure free circulatory serum T_3.

Suffice it to state that serum thyroxin levels can be measured directly. TBG binding sites can be measured by T_3 resin uptake. The combination of the two give reasonable inferential data regarding the amount of free T_4 and the status of thyroid function. When there is true excessive thyroid elaboration, the serum T_4 and T_3 resin uptake will both be elevated. Both will be depressed with hypofunction. However, when the TBG levels are affected by extrathyroidal forces, the serum T_4 and resin T_3 values will move in opposite directions. This constitutes an "out" to the previous dilemma. Simple multiplication of the serum T_4 by the resin T_3 uptake will yield a value that, although it has been called by many names, is essentially equivalent to "the free thyroxin index." (The above points out the misnomer of the commercially popular T_7 determination suggesting T_3 plus T_4 when in reality it should be $T_{12}[T_4 \times T_3]$).

Also available is a single serum T_4 determination that attempts to separate the confusion of TBG changes from true shifts without the necessity of the additional resin uptake determination.

It is impossible to catalogue the almost limitless number of permutations and combinations of procedures commercially available. The only salvation is to try to constantly keep in mind what is being measured and whether the various parameters that affect interpretive judgment are considered in the particular determination. A short "rap-session" with the basement man will help clarify the muddle. (It is wild to discuss this problem with a clinician who works in several different hospitals each employing different techniques with different values.)

To obtain some measure of completeness other determinations must be cited.

Direct T_3 Determination. Employing radio-immunoassay methods (discussed in chapter **8**) the true concentration of T_3 in the serum can be measured. This evaluation has led to improved understanding of the role of the thyroid hormones and has identified a new syndrome referred to as T_3 toxicosis, in which the patient is clinically hyperthyroidal but serum T_4 levels are normal. Except for this special situation, this determination does not seem necessary, routine, or ordinary.

TBG. Thyroxin-binding globulin can be measured directly, if one has little else to do. Although TBG level significantly affects the apparent level of serum T_4, these effects can be deduced if both T_3 resin uptake and serum T_4 values are obtained as previously discussed. Therefore, there is little need to specifically evaluate TBG level.

TSH. It is now possible to measure serum thyroid-stimulating hormone (TSH) levels by radioimmunoassay techniques. This information provides the most sensitive indicator as to the existence of hypothyroidism. All previous thyroid-testing modalities are far more reliable for the euthyroid and hyperthyroid condition, but determination of TSH provides the needed hypothyroid yardstick. Additionally, its use has improved accuracy in monitoring replacement therapy and excessive thyroid medication can be avoided. Although this method of evaluation has diminished the indications for the older TSH stimulatory techniques previously described, such studies may still be necessary to separate the primary from the secondary hypothyroid individual.

therapy

Hyperthyroidism. Despite all efforts to the contrary, the etiology of this problem still eludes absolute capture. Despite reams of literature the absolute single best method of therapy eludes agreement. Thus, each patient must be considered individually and one of the three possible corrective modalities, *i.e.,* antithyroid drugs, surgery, or ^{131}I, chosen.

It would be inappropriate to our avowed purposes to extensively compare and contrast these choices. It will suffice to identify the known pros and cons of ^{131}I management.

It is known that ^{131}I will suppress thyroid function. What is unknown is how much is necessary in each individual problem to suppress only the excessive function and restore the patient to a euthyroid state. Historically the use of radiation to suppress hormone production has decreased as evidence of excessive suppression has increased. Many therapists now strive to achieve a dose of approximately 80μCi ^{131}I/g thyroid tissue. But errors in weight estimation are ever-constant and perhaps more importantly, there is as yet no method of estimating individual sensitivity. So as with

titration to an end point, if one adds enough, neutralization will always occur—but oh, that horrible extra drop! Hypothyroidism!

Time and experience have shown that without exception, regardless of the presenting type of patient with hyperthyroidism (*e.g.,* age, sex, uptake values, nodules, and regardless of the suppression technique employed (*e.g.,* large single doses, small single doses, multiple small), at least 25% (and probably higher) of all treated patients will be hypothyroid in 10 years. This is its single greatest disadvantage. There is no known way at the present time to improve these statistics.

Originally, it was feared that another serious disadvantage, yea hazard, was the possibility of carcinogenesis from the radiation. This hypothesis has been fully exploded. It simply does not happen. Thus the original admonition of reserving therapy only for the elderly because of the concern of eventual malignancy is no longer viable although many therapists are still reluctant to treat the young. Original concern over possibly triggering a "thyroid storm" has also been proven ill-founded. However, a very real concern exists in treating toxic women in the childbearing age. Inadvertent pregnancy shortly after ^{131}I administration may cause irreparable damage to the fetal thyroid. It should also be added that ^{131}I is transferred in the maternal milk, and thus breast feeding is contraindicated for a short time after treatment. And lastly, the length of time between initiation of therapy and clinical response is relatively great—at least 5–8 weeks. It is imperative to forewarn the patient of this delay between treatment and response or she will add both anxiety and depression to her already unhappy state: "Why am I not getting better? Why doesn't anything work on me?" During this latent ^{131}I interval temporary drug therapy can be initiated for symptomatic relief.

Those are the baddies. On the positive side is the absolute simplicity of the technique. A capsule (or liquid) is administered, usually once, on an out-patient basis, and that's it. There is no hospitalization, preoperative preparation, or postoperative morbidity; neither is there daily medication for the rest of the foreseeable future, bouncing hypothyroid and hyperthyroid levels, nor idiosyncratic reactions. And in the long run, it's far, far cheaper.

As initially stated, each diagnosed case should be individually conferenced by the attending, internist, surgeon, and nuclear medicine man for the best therapeutic fit. Most times we think ^{131}I will be best, but we are prejudiced.

Carcinoma. After surgery and pathologic evaluation has established carcinoma ^{131}I may be indicated. If functioning glandular tissue has been left behind (best determined by postoperative scanning) and it is desired to ablate this residuum, massive doses of ^{131}I can accomplish this task. If metastases from thyroid carcinoma are identified and it can be established that they are capable of trapping iodine (best determined by whole body scanning), ^{131}I can be administered for palliative purposes.

In either of these indications the doses required far exceed those usually administered for functional problems. Indeed they are so high that the patient becomes a "radiation hazard" to others and as a consequence must be isolated by hospitalization. Usually, this quarantine does not exceed 2 weeks and is often less. Except for possible salivary gland discomfort, there is no patient morbidity with the treatment.

Although the indications for this type of management are limited, when the right combination of circumstances prevail it is a valuable modality.

Angina Pectoris. It was once thought that if a patient with intractable angina were rendered hypothyroid he would suffer less. For a short historic moment this therapy was invoked. Euthyroid anginal patients were given large suppressive doses of ^{131}I and became hypothyroid. Perhaps 50% of those so treated improved with respect to their chest pain but had to contend with iatrogenic myxedema. With the advent of improved drug management we don't do this anymore.

Table 7-1. Indications, Pharmaceuticals, Methodology and Order of Merit of Radionuclide Study of Thyroid

Why	What	How	Yea–Nay
Masses–nodules	^{131}I, ^{125}I, ^{123}I, ^{99m}Tc pertechnetate	static	+++
Size, shape, position	^{131}I, ^{125}I, ^{123}I, ^{99m}Tc	static	++++
Postoperative	^{131}I, ^{125}I, ^{123}I, ^{99m}Tc	static	++++
Distant metastasis	^{131}I	static	+
Infection	^{131}I, ^{125}I, ^{123}I	static	++
Function			
In vivo			
Uptake			+++
T3 suppression	^{131}I, ^{123}I, ^{99m}Tc pertechnetate	neck count	++++
TSH stimulation			++++
In vitro	^{125}I	well count	++++
Therapy			
Function	^{131}I		++++
Ca and metastasis			++

Table 7-2. More About What

Radiopharmaceutical	Dose (mCi)	Physical Half-life	Energy Peak (keV)
^{131}I	0.005–0.100 (diagnostic)	8.4 days	364
	2–150 (therapeutic)		36
^{125}I	0.05–0.1	60 days	
^{123}I	.30–.50	13 hours	158
^{99m}Tc pertechnetate	1–3	6 hours	140

Why	Preparation	Administration	Time Between Administration and Exam (hr)	Number of Exams	Time for Each Exam (min)	Time for Total Study (hr)	Patient's Position	Instrument
Mass-Nodules	none	oral	24	1 or more	15	24	supine	camera or scanner
Cytomel suppression	T_3—3 to 7 days prior	oral	24	1	15	24	supine	camera or scanner
TSH enhancement	TSH—24 hr prior	oral	24	1	15	24	supine	camera or scanner
Size, shape, position	none	oral	24	1	15	24	supine	camera or scanner
Postoperative	none	oral	24	1	30	24	supine	camera or scanner
Metastasis	none	oral	24	1	60-120	24	supine	camera or scanner
Infection	none	oral	24	1	15	24	supine	camera or scanner
Function In vivo Uptake	fasting	oral	2-6 thru 24 hr	2	5	24	supine	probe
Cytomel	T_3—3 to 7 days prior	oral	2-6 thru 24 hr	2	5	4-8	supine	probe
1° vs 2°	TSH—24 hr prior	oral	2-6 thru 24 hr	2	5	48	supine	probe
In vitro	none	blood sample				3-4		well counter
Therapy Function	none	oral						
Ca and metastasis	none	oral						

 speak to me in nuclear medicine

BIBLIOGRAPHY

GENERAL

Atkins HL et al.: A comparison of technetium ^{99m} and iodine 123 for thyroid imaging. Am J Roentgenol Radium Ther Nucl Med 117:195–201, 1973

Black MB: ^{99m}Tc-pertechnetate flow study for evaluation of "cold" thyroid nodules. Radiology 102:705–706, 1972

Blahd WH: Scanning of the thyroid gland. In Blahd WH (ed): Nuclear Medicine. New York, McGraw–Hill, 1971, pp 227–235

Carpenter GW, Blum AS: A rapid radioimmunoassay for triiodothyronine in unextracted serum (abstr). J Nucl Med 15(6):482, 1974

DeLand FH, Wagner HN: Thyroid. In Reticuloendothelial System, Liver, Spleen, Thyroid. Philadelphia, WB Saunders, 1972, pp 237–287

Halpern S et al.: ^{131}I thyroid uptakes: capsule versus liquid. J Nucl Med 14(7):507–510, 1973

Hamburger JI et al.: Subacute thyroiditis-evolution depicted by serial 131I scintigram. J Nucl Med 6:560–565, 1965

Hamolsky MW, Koplowitz JM, Solomon DH: Measurement of thyroid function. In Blahd WH (ed): Nuclear Medicine. New York, McGraw–Hill, 1971, pp 175–226

Hollander CS, Shenkman L: Radioimmunoassays for triiodothyronine and thyroxine. In Rothfeld B (ed): Nuclear Medicine in Vitro. Philadelphia, JB Lippincott, 1972, pp 136–149

Hurley PJ et al.: The scintillation camera with pinhole collimator in thyroid imaging. Radiology 101:133–138, 1971

James AE, Squire LF: Interpretation of the thyroid scan. In Nuclear Radiology. Philadelphia, WB Saunders, 1973, pp 140–149

Kaplan WD et al.: ^{67}Ga-citrate and the non-functioning thyroid nodule. J Nucl Med 15(6):424–427, 1974

Klinger L: Polyphosphate bone scans, ^{32}phosphorus, and adenocarcinoma of the thyroid. J Nucl Med 15(11):1037–1038, 1974

Krishnamurthy GT, Blahd WH: Diagnosis and therapeutic implications of long-term radioisotope scanning in the management of thyroid cancer. J Nucl Med 13(12):924–927, 1972

Mincey EK et al: An in vitro thyroid function test without alcohol extraction. J Nucl Med 15(11):1032–1034, 1974

Selenkow HA, Karp PJ: An approach to diagnosis and therapy of thyroid tumors. Semin Nucl Med 1(4):461–473, 1971

Shafer RB, Tully TE: Thyroid carcinoma presenting as an isolated bone cyst. J Nucl Med 15(1):50–52, 1974

Silverstein GE et al.: The natural history of the autonomous hyperfunctioning thyroid nodule. Am Intern Med 67:539–548, 1967

Soin JS et al.: Disappearance of autonomous thyroid nodule under TSH stimulation. J Nucl Med 15(12):1209–1211, 1974

Weinstein MB et al.: ^{75}Se selenomethionine as a scanning agent for the differential diagnosis of the cold thyroid nodule. Semin Nucl Med 1(3):390–396, 1971

Woolner LB: Thyroid carcinoma: pathological classification with data on prognosis. Semin Nucl Med 1(4):481–502, 1971

Workman JB: The thyroid. In Freeman LM, Johnson PM (eds): Clinical Scintillation Scanning. Hagerstown, Harper & Row, 1969, pp 446–468

RADIOTHERAPY

Blumgart HL et al.: Treatment of incapacitated euthyroid cardiac patients with radioactive iodine. In Blahd WH (ed): Nuclear Medicine. New York, McGraw–Hill, 1971, pp 751–759

Chapman EM: Treatment of hyperthyroidism with radioactive iodine. In Blahd WH (ed): Nuclear Medicine. New York, McGraw–Hill, 1971, pp 711–734

Hagen GA et al.: Comparison of high and low dosage levels of 131-I in the treatment of thyrotoxicosis. N Engl J Med 277:559–562, 1967

Lewitus Z et al.: Treatment of thyrotoxicosis with ^{125}I and ^{131}I. Semin Nucl Med 1(4):411–421, 1971

Nishiyama H et al.: Evaluation of clinical value of ^{123}I and ^{131}I in thyroid disease. J Nucl Med 15(4):261–265, 1974

Rawson RW, Leeper RD: Treatment of thyroid cancer with radioactive iodine. In Blahd WH (ed): Nuclear Medicine. New York, McGraw–Hill, 1971, pp 735–750

Siemsen JK et al.: Early results of ^{125}I therapy of thyrotoxic Graves' disease. J Nucl Med 15(4):257–260, 1974

Who does not remember with joy the day, when under the protective aura of "scientific wunder kind," he dissected the family alarm clock to see what made it tick and ring? And who does not remember that sensation of horror when having carefully replaced what seemed like all of the essential components there were still pieces left over on the table?

At the end of a dissertation, after neatly packaging what seems like all of the essential components into their proper chapters, boxes still left on the table are an assortment of pieces. For some nuclear clocks they are unessential to either the tick or ring, but to others, at least some, are absolutely critical. The unboxed pieces represent a wide variety of procedures and techniques. Some may never—or only rarely—be called for in some departments, while some, perhaps even many, represent commonly requested studies. Each, however, in our prejudiced judgment, does not warrant an individual chapter, and so they are lumped together under the ubiquitous umbrella called miscellany. Our categories ETC. Etc. etc. define the order of merit assigned. The first group consists of well-established, proven, and often indispensable techniques. The second classification blankets the more controversial, less generally accepted examinations, and the last those in which the jury is still out.

ETC.

radioisotope therapy

If the founding fathers of nuclear medicine were reconvened and permitted an historic retrospective, undoubtedly their only disappointment referable to their original expectations would be in the realm of therapeutics. Initially, anticipations were high that radioactive materials would contribute significantly to treatment, particularly in problems oncologic. Theoretically, all of the advantages of ionizing radiation should be obtained with none of the major disadvantages. The major deterrent to radiation therapy from external sources is the volume of normal tissue violated in reaching the seat of pathology. With radioisotopes this problem was obviated. The therapeutic agent could be delivered selectively to the site, and radiation would be localized and specific. Obviously these remarks exclude all external forms of radiation even though some are from radioactive nuclides

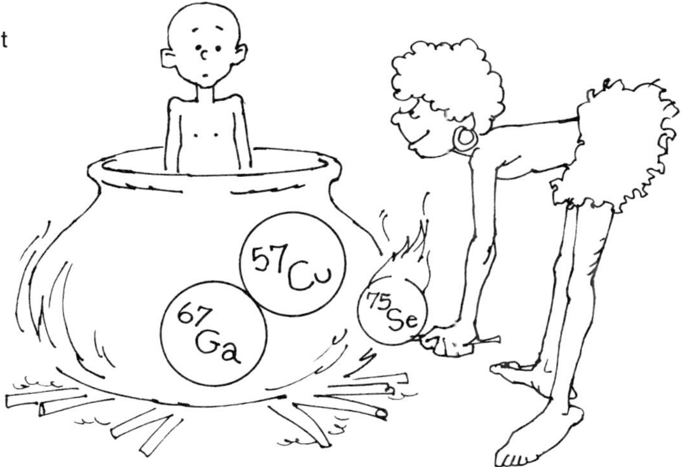

chapter 8

ETC. Etc. etc.

in sealed sources. But as with other "best laid plans," it has, with only few notable exceptions, yet to be achieved. Those isolated pathologic states that do respond to radioisotopic management will be discussed, but the larger dream of one-to-one radionuclide-to-tumor specificity remains unrealized.

This is not to suggest that the original expectations or anticipations were ill-founded. The hopes are still viable because the concepts are still sound, and it is still rational to expect that the not too distant future will yield tumor-specific therapeutic nuclides.

Thyroid. Disease of the thyroid gland, both benign as hyperfunctional aberrations and certain types of malignancies can be treated successfully with ^{131}I (see chapter 7).

Polycythemia Vera. Polycythemia vera responds to radioactive phosphorus (^{32}P), which is a pure beta emitter. In adhering to our previously agreed promise of keeping to a minimum of nuclear physics, it suffices here to explain beta emission, in contradistinction to gamma emission, as a radiation form in which all ionizing effects are spent within a few centimeters of tissue. This is most advantageous in therapy since it provides a very localized effect in the patient and avoids the hazards of exposure to others. Gamma emissions are so energetic that most escape from the body, which is what makes scanning possible only with the big G and not with beta-emitting nuclides. Thus, patients treated with therapeutic doses of gamma-emitting nuclides must be isolated and prevented from becoming unwitting sources of irradiation to others until the dosage is spent. Additionally, any inadvertent loss of these gamma agents from the body through fluid leakage, urine, vomit, and so forth constitutes another hazard and contaminated bed linens, dressings, and clothing must also be isolated. None of these prohibitions exist with the beta emitters. The treated patients need not be hospitalized.

Whether or not ^{32}P is better in this condition than other chemotherapeutic agents is unresolved. Leukemia as a potential sequela in isotopically managed patients, a persistent specter raised against the use of ^{32}P, is still to be proven since leukemia is not uncommonly part of the natural history of polycythemia. In those case histories cited of polycythemia–^{32}P–

leukemia, the dosages employed approached 20 mCi. Few cases have been described where the dosage range was lower. An unrestricted regimen of 5 mCi doses as needed is now recommended, but with a retreatment interval between doses of at least 3 months. The route of administration may be oral or IV. The morbidity of phlebotomy is usually avoidable, and neither hospitalization nor other radiation precautions are necessary.

Bone Metastasis. In proven skeletal metastasis from both the breast and prostate, palliation of pain is often possible with ^{32}P. It is usually reserved for those advanced problems where localized radiation or even neurosurgical relief is no longer tenable and where hormonal or chemotherapeutic response, or both, has become ineffective. Various protocols exist as to its administration. Some advocate daily doses for some prescribed interval, such as 7 days, whereas others suggest a more protracted course over a 4- to 6-week period. Most employ a priming dose of testosterone or parathormone to enhance ^{32}P uptake in the bone. All carry the potential hazard of aplastic anemia since there may be extensive depression of the marrow from the combination of neoplastic invasion and radiation effect.

Although palliation of pain is not always achieved, in isolated cases there are spectacular results, and when all else has failed ^{32}P is certainly worth a trial.

Malignant Effusion. Recurrent malignant effusion may respond to the local instillation of radioactive colloidal suspensions. Gold (^{198}Au) has been used with success, but this has all of the above-discussed disadvantages of a gamma emitter. Thus again, ^{32}P as chromic phosphate is the nuclide usually employed.

It is hoped in these problems that the colloidal particles will "plate out" on either the pleural or peritoneal surfaces and irradiate the metastatic implants responsible for fluid elaboration. Success, again palliative in degree, is reportedly achieved in some 50%–60% of cases. Care must be exercised that the suspension is not instilled into a loculated cavity since the confined radiation dose, being excessive, may create fistulas, particularly into the GI tract. This may be avoided by first instilling a suspension of ^{99m}Tc sulfur colloid and scanning the abdomen. The distribution pattern will confirm or deny loculation. If free, the therapeutic agent can then be instilled.

Obviously a procedure that promises only a 50%–60% temporary success yield cannot be heralded as a major weapon, but these are desperate problems and since the technique adds little morbidity to the already tragic patient, it should be attempted in appropriate situations.

Lymphatics. It is not surprising that, shortly following the introduction and acceptance of lymphangiography as a diagnostic technique, the same route of introduction was employed for a radioactive agent, [198]Au colloid. The procedure requires a meticulous minor surgical feat of cannulating a lymphatic, usually of the foot. Once accomplished (the failure rate of 5%–50% varies with the skill, patience, and tenacity of the operator), either a radiopaque agent, if for diagnostic purposes, or a radionuclide, if for therapeutic, is pressure injected. The radiopaque material ascends and defines the afferent and efferent lymphatic channels and by incorporation into the lymph nodes permits their visualization. It was this incorporation of a colloidal agent that suggested its use for therapeutic purposes. Conceptually, both primary and secondary lymph node involvement could be irradiated *in situ.*

Unfortunately, all that is radioactive gold does not glitter. It was quickly discovered that nodes involved by a disease process do not incorporate, or rather do not incorporate uniformly. It was also noted that extraction of the injected colloid was greater in the first nodal station encountered by the ascending agent and lower with cephalad progress. The consequence of these and additional radiation dosimetry and handling problems have dampened the original enthusiasm. Although some reported success in seminomas and melanomas has been described, the procedure has not been accepted as routine.

nonimaging studies

All of the previous chapters and pages to the contrary (which might have suggested it ain't so) there are important and valuable isotopic procedures other than scanning. From an historic perspective, when the final judgment is rendered it is not inconceivable that the nonimaging studies, such as the radioimmunoassays, may be considered a more important contribution to the grand medical design than

organ imaging. These modalities, in general, measure functions or body components. They can be roughly classified as *in vivo* (those in which a tracer must be administered) and *in vitro.* *In vivo* techniques are used to measure blood volume, GI bleeding losses, GI protein losses, vitamin B_{12} malabsorption (Schilling test), and ferrokinetics. *In vitro* procedures consist of thyroid studies and immunoassays. Detailed methodology will not be discussed. General concepts of indications and anticipations with orders of merit are more appropriate to our purposes.

Blood Volume. The two components that equal blood volume, *i.e.,* the red cell mass and plasma volume, can each be individually measured and added together to obtain a true volume, but in practice this is rarely done. As a rule, the plasma volume is determined since it is the easier and faster of the two techniques. If corrections are applied to the peripheral hematocrit value to have it more closely reflect a central hematocrit, then a reasonable approximation of red cell mass can be obtained. However, if the definitive red cell mass value is critical, as in differential problems of primary versus secondary polycythemia, then it should be calculated directly.

When plasma volume is determined, either ^{131}I or ^{125}I as serum albumin is injected directly into the patient and following a 10- to 20-min mixing time, blood samples are obtained and their activity compared to the activity of the initial dose. The difference represents the dilution factor or the volume. A simple analogy is dropping a few drops of ink into a bathtub. The resultant color will be porportionate to the amount of water in the tub—deeper with a smaller volume, paler with a greater.

When red cell mass is measured directly, ^{51}Cr is tagged to the patient's own cells by an *in vitro* method (similar to that described in chapter 2, but the cells in this study are not damaged), reinjected, and then sampled.

Blood volume determinations by either technique, can, when care is exercised, be most accurate. The study has failed to gain total acceptance because errors of performance are common and the resultant values bizarre. The most common problem is dose infiltration. Often the patient requiring the determination is in a state of vascular collapse. Veins are difficult to cannulate and a resultant tap is less than optimal. Since the injection volume is small, 1–10 cc, and this volume is compared to the patient's 2000–4000 cc, even a minute infiltration loss can build a mighty error. Often to avoid this problem the uninitiated will inject the tracer into infusion tubing already in use. Unfortunately, albumin will bind to the rubber or plastic to some variable degree, and this again results in error. However, assuming scrupulous technique and faultless calculations, what do the obtained numbers mean? What is normal for that particular patient? Standard tables of expected normal volume based on sex, height, and weight can be consulted, but the values of one investigator do not agree with the values of another, which is why there are so many different tables. Assuming that the correct table is chosen, none build in such clinical problems as congestive failure with edema, cirrhosis with ascites, or recent weight loss.

In elective situations when blood volume may become a necessary determination, *i.e.,* prior to extensive surgery, particularly in the elderly, it is recommended that baseline determinations be made. Subsequent studies can then be compared against the patient himself. When this is not clinically possible and the first determination is evaluated against a standard, subsequent serial studies can still be equated against the previous and a sensitive monitor is thus available.

When all of the above are appreciated and technical performance is scrupulous, the study has definite merit.

GI Bleeding. Evidence and detection of GI blood loss is obtained without too much difficulty by routine chemical techniques. These techniques, unfortunately, cannot quantitate the volume of loss, but merely establish its existence. Determination of the amount can be done isotopically.

The procedure again is initiated by labeling the patient's red blood cells with ^{51}Cr, reinjecting, and then collecting all of the stools for at least 72–96 hours. The volume of ^{51}Cr-tagged erythrocytes in this collection can be determined down to the cubic centimeter.

There is no question that the information is obtainable. The only question is why? Having established the presence of blood loss and grossly estimated its category, *e.g.,* trace, moderate, massive, few clinicians seem to care whether the volume is 11 or 63 cc. No technique that has a stool collection, and particularly one requiring care that there be no urinary contami-

nation, can be considered noninvasive either to the patient or technologist. So when push comes to shove if the volumetric data is essential, the study should be performed and is valuable, but when the question is simply is there or ain't there blood, use chemical indicators.

GI Protein Loss. Confirmation and even quantitation of GI protein loss can be performed in a fashion similar to the blood loss determination. For this evaluation ^{51}Cr albumin is currently considered the best of a not too perfect group of nuclides.

There are close to 100 established etiologies for protein-losing enteropathies. It has become evident that the abnormal loss of serum proteins into the GI tract is not uncommon. Usually, GI disease can be identified by the diagnostic techniques for these disorders and the hypoproteinemia is then explained. However, situations do exist in which there is hypoproteinemia without liver or obvious GI disease. Proof that the loss is from the digestive tract then becomes clinically significant. In these situations the study is indicated and valuable.

Schilling Test. The existence of B_{12} malabsorption can be determined with accuracy, and if present, its etiology can be identified. The ingested vitamin combines with a glycoprotein, intrinsic factor, in the stomach whence it is elaborated, transported to the ileum, and there absorbed. Aberrations either in the stomach, small bowel, or—occasionally—the pancreas can result in malabsorption. The determination is usually initiated when pernicious anemia is suspected.

Vitamin B_{12} can be tagged with an isotope of cobalt (^{57}Co, ^{58}Co, ^{60}Co). Following ingestion and absorption, 6% plus will normally be excreted in the urine if there has not been unusual storage in the liver. The latter contingency is obviated by administering an IM dose of cold B_{12} which acts to saturate the liver and flush the excretion of the tagged material. If the 24-hour urine collection (occasionally carried to 48) yields the anticipated amount, the test is normal and is terminated. If, however, the yield is low, malabsorption does exist, but its etiology is still unknown. The determination is then repeated, but now intrinsic factor is also given. If the urinary B_{12} volume is increased to normal levels, the original malabsorption can be attributed to a deficiency of intrinsic factor and the mechanism of this deficiency at the gastric level identified. If the addition of intrinsic factor does not improve the excretion, the malabsorption is a function of small bowel, usually ileal, dysfunction. However, small bowel etiologies are frequently (as high as 40%) associated with concurrent intrinsic factor defects. Thus when part II of the Schilling determination is still abnormal, *i.e.,* no improvement with intrinsic factor, some recommend a part III, which is a determination for intrinsic factor. (Determination of intrinsic factor levels is not an isotopic technique.) The malabsorption can then be characterized as purely small bowel or small bowel plus intrinsic factor deficiency.

Numerous modifications of this basic determination exist. Some include blood sampling. However, all are predicated on the above-described principles. The determination is reasonably simple to perform, although occasionally an indwelling catheter through the 24-hour period is required to ensure an accurate urine collection. It is a good and useful technique.

Ferrokinetics. It is possible to study the disappearance rate of iron from the plasma and its subsequent incorporation into maturing red blood cells in the marrow. Iron 59 is the nuclide employed. However, the simple plotting of plasma iron clearance (PIC) or the graphing of ascending levels of iron incorporation into the marrow (usually estimated over the sacrum) is not true ferrokinetics. True kinetic studies are highly complex research-oriented procedures that are rarely done in the average clinical laboratory.

Thyroid. The *in vitro* thyroid studies are described in chapter 7.

Immunoassays. The conceptualization and ultimate methodology that permit the labeling of antibodies with a radioactive nuclide ranks high on the All Time All Time Nuclear Medicine Man Super Star Achievement Charts (or for simplification A.T.A.T.N.M.M.S.S.A.C.). It is not inconceivable that at some time in the future when isotopic organ imaging has been replaced by other modalities, perhaps ultrasonics (?), perhaps computerized radiation absorption modalities (?), perhaps (?), the immunoassay laboratories will still remain to remind us that once there was a nuclear Camelot.

The exact number of possible determinations is indeterminable. It changes almost minute by minute. All of the evaluations are similarly structured. The methodology varies only to accommodate the characteristics of the particular substance being evaluated. Hormones, vitamins, innumerable biologic materials, and pharmaceuticals are being measured by "simple" antibody–antigen reactions.

This "simple" reaction deserves some simple generalizations. Assays are predicated on the assumption that when antigens are in a system with their own antibodies, binding of antigen to antibody to form complexes will occur to the extent of available antibody-binding sites. If the amount of antibody in the system and the amount of antigen are both known, the complex formation is equally predictable. So, if a measuring device is established to monitor this reaction, quantitation is possible.

Antiserum is elaborated in a test animal to an antigen later to be quantitated. A radioactive label is then applied to that antigen, usually ^{125}I or ^{131}I for most clinical situations. A known quantity of labeled antigen is then mixed with a known volume of the patient's serum containing an unknown quantity of antigen (unlabeled); this mixture in turn is incubated in a known amount of antiserum. The labeled and unlabeled antigen will compete for the existing binding sites on the antibodies. The amount of labeled antigen binding is a function of the amount of existing unlabeled antigen in the system. Once the reaction has occurred, the bound (labeled) antigen–antibody complex can be separated from the unbound or free (labeled) antigen and a bound to free ratio (B:F) computed. If standards have previously been prepared in which the same reaction is calculated against various known quantities of added antigen, the B:F curves will identify the amount of "unknown" antigen that had to exist to result in the obtained ratio. Orders of magnitude down to 10^{-12} moles/liter have been derived by this system.

The adjective "simple" used to describe the methodology was directed to the concept, not the performance. The techniques demand scrupulous skill and attention by the technologist, and it is desirable that the supervision be by one with the advantage of a laboratory background. More often than not the clinical nuclear person who over the years has clogged all or most synaptic junctions with matters imaging is both ill equipped and ill disposed to gear up and accept responsibility for a sophisticated radioimmunoassay laboratory. So, it may be logical and expedient in many departments to separate the nuclear services, with the immunoassay determinations becoming the domain of the department of laboratories. But this debate and decision is hardly germane to our discussion, and it is added only as a possible insight as to why the general acceptance and utilization of this most valuable modality is dragging. Although such a lag is often common prior to major innovations, it is to be anticipated that radio-immunoassay techniques will become an indispensable laboratory service.

Already the list of quantifiable hormones and nonhormonal substances is formidable and sounds a rousing testimonial to the genius and tenacity of the investigators. Although almost meaningless in such an ever-changing, ever-expanding area, a small catalogue sampling is listed just to identify the scope of what can be measured: cortisone, testosterone, triiodo-thyronine, insulin, growth hormone, TSH, calcitonin, digoxin, morphine, Australia antigen, and many, many more!

Etc.

pancreas

Some people, ideas, and things have the capacity to stir the emotions so that there is no middle ground or position. One loves—or hates: *e.g.,* Richard Nixon, Mao Tse-tung, cold showers, olives, halvah. So it is, too, with pancreas imaging. Either one is for it or "agin" it! Why? Considering the severe paucity of reliable and sensitive diagnostic techniques for identifying early pancreatic disease and considering, too, the horrendous 5% 5-year survival rate in these malignancies, any technique that improves detection should come on like "gang busters." The ability to image the pancreas has been available for more than a dozen years, it still has not been universally accepted as a reliable technique. Why?

The pancreas, as part of its exocrine function elaborates and secretes certain proteins essential to the hydrolysis of certain food materials. Methionine is one amino acid utilized in the enzymatic synthesis. Methionine contains a sulfur radical which under proper conditions and coaxing can be replaced by a radioactive isotope of selenium (^{75}Se). Thus, a radiopharmaceutical is available which has eyes for the pancreas.

Unfortunately, the pancreas is not the only organ that "trips" on the amino acid. The liver,

too, is "strung out" and clears it with equal affinity. Since the liver weighs approximately 10 times more and is so much larger, almost 4 times as much tracer is concentrated in it than the pancreas. Only 6%–10% of the administered dose appears in the pancreas. The remainder, in addition to the liver localization is distributed in the plasma, GI tract, and kidneys. Innumerable ingenious methods have been devised in attempts to increase pancreatic uptake both actually and relative to the liver. These techniques can be categorized as physiologic and technologic. Physiologic efforts have centered on measures to increase methionine uptake by the pancreas at the front end and delay its discharge at the back. Numerous dietary protocols have been designed to stimulate methionine dumping so that uptake of the subsequently introduced tagged amino acid by the depleted organ will be increased. Morphine and propantheline bromide (Pro-banthine) have each been utilized to constrict the sphincter of Oddi and thus impede excretion. Additionally, efforts have been expended to block uptake by the liver. None of these has, to date, proven of particular value. A recent report utilizing both bethanecol and pancreozymin offers promise of a positive enhancement modality but this too must be measured by the rigors of clinical trial.

Fig. 8-1. Pancreas
Diagnosis: Normal pancreas
A. The "pistol-shaped" band of activity is clearly separated from the activity in the liver bed. There is a slight decrease in the intensity at the site of aortic crossing (arrow). Normal image
B. The head of the pancreas is inseparable from the liver but is probably definable. Normal image
Diagnosis: Carcinoma of the body of the pancreas.
C. The single arrow identifies the head of the pancreas. The double arrow identifies a possible defect in the proximal portion of the body.
(Courtesy of G. Jackson, Harrisburg Hospital, Harrisburg, Pa.)

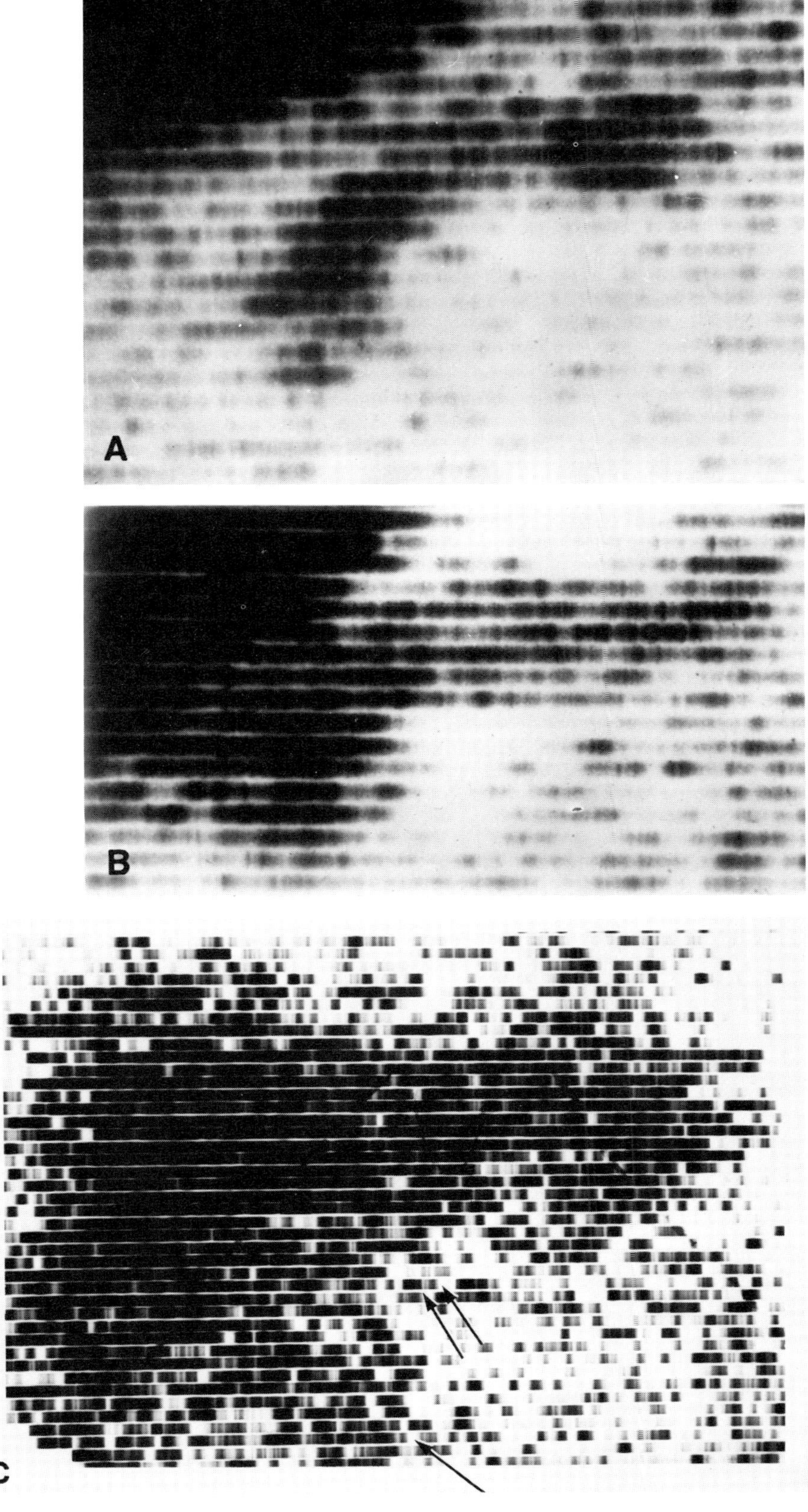

A
B
C

Technologic attack has ranged from a simplistic lead blocking of the liver to a sophisticated dual electronic scanning system that permits the subtraction of the liver image, leaving only the pancreas. At this time, too few instruments possess this dual scanning ability to permit its consideration as a routine technique. Obtaining serial 10-min images with the gamma camera through 1 hour after dose injection has become the recommended technique of many. But none of these methods is routinely or consistently satisfactory.

All of the above contribute to answer the question why. The pancreas can be imaged, but only sometimes (Fig. 8-1). Different series report different success and failure figures, but too many identify a false positive range of 20%– 30%. False positive is defined as those cases in which no pancreatic image is obtained but no pancreatic disease exists. Failure of the organ to image is the signature of pathology, thus, when a high percentage of "normals" behaves like "abnormals" an unacceptable or unreliable label is applied.

Advocates of the study suggest that the high failure rate can be attributed in large measure to less than careful physician attention and patient selection. Pancreatic response, they state, is dependent on a combination of conditions including the pH of the upper GI tract, vagal innervation, and the state of nutrition. Failure to screen patients who may be suffering from inflammatory conditions (*e.g.,* peptic ulcer or infiltrative gastric mucosa), patients with ante- cedent gastrectomy with or without vagotomy, patients receiving drugs that may affect intestinal motility or acid secretion, all help to explain the high failure rate in imaging. Thus, if proper selection were utilized, the false positive rate would fall into acceptable limits.

Additionally, and perhaps crucial to their argument, is that when the organ is positively imaged and interpreted as "within normal limits" the probability of undetected pathology is negligible or nonexistent. Thus, the false negative yield is almost zero. When the differen- tial diagnosis includes pancreatitis or carcinoma and the scan is negative, *i.e.,* there is a normal image, these diseases have been ruled out.

And, as a parting shot—"what else is there for early detection or screening. The yield from x ray and the laboratory is poor even in advanced diseases." The anti's respond "exple- tive deleted!" Any procedure which has as inordinately high a false positive yield as this technique is unreliable, unacceptable, and must be consigned to an experimental position. The figure of false positive becomes even higher if less than optimal imaging is added to the nonvisualized group. Less than optimal refers to those cases in which the organ is identified, but the interpreter is not certain as to its integrity. Often this is due to the adjacent and overlapping liver activity or the pressure produced by the aorta crossing the midportion of the body. The percentage of absolutely normal may then be hardly more than 50%. Thus, whereas the positive 50% can be excluded from the differential, the other group must be considered as potentially positive.

We stand with our feet planted solidly in mid-air on this one. If there were anywhere else to go, we would absolutely agree that the existing study is a "no-no." But there isn't. Celiac and superior mesenteric angiography hardly represent the routine, simple, noninvasive screening technique so desperately needed. Duodenal endoscopy with pancreatic ductal catheterization and opacification requires skill possessed by a rare few, and successful diagno- sis is even rarer. The technique has a high failure rate and significant patient morbidity, but perhaps time and experience will improve its potential. Again, ultrasonics may be considered as a possible answer. But, again, there are too little data as yet to know whether or not sonography will fill the breach. So, we conclude, if everyone knows the serious limitations of pancreatic imaging and will accept a positive study, *i.e.,* one in which the organ is not visualized or poorly identified as only possibly positive, then we feel the procedure has value because the negative study (regardless of how few of them there may be) is sufficiently reliable to improve the diagnostic deliberation.

tumor-scanning agents

The ancient alchemists sought the philosophers' stone which would change base metals into gold. The modern radiopharmacologist seeks the philosophers' nuclide which will localize only in malignant tissue. They are close, but still no cigars.

Serendipity probably was the first robin of the spring. Early on in the nuclear game the keen observers realized that certain nuclides had a higher affinity than others for tumor localization.

First ^{203}Hg and then ^{197}Hg were examined for this tumor localization potential and found wanting. Soft tissue tumor localization was found to be a property of ^{99m}Tc polyphosphate, ^{87}Sr and ^{111}In, but none of these had sufficient specificity to be considered a reliable agent.

Later, ^{67}Ga citrate while being investigated as a bone-scanning radionuclide was observed to have tumor-localizing potential. Unquestionably, the urgent need for such an agent explains the subsequent events. Few nuclides receive the public relations treatment given this material. Even the hospital orderlies sing the litany "when in doubt get the gallium out." Unfortunately, it was not, and is not, the answer. Yes, ^{67}Ga citrate will localize in neoplastic tissue, but it will also localize in inflammatory tissue with equal or greater avidity. It has even been identified in an acute cerebral infarct. Therefore, except in special situations it is hardly the sought after tumor specific. Its mode of localization is still uncertain, but in malignant cells its concentration appears highest in the lysosomes whereas in inflammatory tissue it is distributed in the neutrophilic leukocytes. Experience has also shown sensitivity to be low in adenocarcinoma. Thus another hope was dashed. Gallium is neither tumor specific nor uniformly sensitive to all tumor types. Additionally, it clears slowly from the blood and is excreted primarily through the GI tract (renal excretion does occur in the first 24 hours) so that rigorous bowel cleansing is essential when the abdomen is to be imaged. Imaging is optimally performed 48–72 hours after the dose (another potential hassle with the Utilization Committee).

But, there are definite pluses to be obtained, albeit they are nonspecific and unpredictable. An occasional occult neoplasm will be identified, particularly when imaging lesions of bronchogenic origin (see Fig. 6-16).

Positive uptake has also been identified in adjacent mediastinal nodes later found to be metastatic. This finding may prove to be of future value as a staging modality. Numerous independent studies agree that an 85% accuracy rate can be anticipated in bronchogenic carcinoma.

Melanomas, anaplastic thyroid carcinoma, and certain malignancies of the stomach have all been found with high sensitivity. On the other hand, ^{67}Ga citrate imaging in adenocarcinoma lesions offers a low correlative yield.

Its value in lymphoma staging is undergoing extensive investigation. A consortium of coopering universities is pooling their data. In patients with untreated Hodgkin's disease the scans correctly recognized 90% of the cases. Best results were found where the involvement was in the neck or thorax. When only abdominal disease was present, detection dropped to approximately 50%. The data that proved most disturbing was that although the scan could correctly identify a patient with nodal disease, when the particular scan lesion was subjected to histologic analysis only a 70% correlation existed. Therefore, opinion is still unsettled as to the value of scanning as a staging yardstick.

The same group reporting initial findings in patients with untreated malignant lymphoma identified an overall 78% positive yield. They concluded that although a positive examination almost always signifies disease, a negative study does not exclude it.

The indications for gallium-imaging in focal lesions of the liver has been discussed in chapter 2, where an example (Fig. 2-9) of incorporation in a malignant process was cited. Uptake can also occur in inflammatory defects (Fig. 8-2).

The known sensitivity for localization in inflammatory tissue is being explored. The search for the possible postoperative abdominal abscess is being aided and abetted by gallium. One series reported that 19 of 28 patients strongly suspected of harboring a postsurgical abscess had positive gallium localization. Of these 15 were reoperated and an abscess was found in all. Maximum uptake was found in the abscess wall, but activity was also present in the supernatant and pus cells.

A very small reported series suggests that acute cholecystitis can be diagnosed in symptomatic patients with nonvisualized gall bladders on conventional x ray since these gall bladders demonstrate increased radioactive localization. Also being touted is a technique to identify pyelonephritis. Normally, all injected ^{67}Ga citrate is cleared by the kidneys within 24 hours. Retention, and thus positive renal imaging beyond 24 hours has been proven in a series of cases to be due to pyelonephritis.

Another, and perhaps more promising, avenue of investigation has been to label available chemotherapeutic compounds. Bleomycin, labeled with ^{111}In, ^{57}Co, or ^{67}Ga is currently receiving the most attention. Although, it is still

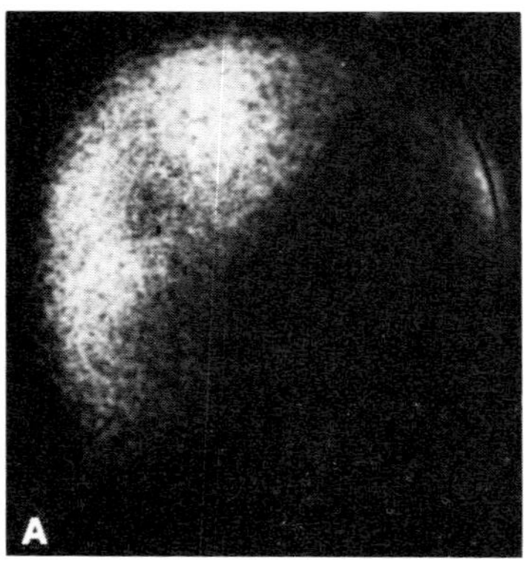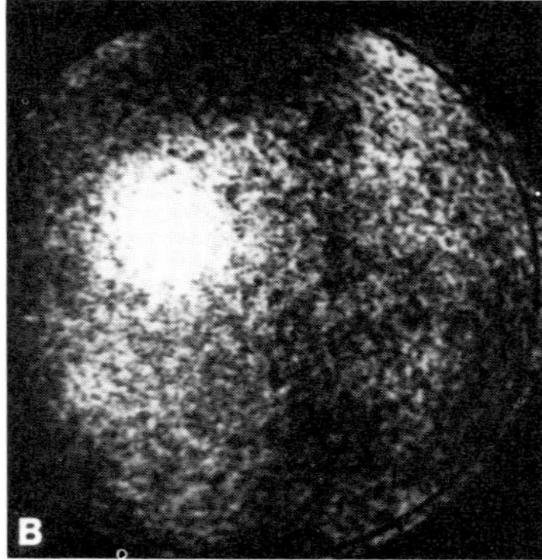

Fig. 8-2. Gallium
Diagnosis: Liver abscess
A. Scan, posterior view, ^{99m}Tc sulfur colloid. Liver scan identifies a prominent focal defect.
B. Scan, posterior view, ^{67}Ga citrate. Liver scan 72 hours following **A** identifies trapping activity of the previous site of defect.

too early to be certain, certain findings have appeared early. The first, and most critical for the search is that the agent is not tumor specific —it will localize equally in inflammatory tissue. It appears, at least to some investigators, that the ^{57}Co tag is the superior and that as a choice between it and ^{67}Ga citrate, the bleomycin is a better seeker. Additionally, scanning can be done 6 hours after injection since there is more-rapid blood clearance and no bowel prep is needed since it behaves like a metal chelate and is excreted by the kidneys.

And still another promising avenue of investigation is in the tagging of antibodies of tumor antigens. It is hoped that the antigen will capture and localize the antibody. This has been done with carcinoembryonic antibody (CEA), produced by the CEA antigen found to be present in human colonic tumors, which was tagged with ^{131}I. The tumor localization with this approach exceeded that of all other agents utilized, ^{111}In bleomycin, ^{67}Ga, and ^{111}In chloride, in a group of patients with colon carcinoma.

This approach is as yet too new to permit judgment. But unlike the alchemist who never did find the magic it would seem most realistic that our magic bullet will be discovered in the very near future.

synovial membrane–joint scanning

It has been noted that both ^{131}I and ^{99m}Tc compounds localize in joints suffering with synovial inflammation in far higher concentrations than in uninflamed joints. Synovitis from any etiology will invoke a "hot joint" (Fig. 8-3). Thus another diagnostic technique becomes

available to evaluate these areas. The positive scan occurs only because of synovial change. If there is no synovitis with resultant increased membrane permeability and increased vascularity, the study will be normal. Osseous and cartilagenous components are not evaluated.

The proponents of the study suggest that early disease is more readily detected and is more sensitive than either physical or x ray examination. They also suggest that pain in the region of joints may be differentiated as to the presence or absence of synovial infection and the effects of therapy may be monitored more objectively. Occasionally the pattern of distribution may help in the differential diagnosis of the type of arthritis, *e.g.*, positive uptake in the region of the Achilles tendon insertion and the sole of the foot may distinguish Reiter's disease from rheumatoid arthritis—but this is the exception, not the rule. The type and extent of arthritis is not being evaluated, only the presence or absence of synovial inflammation.

lymphangiography

Lymphangiography by isotope techniques must be distinguished from lymph node scanning. The latter can be accomplished with the tumor-seeking nuclides when there is primary or secondary involvement (sometimes, as these agents are not specific for the lymphatics). Isotopic lymphangiography is a technique analogous to contrast lymphangiography and is specific for the system. The radionuclide, usually ^{198}Au or sometimes ^{99m}Tc sulfur colloid, is injected subcutaneously, usually in the webbed space between the toes; it enters the

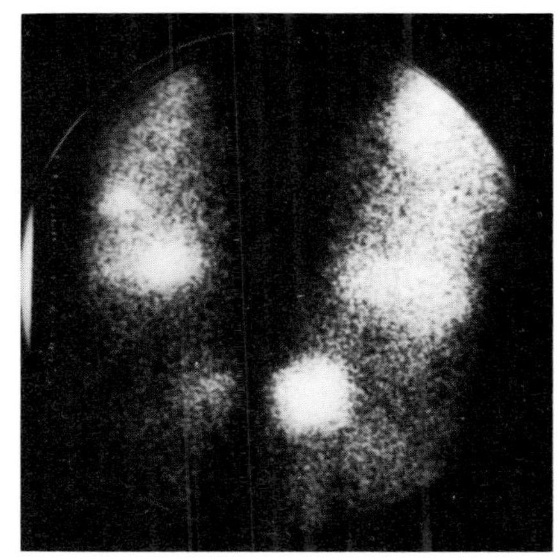

Fig. 8-3. Synovial membrane. Diagnosis: Degenerative arthritis with acute synovitis. There is marked increase of uptake in the region of the metatarsophalangeal joint. X rays revealed only a mild hallux valgus deformity and degenerative arthritis, with similar changes in the right. The patient complained of acute pain in the left great toe.

lymphatic channels and is transported through the system. Scanning will identify the pathway and the nodal stations.

In concept isotopic lymphangiography presents many attractive alternatives to the tedious contrast study. The latter is attended with the necessity of identifying a lymphatic, cannulating it, and then injecting an iodinated opaque agent. Since the average peripheral lymphatic vessel approximates the diameter of a gnat's penis, cutdown techniques are required and injection must be performed under pressure. The time of needle placement may vary from minutes to hours and—when successful—the opaque instillation time adds another hour. Added to this is the occasional patient who is allergic to the medium and who has pulmonary embarrassment secondary to the eventual microembolization of the oily opaque in the lungs. There are many radiologists who define happiness as "a day without a lymphangiogram."

When the isotopic procedure is elected, only the subcutaneous instillation is required. There is no patient morbidity, no extended procedure time, no allergy, and no oil emboli. Unfortunately, too often, there is also no diagnostic picture. Obviously, if the isotopic study were equivalent to the contrast, there would be no discussion as to choice, but the incidence of technical failure, false positive, and false negative results is high, and for this reason the procedure has not achieved universal acceptance. However, those who advocate its use assert that experience both diminishes the technical failure to negligible figures and sophisticates the diagnostic accuracy to acceptable levels. They do not recommend an either—or approach, but one of complemen-

tary studies. When the isotopic procedure is unequivocally negative, the contrast study need not be done. When, on the other hand, the imaging is either questionable or positive, then the more-definitive contrast modality is added. Additionally, once a baseline image is obtained, sequential monitoring to evaluate response to therapy is accomplished more easily than the second-and-third look contrast studies.

The arguments are difficult to refute, and the technique deserves greater attention (Fig. 8-4).

etc.

marrow scanning

The distribution of active marrow sites can be imaged with radioactive colloids. The existence of expansion or contraction or even depletion of these sites is detectable. Following the IV introduction of a radioactive colloid, ^{99m}Tc sulfur colloid is the most commonly used, the axial and appendicular skeleton is imaged and the active trapping marrow space plotted. Normally only the axial structures will be active. When as in the chronic leukemias, polycythemias, and hemolytic anemias, cellular proliferation results in an expansion of the red marrow, activity is also found in the appendicular structures. Conceivably, the degree of expansion correlates with the severity of the pathologic process (Fig. 8-5). Conversely, myelofibrosis, certain metastatic diseases, and certain stages of leukemia will result in patterns of depletion. Focal depletion may also be identified in osteomyelitis, sickle cell disease, and meta-stasis.

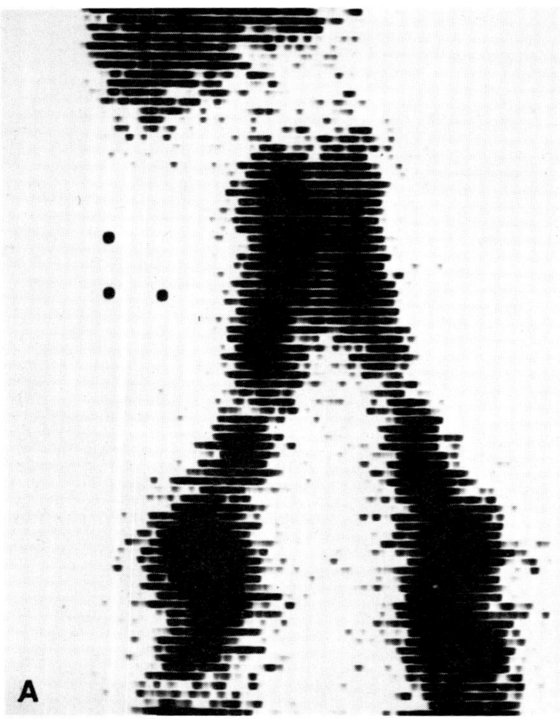

Fig. 8-4. Lymph scan
Diagnosis: Normal lymph scan
A. Scan, [198]Au. Distribution of activity assumes an inverted "Y" shape. The limbs represent trappings in the iliofemoral and iliac nodes; the stem represents trapping in the paraaortic group. The activity in the upper right hand corner is the liver.
Diagnosis: False positive lymph scans in Ewing's sarcoma
B. Scan, [198]Au. Gross ballooning of the iliac group, irregular activity in the paraaortic, and diminished liver uptake. The findings suggest an incomplete obstructive process in the paraaortic nodes. The patient had a known Ewing's sarcoma of the right femur. The scan suggested metastatic nodal invasion, which is probably incorrect since the patient is still alive six plus years after diagnosis and therapy.
(Courtesy of R. Wallner, Hahnemann Medical College, Philadelphia, Pa.)

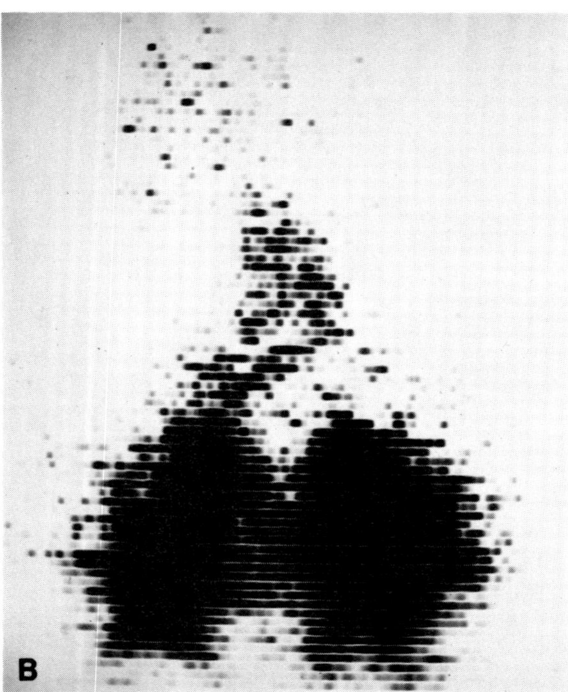

But after doing all that is required to bring about these chartings and mappings, the big and embarrassing question is "so what?" Rarely does marrow scanning discover what is not already known, nor does it even, as a rule, modify the program of management. So at this time it remains in limbo. Just as the mountain climber must scale a peak because it is there, the scanner must image whatever he or she can. Perhaps the future will bring other nuclides or instrumentation, or both, that will be productive of data to warrant the routine use of this technique.

parathyroid

Primary hyperparathyroidism is usually caused by an adenoma of the gland. But which gland and in what location is frequently unknown preoperatively. It has been reported that even at surgery as many as 20% of cases go undetected. Ectopic mediastinal localization is not rare. And so, like the instructions to the Mission Impossible Team: "your assignment is to develop a procedure which will reliably image the parathyroid and confirm or deny the existence of an adenoma(s) and its location." (The mission proved almost impossible—but not quite.)

Fig. 8-5. Marrow. Diagnosis: Myelogenous leukemia
    A. Scan. Liver–spleen image employing 99mTc sulfur colloid in a patient with myelogenous leukemia. The spleen is particularly enlarged.
B and C. Scan. The same patient 2 years later. (Splenectomy because of spontaneous rupture has been necessary since the original study.) 99mTc sulfur colloid is again employed, revealing gross hepatomegaly and no splenic uptake. Activity is prominent in the lungs but diminished in the axial skeleton. Increased trapping is, however, noted in the appendicular structures of the tibia and feet.

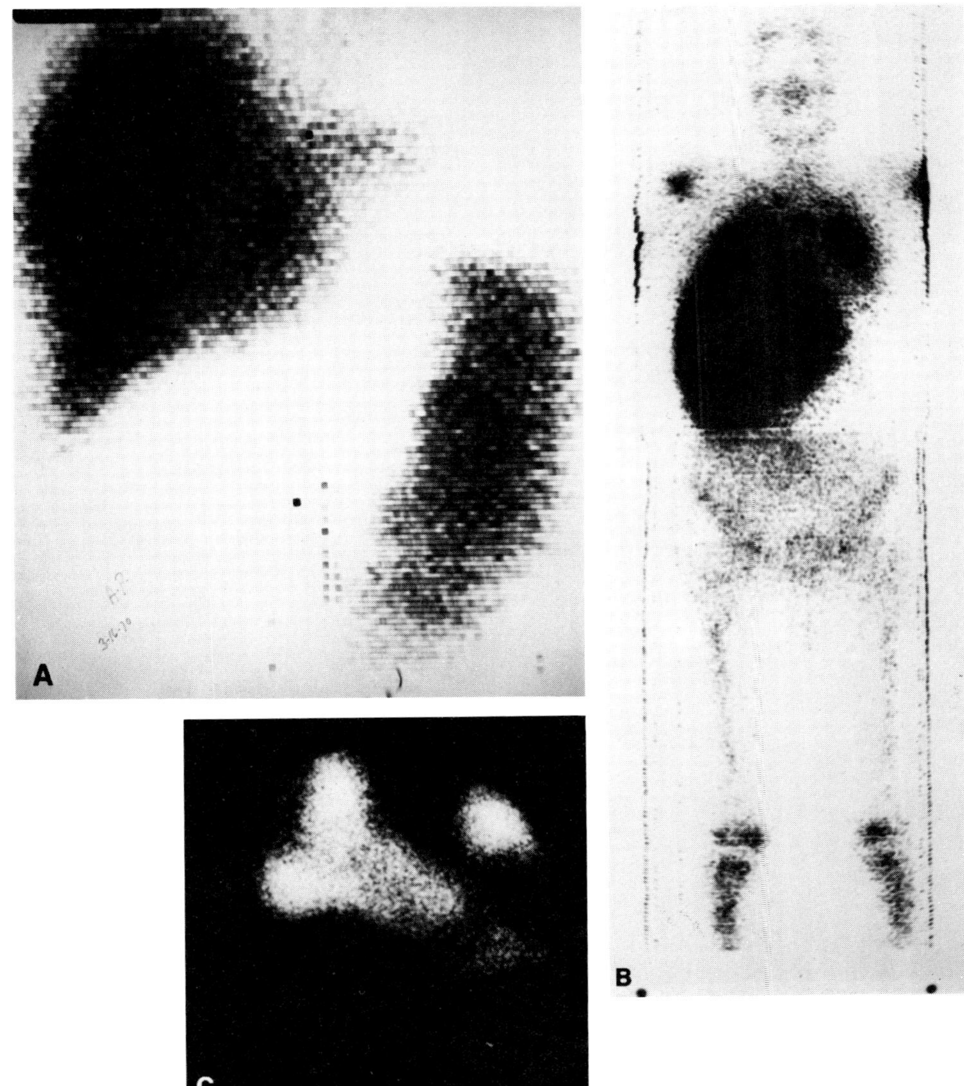

Parathyroid imaging has been accomplished using selenomethionine [75]Se. The rationale is similar to that behind the use of this nuclide in pancreatic imaging, *i.e.*, the parathyroid proteins also contain methionine. The procedure, unfortunately, has not attained the reliability necessary to consider it as a routine study. Diagnostic accuracy is below acceptable standards, but the team has never failed in the past and it will only be a matter of time until the right combination is identified.

salivary glands

The diagnostic armamentarium for salivary glandular disturbances is less than super. Cytology has been notoriously disappointing, biopsy may be contraindicated and function studies of little value except in advanced disease states. X ray (sialography) offers the best attack. Except for those obvious problems caused by an opaque calculus, direct ductal cannulization and instillation of an opaque medium is necessary. The examination may be technically difficult to obtain and often induces patient discomfort.

It is known that since radioiodine and ^{99m}Tc as pertechnetate localize in the salivary glands, scanning is possible (Fig. 8-6). Those who have

studied the potentials of the technique offer mixed reviews. Although simple to do and noninvasive, all lesions are cold except for Warthin's tumor, which may hyperconcentrate the nuclide. Since, as of now, the study merely provides a nonspecific result to complement the already palpably established existence of a lesion, it does not win a Go.

adrenal imaging

Unlike some of the other topics in this section adrenal imaging carries promise of moving out of the little "etc." and into the big time of Routine. The jury is still out because experience is still so limited, but there are reports of successful presurgical localization of cortical lesions and ectopic tissue.

Because of duality of function, the cortex and medullary portions must be attacked separately. For each, a precursor necessary to the elaboration of its secretory product is labeled. Cholesterol, a major precursor of adrenocortical steroids, has been successfully tagged with ^{131}I and has proven capable of selective uptake in the cortex. Dopamine, essential in the elaboration of epinephrine has been found experimentally to localize selectively in the adrenal medulla. The laboratory label is [14]C. Unfortunately, this radionuclide is unacceptable for human use. Although its long half-life is economical with reference to shelf life (5570 years), it is a touch long for clinical consideration. Additionally, it is a pure beta emitter, which is useless for external scanning. Thus when a suitable gamma emitter with which to tag dopamine is found, adrenal medullary scanning will also be a realized procedure.

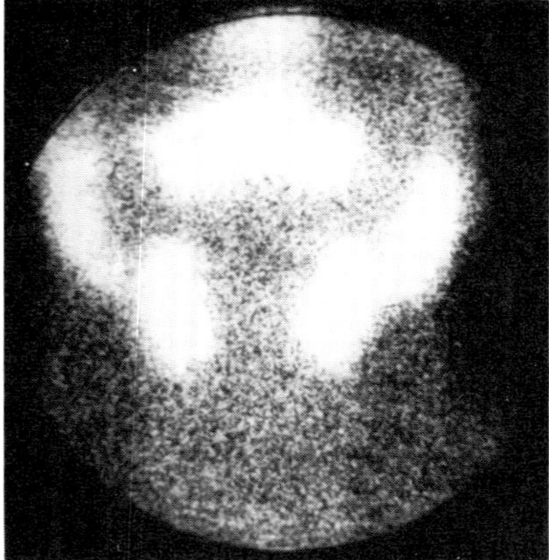

Fig. 8-6. Normal salivary glands. Scan, 30 min following IV injection of 3 mCi [99m]Tc. Salivary glands are visualized. The submaxillary and parotids are bilaterally symmetric. The activity centrally located is nasopharyngeal trapping.

BIBLIOGRAPHY

RADIOTHERAPY

Ariel IM et al.: The intralymphatic administration of radioactive isotopes for treating malignant melanoma. Surg Gynecol Obstet 124:25–39, 1967

Blahd WH: Treatment of malignant disease with radio-colloids. In Blahd WH (ed): Nuclear Medicine. New York, McGraw–Hill, 1971, pp 775–787

Ching TT, Han SY: Intracavitary radiogold therapy, a critical appraisal of its value. Am J Roentgenol Radium Ther Nucl Med 85:62–68, 1961

Dennis JM et al.: Radioactive colloidal gold in the control of malignant effusions: report and analysis of 60 patients. Am J Roentgenol Radium Ther Nucl Med 75:1124–1128, 1956

Hollander L: Treatment of malignant blood diseases with radioactive phosphorus. In Blahd WH (ed): Nuclear Medicine. New York, McGraw–Hill, 1971, pp 760–774

Jaffe HL: Treatment of malignant serous effusions with radioactive colloidal chromic phosphate. Am J Roentgenol Radium Ther Nucl Med 74:657–666, 1955

Muller JH: Curative aim and results of routine intraperitoneal radiocolloid administration in the treatment of ovarian cancer. Am J Roentgenol Radium Ther Nucl Med 89:533–540, 1963

Taylor A Jr et al.: Loculation as a contraindication to intracavitary ^{32}p-chromic phosphate therapy. J Nucl Med 16(4):318–319, 1975

Teates CD, Constable WC: Letter: Intraperitoneal ^{99m}Tc-sulfur colloid distribution. J Nucl Med 15(11):1067–1068, 1974

Tully TE et al.: The use of ^{99m}Tc-sulfur colloid to assess the distribution of ^{32}p-chromic phosphate. J Nucl Med 15(3):190–191, 1974

NONIMAGING TECHNIQUES

Blood Volume
Albert SN: Blood Volume and Extracellular Fluid Volume, 2nd ed. Springfield, Ill, CC Thomas, 1971

Albert SN: Blood volume in clinical practice. In Rothfeld B (ed): Nuclear Medicine in Vitro. Philadelphia, JB Lippincott, 1974, pp 52–68

Gastrointestinal
Berquist TH et al.: Diagnosis of Barrett's esophagus by pertechnetate scintigraphy. Mayo Clin Proc 48:276–279, 1973

Chaudhuri TK: Use of ^{99m}Tc-DTPA for measuring gastric emptying time. J Nucl Med 15(6):391–395, 1974

Chen I-W et al.: ^{14}C-tripalmitin breath test as a diagnostic aid for fat malabsorption due to pancreatic insufficiency. J Nucl Med 15(12):1125–1129, 1974

Czerniak P et al.: Usefulness of radionuclides in evaluation of stomach disorders. Semin Nucl Med 2(3):288–301, 1972

Friedman BI: Radionuclide determination of gastrointestinal blood loss. Semin Nucl Med 2(3):265–269, 1972

Herbert V: Detection of malabsorption of vitamin B_{12} due to gastric or intestinal dysfunction. Semin Nucl Med 2(3):220–234, 1972

Kilpatrick ZM, Aseron CA: Radioisotope detection of Meckel's diverticulum causing acute rectal hemorrhage. N Engl J Med 287:653–654, 1972

Mark R et al.: Diagnosis of an intrathoracic gastrogenic cyst using ^{99m}Tc-pertechnetate. Radiology 109:137–138, 1973

Marsden DS et al.: The use of ^{99m}Tc to detect gastric malignancy. Am J Gastroenterol 59:410–415, 1973

Rosenthall L et al.: Radiopertechnetate imaging of the Meckel's diverticulum. Radiology 105:371–373, 1972

Schwabe AD: Gastrointestinal tract function and disease. In Blahd WH (ed): Nuclear Medicine. New York, McGraw–Hill, 1971, pp 350–366

Waldmann TA: Protein-losing enteropathy and kinetic studies of plasma protein metabolism. Semin Nucl Med 2(3):251–264, 1972

Red Cell Survival
Weinstein IM: Measurement of red cell life span. In Biahd WH (ed): Nuclear Medicine. New York, McGraw–Hill, 1971, pp 426–439

Pernicious Anemia
Schilling RF: Diagnosis of pernicious anemia and other vitamin B_{12} malabsorption syndromes with radioactive vitamin B_{12}. In Blahd WH (ed): Nuclear Medicine. New York, McGraw–Hill, 1971, pp 444–447

Ferrokinetics
Friedman BI: Radionuclide studies associated with abnormalities of iron. In Rothfeld B (ed): Nuclear Medicine in Vitro. Philadelphia, JB Lippincott, 1974, pp 85–95

Weinstein IM: Measurement of iron metabolism and erythropoiesis. In Blahd WH (ed): Nuclear Medicine. New York, McGraw–Hill, 1971, pp 416–423

Immunoassay
Goldsmith SJ: Basic principles of competitive radioassay. In Rothfeld B (ed): Nuclear Medicine in Vitro. Philadelphia, JB Lippincott, 1974, pp 96–119

Goldsmith SJ: Radioimmunoassay: review of basic principles. Semin Nucl Med 5(2):125–152, 1975

Hollander CS, Shenkman L: Radioimmunoassays for triiodothyronine and thyroxine. In Rothfeld B (ed): Nuclear Medicine in Vitro. Philadelphia, JB Lippincott, 1974, pp 136–149

PANCREAS

Agnew JE et al.: The false–positive pancreas scan: does it reflect "low–normal" pancreatic function? J Nucl Med 15(2):90–93, 1974

Bachrach WH et al.: Pancreatic scanning: a review. Gastroenterology 63: 890–910, 1972

Chandra S, Prezio JA: Successful modification for pancreatic imaging. J Nucl Med 15(11):935–937, 1974

Cho KJ, Doust BD: Experimental suppression of hepatic uptake of ^{75}Se-selenomethionine. J Nucl Med 15(12):1171–1173, 1974

Cottrall MF et al.: Investigations of ^{18}F-fluorophenylalanine for pancreas scanning. Br J Radiol 46:277–288, 1973

Haynie TP: The pancreas. In Freeman LM, Johnson PM (eds): Clinical Scintillation Scanning. New York, Harper & Row, 1969, pp 384–396

Mattar AG, Laor Y: Improvement of pancreatic imaging. J Nucl Med 15(8):707–708, 1974

Miale A Jr et al.: Pancreas scanning after ten years. Semin Nucl Med 2(3):201–219, 1972

Spencer RP: The role of radionuclides in the evaluation of pancreatic blood flow, size, and exocrine function. Semin Nucl Med 2(3):191–200, 1972

Steven LW et al.: Experience with radioisotope scanning of pancreas. Med J Aust 2:867–873, 1972

Webber MM et al.: Pitfalls in ultrasonic diagnosis of pseudocysts of pancreas (abstr). J Nucl Med 15(6):543, 1974

Winston MA et al.: Enhancement of pancreatic concentration of ^{75}Se-selenomethionine. J Nucl Med 15(8):662–665, 1974

Tumor-scanning Agents

Chaudhuri TK et al. Tumor uptake of ^{99m}Tc-polyphosphate: its similarity with [87m]Sr citrate and dissimilarity with ^{67}Ga-citrate. J Nucl Med 15(6):458–459, 1974

Deland FH et al: ^{67}Ga-citrate imaging in untreated primary lung cancer: preliminary report of cooperative group. J Nucl Med 15(6):408–411, 1974

Eckelman WC et al.: Early detection of mammary carcinoma with radiolabeled bleomycin (abstr). J Nucl Med 15(6):489, 1974

Frankel RS et al.: Renal localization of gallium-67 citrate (abstr). J Nucl Med 15(6):491, 1974

Fratkin MJ et al.: Ga-67 localization of postoperative abdominal abscesses (abstr). J Nucl Med 15(6):491, 1974

Greenlaw RH et al.: ^{67}Ga-citrate imaging in untreated malignant lymphoma: preliminary report of cooperating group. J Nucl Med 15(6): 404–407, 1974

Grove RB et al.: Clinical evaluation of radiolabeled bleomycin (bleo) for tumor detection. J Nucl Med 15(6):386–390, 1974

Hayes RL et al.: A comparison of the tissue distribution of ^{67}Ga and the rare earth radionuclides (abstr). J Nucl Med 15(6):501, 1974

Higasi T et al.: Clinical evaluation of ^{67}Ga-citrate scanning. J Nucl Med 13(3):196–201, 1972

Hoffer PB, Gottschalk A: Tumor scanning agents. Semin Nucl Med 4(3):305–316, 1974

Hoffer PB et al.: Use of ^{131}I-CEA antibody as a tumor scanning agent. J Nucl Med 15(5):323–327, 1974

Johnston G et al.: ^{67}Ga-citrate imaging in untreated Hodgkin's disease: preliminary report of cooperative group. J Nucl Med 15(6):399–403, 1974

Kaplan WD et al.: ^{67}Ga-citrate and the non-functioning thyroid nodule. J Nucl Med 15(6):424–427, 1974

Kinoshita F et al.: Scintiscanning of pulmonary diseases with ^{67}Ga-citrate. J Nucl Med 15(4):227–233, 1974

Langhammer H et al.: [67]Ga for tumor scanning. J Nucl Med 13(1):25–30, 1972

Rao DV et al.: Erbium-165: a possible tumor-localizing agent with ideal imaging properties (abstr). J Nucl Med 15(6):526, 1974

Wallner RJ et al.: [67]Ga localization in acute cerebral infarction. J Nucl Med 15(4):308–309, 1974

Waxman AD et al.: Gallium scanning of the gall bladder (abstr). J Nucl Med 15(6):543, 1974

Yea E–L: Extraosseous tumor uptake of [85]Sr and [67]Ga. J Nucl Med 15(5): 361–362, 1974

Synovial Membrane–Joint Scanning

Desaulniers M et al.: Radiotechnetium polyphosphate joint imaging. J Nucl Med 15(6):417–423, 1974

Hays MT, Green FA: In vitro studies of ^{99m}Tc-pertechnetate binding by human serum tissues. J Nucl Med 14(3):149–158, 1973

Maxfield WS et al.: Synovial membrane scanning in arthritic disease. Semin Nucl Med 2(1):50–70, 1972

Lymphangiography

Fairbanks VF et al.: Scintigraphic visualization of abdominal lymph nodes with ^{99m}Tc-pertechnetate-labeled sulfur colloid. J Nucl Med 13(3):185–190, 1972

Glassburn JR et al.: Correlation of [198]Au abdominal lymph scans with lymphangiograms and lymph node biopsies. Radiology 105:93–96, 1972

Hauser W et al.: Lymph node scanning with ^{99m}Tc-sulfur colloid. Radiology 92:1369–1371, 1969

Herting SVE et al.: Lymph node scanning with colloidal radioactive gold. Acta Radiol [Diagn] (Stockh) 10:359–368, 1970

Kazem I et al.: Clinical evaluation of lymph node scanning utilizing colloidal gold[198]. Radiology 90:905–911, 1968

PARATHYROID

Potchen EJ: Scanning of the parathyroid glands. In Blahd WH (ed): Nuclear Medicine. New York, McGraw–Hill, 1971, pp 526–532

Potchen EJ et al.: Parathyroid scintiscanning. Radiol Clin North Am V(2):267–275, 1967

SALIVARY GLAND

Schall GL, DiChiro G: Clinical usefulness of salivary gland scanning. Semin Nucl Med 2(3):270–277, 1972

BONE MARROW SCANNING

DeLand FH, Wagner HN: Reticuloendothelial system. In Atlas of Nuclear Medicine, Vol 3. Philadelphia, WB Saunders, 1972, pp 1–61

Feigin DS et al.: Detection of osteomyelitis by bone marrow scanning (abstr). J Nucl Med 15(6):490, 1974

Kniseley RM: Marrow studies with radiocolloids. Semin Nucl Med 2(1):71–85, 1972

Lilien DL et al.: ^{111}In-chloride: a new agent for bone marrow imaging. J Nucl Med 14(3):184–186, 1973

McNeil BJ et al.: Use of indium chloride scintigraphy in patients with myelofibrosis. J Nucl Med 15(8):647–651, 1974

ADRENAL IMAGING

Anderson BG et al.: Labeled dopamine concentration in pheochromocytomas. J Nucl Med 14(11):781–784, 1973

Beierwaltes WH et al.: Visualization of human adrenal glands in vivo by scintillation scanning. JAMA 216:275–277, 1971

Blair RJ et al.: Radiolabeled cholesterol as an adrenal scanning agent. J Nucl Med 12(4):176–182, 1971

Counsell RE et al.: Potential organ or tumor-imaging agents. 12. Esters of 19-radioiodinated cholesterol. J Nucl Med 14(11):777–780, 1973

Ravasini RG et al.: Adrenal scanning: its use in medical and surgical routine (abstr). J Nucl Med 15(6):526, 1974

Sturman MF et al.: Uptake of radiolabeled estradiol by the canine adrenal. J Nucl Med 16(1):77–79, 1975

index

Infarction *(continued)*
  myocardium, 31f
  pulmonary, 158f, 160f
Innominate vein, imaging, 7, 12, 16f, 30f
Iodine. *See* [123]I; ^{125}I; [131]I
Iron hydroxide, labeled, lung scanning, 149, 173
Isotope drip, inferior vena cavagraphy, 19, 20

Jaundice, 38, 39, 40, 50, 51f, 52, 58t, 59t

Kidney scanning, 61—85
  acute tubular necrosis, 62t, 63t, 79—80
  agents, 62, 63t
  aneurysm, 76f
  arterial stenosis, 77, 79
  congenital abnormalities, 62t, 63t, 85
  cyst, 65f, 68f, 69f, 71f
  ectopic, 84f
  horseshoe, 85f
  hydronephrosis, 81, 83f
  hypertension, 62t, 63t, 70—71, 77
  infarction, 78f, 79
  inflammatory disease, 62t, 63t, 80, 81f
  mass, 62t, 63t, 64—70
    angiography, 68, 72f, 73f
  obstruction
    arterial, 80
    mechanical, 62t, 63t, 81, 85
  occlusion, 77, 79
  parenchymal disease, 71
  perfusion study, 74f, 77
    normal, 73f
  technique, 62, 63t
  transplant rejection, 62t, 63t, 79—80
  trauma, 62t, 63t, 84f, 85
  urinary tract obstruction, 71, 80, 82f

Leukemia, 12, 56f, 211f
Liver scanning, 37—55, 58t, 59t
  abscess, 39, 40, 44, 208f
  agents, 38—39, 58t
  atresia, neonatal, 52
  blood flow, 47—48
  cirrhosis, 42f, 44, 45, 47, 48—49, 58t
  clearance, 52
  cyst, 44
  diffuse defects, 47—50, 58t, 59t
  displacement, 52, 53, 55
  enlargement, 41f, 52, 56f, 58t, 59t

Liver scanning *(continued)*
  extrahepatic obstruction, 50, 52
  flow study, 44—45
  focal defects, 39, 40—47, 58t, 59t
    "cold," 42f, 44
    "hot," 43f, 44
  hemangioma, 44
  hepatitis, 50
  hepatoma, 44, 45
  infection, 55, 58t, 59t. *See also* Hepatitis
  jaundice, 38, 39, 40, 50, 51f, 52, 58t, 59t
  normal, 40, 52
  obstruction, intrahepatic, 50
  polycystic disease, 42f
  position, abnormal, 53f
  radiation trauma, 52
  technique, 39—40, 59t
  trauma, 52, 54f, 58t, 59t
  tuberculosis, miliary, 48f
Lung scanning, 147—174
  agenesis of pulmonary artery, 169, 173t
  agents
    perfusion, 149, 173t
    ventilatory, 150, 173t
  bronchial asthma, 152, 163. *See also* chronic obstructive
      lung disease
  chronic obstructive lung disease, 161, 163, 164f, 165,
      173t, 174t
  cirrhosis and, 49—50
  congestive failure, 172, 173t
  edema, 172
  effusion, 169, 171f, 173t
  embolism, 147—148, 152, 154f, 155f, 158f, 159, 160f,
      161, 162f, 163, 173t, 174t
  emphysema, 161, 163. *See also* chronic obstructive lung
      disease
  "fissure sign," 172
  hypertension, 172
  infarction, 148, 152, 158f, 159, 160f, 161, 173t, 174t
  lymphatic drainage, 13f
  mass, 7, 12, 27f, 153f, 165, 167f, 168, 169, 173t, 174t
  mitral valvular disease, 172
  perfusion, 148, 149, 150
    normal, 152f
  shunts, 169, 172, 173t
  subdiaphragmatic abscess, 173, 173t, 174t. *See also under*
      Liver scanning
  techniques, 148, 149, 150, 173t, 174t
  ventilatory, 148, 149, 150
    normal, 152f
Lymphagiography, 209—210
  lung drainage, 13f
  therapy, 201

Marrow invasion, bone scanning, 128
Marrow scanning, 209, 211f
Mediastinum, adenopathy, 12

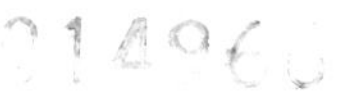